This Book

was presented to

The E.N.T Department

by R. Chignell

A.Y....

Date 1 July 1980

DG 2107

Scott-Brown's
Diseases of the Ear, Nose and Throat

Volume 3
The Nose and Sinuses

Titles of other volumes

Volume 1 Basic Sciences
Volume 2 The Ear
Volume 4 The Pharynx and Larynx

Scott-Brown's
Diseases of the Ear, Nose and Throat
Fourth Edition

Volume 3

The Nose and Sinuses

Editors

John Ballantyne, FRCS, HON FRCS (I)
Consultant Ear, Nose and Throat Surgeon,
The Royal Free Hospital and King Edward VII Hospital for Officers, London;
Civilian Consultant in Otolaryngology to the Army

John Groves, MB, BS, FRCS
Consultant Ear, Nose and Throat Surgeon,
The Royal Free Hospital, London

Butterworths
London Boston
Sydney Wellington Durban Toronto

United Kingdom London	**Butterworth & Co (Publishers) Ltd** 88 Kingsway, WC2B 6AB
Australia Sydney	**Butterworths Pty Ltd** 586 Pacific Highway, Chatswood, NSW 2067 Also at Melbourne, Brisbane, Adelaide and Perth
Canada Toronto	**Butterworth & Co (Canada) Ltd** 2265 Midland Avenue, Scarborough, Ontario, M1P 4S1
New Zealand Wellington	**Butterworths of New Zealand Ltd** T & W Young Building, 77–85 Customhouse Quay, 1, CPO Box 472
South Africa Durban	**Butterworth & Co (South Africa) (Pty) Ltd** 152–154 Gale Street
USA Boston	**Butterworth (Publishers) Inc** 10 Tower Office Park, Woburn, Massachusetts 01801

First edition 1952
Second edition 1965
Reprinted 1967
Reprinted 1968
Third edition 1971
Reprinted 1977
Fourth edition 1979

© Butterworth & Co (Publishers) Ltd, 1979

ISBN 0 407 00149 2   Individual volume
ISBN 0 407 00143 3   Set of four volumes

British Library Cataloguing in Publication Data

Scott-Brown, Walter Graham
   Scott-Brown's diseases of the ear, nose and throat—4th ed.
   Vol. 3: The nose and sinuses
   1. Otolaryngology
   I. Ballantyne, John II. Groves, John
   616.2'1   RF46   79–41008

   ISBN 0-407-00149-2
   ISBN 0-407-00143-3 Set of 4 vols

Typeset by CCC and printed and bound at
William Clowes & Sons Limited, Beccles and London

Introduction to the Fourth Edition

Some eight years after the last edition of this work appeared it may now seem to the practising clinician that the present decade has been a relatively quiet one in the history of our specialty. In fact, there has been a steady growth in the scientific foundations upon which an increasing amount of our practice is built, and it is therefore not surprising that the first volume, *Basic Sciences*, has now been considerably enlarged.

There has also been a steady expansion of clinical knowledge, and in planning this new edition we quickly became aware that no single volume from the last edition could stand without revision.

Sadly, the list of authors has been depleted by deaths and retirements of old friends and colleagues, whose contributions to British otolaryngology will never be forgotten. We thank sincerely all our colleagues, both old and new, who have spared no effort in preparing their manuscripts for this new presentation. The connoisseur will notice that a number of distinguished contributors from overseas have again been invited; we hope that this broadening of outlook will be welcomed by readers, and it is in keeping with the concepts of Mr W G Scott-Brown who originated the text nearly 30 years ago and who continues to flourish and to practice.

In some parts of the work, notably in Volume 2 (*The Ear*), advances in academic research have out-paced our ability to classify neatly a plethora of theories, facts (and sometimes fancies) for clinical application. Retaining the clinical approach as far as possible has compelled us, therefore, to commission chapters (for example in the field of sensorineural deafness) which overlap one another very considerably in content, while differing widely in emphasis. We hope that the reader will bear with this, and that the overall presentation will form a wider basis for learning than could be achieved by a more rigidly structured approach.

As far as we could we have used metric and SI units of measurement, even though a sense of humour is needed to accept some of the numerical absurdities which result. We are increasingly aware, too, that the SI system has brought upon us a hybrid and irrational system, heavily be-spattered with eponymously named units, at a time when eponyms are discouraged in the basic scientific disciplines. We are confident that the present generation will continue to honour Eustachius, Morgagni, Paget, Pott, Rosenmüller, and a hundred and one other great names, however the winds of pseudo-change may blow.

It is a great pleasure to thank and acknowledge all those who have helped so much in the preparation of this edition. We are grateful to those many colleagues who have lent us illustrations; to our registrars who have read proofs, criticized, advised and encouraged; and to those artists who have drawn new illustrations. Among the latter we thank especially Mr Frank Price for his unfailing generosity and technical skills. Equally we thank Mr Cedric Gilson and the Photographic Department of the Royal Free Hospital for their tremendous and willing efforts to provide so many of the new photographs.

Finally our gratitude goes to our publishers, Butterworths, who have done so much to lighten our editorial tasks.

London, 1979
John Ballantyne
John Groves

Introduction to the Third Edition

A radical new departure is made in the presentation of this work in four separately available volumes. This has been done for two main reasons. First, there is a real need, we feel, to recognize the diverse requirements of different readers—the newcomer to the specialty who needs a compact presentation of the special anatomy, physiology and radiology (for preparation for the DLO Part I and Primary FRCS examinations), and the specialist who is more interested in, say, the ear than in the throat. Secondly, advances are more numerous and more rapid in some sub-divisions of the specialty than in others so that it will be advantageous in the future to revise one volume at a time. The reduction in bulk of the individual volumes results, we hope, in easier handling and more pleasant reading.

A consequence of this change in format and policy is that page and chapter cross-references between different volumes cannot be given, nor is it practicable any longer to compile the symptom index featured in the last edition. To offset the former disadvantage some overlapping of subject material has been deliberately introduced wherever it was felt that too frequent referral to another volume would otherwise be necessary. Each volume has its own Table of Contents and Index, the latter compiled on the basis of noun-entries only.

The text throughout has been comprehensively revised. As a matter of general editorial policy, for this and for any subsequent editions which may appear under our direction, we have invited contributions only from those of our colleagues who are still actively engaged in hospital, university or college practice; and it has been our pleasure to welcome several new contributors. By including several new chapters, we have been able to remedy some of the omissions from earlier editions (for example, 'Congenital Diseases of the Larynx'), and also to give due emphasis to such topics as 'Acoustic Trauma' and 'Acoustic Neuroma', each of which now demands a separate chapter. The weights and liquid measures of all drugs, as well as the measures of distance, are all given in the metric system.

We are grateful to all the authors for submitting their work on schedule so that the production can be uniformly up-to-date. We warmly appreciate the efforts and enthusiasm of the Publisher's Editorial Staff, and the kind help we have received from colleagues, artists, and many friends too numerous to be named. It has been a tremendous encouragement to have the continuing interest of Mr W G Scott-Brown,

CVO, MD, FRCS, who has read and contributed substantially to the editing of a large part of this edition. We wish to thank him for the honour of his invitation to join in the Editorship of this standard textbook, which was established solely by him in the First Edition of 1952. Although he has now handed over completely the pleasant duties of joint Editorship to us and our successors, it remains his book and it retains his name.

London, 1971
John Ballantyne
John Groves

Introduction to the Second Edition

The objects set out in the Introduction to the First Edition have been the guiding principles in the present work. In order to make this new edition authoritative and contemporary in outlook, I asked two of my colleagues to join me as co-editors and I have been most fortunate in having the help and inspiration of John Ballantyne and John Groves. We have together re-cast the main sections, sub-sections and chapters and have given more emphasis to those departments of the specialty which have undergone the greatest changes. We have also made great efforts to have all contributions written and despatched to the printer within one year of starting the project, in order that all the articles shall be finished at the same time and be up-to-date when published. This object has been achieved thanks to the cooperation of our contributors.

It will be seen that the sections on physiology have been extended and improved and the chapters on the ear have been considerably altered and enlarged to include the many fresh ideas and techniques associated with both infective and non-infective ear conditions. The sections on endoscopy have been re-arranged to make the subject as practical as possible for our specialty. It is hoped that the necessary curtailment has not given rise to any major omissions. Neoplasms of the larynx and pharynx have been separated and new chapters on voice and speech have been introduced.

The index has been completely revised, and an innovation in a textbook of this size is an additional index—a symptom index—which is complete for the whole work at the end of each volume. It is hoped that this may be particularly useful to candidates for higher examinations and to general practitioners looking for causes of particular symptoms.

It is a pleasure to acknowledge the generous help which has been given by all the contributors, a number of them new to this book, and to artists and friends, for their kindly and stimulating interest. It is not possible here to record individual acknowledgments, but a special word of thanks must be made to the Editorial Staff of the Publishers.

London, 1965
W G Scott-Brown

Introduction to the First Edition

This work has been compiled with the object of presenting a textbook on Diseases of the Ear, Nose and Throat which would include most of the subject matter required by students and post-graduates with sufficient detail for those taking the higher specialized qualifications. It should also be a suitable reference book for general practice.

To achieve this it was decided to ask a number of teachers, examiners and other well-recognized authorities in the specialty to contribute articles on this general plan while leaving them free to put forward their own views of the particular subject in their own way. This has in some cases meant the presentation of individual preferences, classifications or theories, but as far as possible these have been integrated with the more usual views to give a balanced appreciation of the subject. It is hoped that this individuality of articles will give a more stimulating approach to the subject in spite of some overlapping of subject matter and differences of opinion.

Each section is prefaced by its anatomy and physiology as an essential basis to the understanding of the subject, and also to include in a concise manner the material necessary for the examinee. Methods of examination on the other hand have been cut to a minimum as they can only be learnt by the practical examination of patients. After considerable deliberation it was decided to include a chapter on plastic surgery of the nose and ear which should set out what can be done rather than entering into details of technique which are largely the province of the plastic surgeon.

My thanks are due in the first place to all the contributors who have lightened the editorial burden: they have all been most cooperative and have given freely of their time, knowledge and, in many cases, helpful criticism. Acknowledgement is made in the text for opinions and illustrations used.

I must particularly thank the Publisher's team, all of whom have been not only helpful but also encouraging during the many unavoidable delays and difficulties in the production of a new work.

London, 1952
W G Scott-Brown

Colour plates in this volume

Plate 1   *facing page 16*
(a) Bifid nose;
(b) nasal dermoid;
(c) deviated nasal septum with vestibulitis;
(d) examination of the anterior nares to demonstrate the inferior
     turbinate

Plate 2   *facing page 16*
(a) Unilateral vestibulitis in a child with a nasal foreign body;
(b) herpes zoster;
(c) alar destruction from lupus vulgaris;
(d) gross alar destruction from lupus vulgaris;
(e) destruction of the external nose from tertiary syphilis (patient of
     Mr Charles Heanley);
(f) carcinoma of the external nose;
(g) carcinoma of the external nose and columella;
(h) fractured nasal bones

Plate 3   *facing page 16*
(a) Osler's disease (hereditary haemorrhagic telangiectasia);
(b) sarcoidosis;
(c) orbital cellulitis complicating acute ethmoiditis

Contributors to this volume

John Ballantyne, FRCS, HON FRCS (I)
Consultant Ear, Nose and Throat Surgeon, The Royal Free Hospital and King Edward VII Hospital, London; Civilian Consultant in Otolaryngology to the Army

David Brain, MB, CHB, FRCS
Senior Clinical Lecturer in Otolaryngology, University of Birmingham; Consultant Surgeon, The Birmingham Ear, Nose and Throat Hospital; Consultant Ear Nose and Throat Surgeon, The Walsall Group of Hospitals; Member of Council, European Rhinologic Society; Regional Vice-President, Josef Society

T R Bull, FRCS
Consultant Surgeon, Royal National Throat, Nose and Ear, Hospital, Metropolitan Ear, Nose and Throat Hospital; Lecturer, Institute of Laryngology and Otology, University of London

J D K Dawes, BSC, MD, BS, FRCS
Reader in Otolaryngology, University of Newcastle upon Tyne; Consultant Ear, Nose and Throat Surgeon, Newcastle Area Health Authority (Teaching)

R L G Dawson, MB, FRCS
Plastic Surgeon, The Mount Vernon Centre for Plastic Surgery, Northwood, Middlesex

Ellis Douek, FRCS
Consultant Ear, Nose and Throat Surgeon, Guy's Hospital, London

Philip H Golding-Wood, BSC, FRCS, DLO
Consultant Ear, Nose and Throat Surgeon, Kent County Ophthalmic and Aural Hospital, Maidstone; Member of Council, European Rhinologic Society; Honorary Member, American Rhinologic Society

D F N Harrison, MD, MS, FRCS, HON FRACS
Professor of Laryngology and Otology, University of London; Head, Surgical Unit, Royal National Throat, Nose and Ear Hospital, London

R Pracy, MB, BS, FRCS
Consultant Surgeon, The Royal National Throat, Nose and Ear Hospital and The Hospital for Sick Children, Great Ormond Street, London

Joselen Ransome, MB, BS, FRCS
Consultant Otolaryngologist, Kensington, Chelsea and Westminster Area Health Authority (Teaching)

Stephen H Richards, MB, BS(LOND), FRCS(ENG), DLO
Senior Consultant Ear, Nose and Throat Surgeon, University Hospital of Wales, Heath Park, Cardiff

O H Shaheen, MS, FRCS
Consultant Surgeon, Ear, Nose and Throat Department, Guy's Hospital; Director, Head and Neck Oncology Clinic, Guy's Hospital; Consultant, Royal National Throat, Nose and Ear Hospital, London

Neil Weir, MB, FRCS
Consultant Ear, Nose and Throat Surgeon, Royal Surrey County Hospital, Guildford

David Wright, MA, MB, BCHIR, FRCS
Consultant Ear, Nose and Throat Surgeon, The Royal Surrey County Hospital, Guildford

Contents

1 Examination of the nose   1
  T R Bull

2 Conditions of the external nose   13
  T R Bull

3 Injuries of the facial skeleton   21
  R L G Dawson

4 Cosmetic surgery of the nose   47
  R L G Dawson

5 Congenital diseases of the nose   73
  R Pracy

6 The nasal septum   83
  David Brain

7 Foreign bodies in the nose: rhinoliths   141
  Joselen Ransome

8 Epistaxis   147
  O H Shaheen

9 Acute and chronic inflammations of the nasal cavities   163
  Neil Weir

10 Vasomotor rhinitis—allergic and non-allergic   209
  Neil Weir

xv

11 Nasal polyposis   225
    John Ballantyne

12 Abnormalities of smell   235
    Ellis Douek

13 Acute sinusitis   243
    David Wright

14 Chronic sinusitis   273
    David Wright

15 Complications of acute and chronic sinusitis   315
    J D K Dawes

16 Non-healing granulomas of the nose   351
    D F N Harrison

17 Tumours of the nose and sinuses   357
    D F N Harrison

18 Facial pain   385
    Philip H Golding-Wood

19 Trans-ethmoidal hypophysectomy   425
    Stephen H Richards

20 Surgery of the pterygo–palatine fossa   447
    Philip H Golding-Wood

    Index   483

1 Examination of the nose
T R Bull

The exterior of the nose requires no special apparatus for examination. The nasal fossae, however, are not easy to examine without good lighting, special instruments and, occasionally, the topical use of a vasoconstrictor to shrink the nasal mucosa.

A head mirror or head light is necessary for a thorough examination and leaves both hands free for using instruments: a hand-held light is adequate to demonstrate the nasal vestibule. In children, an auriscope with a wide speculum is a useful additional instrument for examining the nasal fossae. A nasal speculum is necessary in adults to dilate the vestibule and elevate the tip of the nose. In children, however, where the use of instruments is best avoided, simple pressure on the tip of the nose will suffice (*Figure 1.1*). A child may require to be held firmly during this examination, if any instrumentation is needed, for example for removal of a foreign body.

The Thudicum nasal speculum is in common use (*Figure 1.2*). Several sizes are

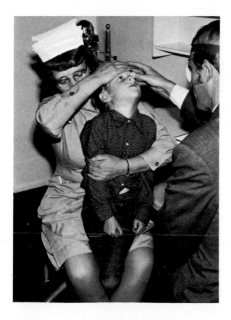

Figure 1.1 Examination of the nose in a child. (If a foreign body is to be removed a child may have to be held firmly as shown)

needed, with blades of varying lengths. The spring action should be gentle and the blades smooth. The speculum is inserted into the skin-lined, relatively insensitive vestibule and the blades are opened slowly: if the blades are allowed to spring apart or if the speculum is opened forcibly, it is an uncomfortable experience for the patient.

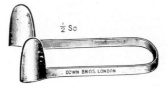

Figure 1.2   Thudicum's speculum. (Reproduced by courtesy of Down Bros.)

The blades are opened just sufficiently to give an adequate view of the nasal fossae. To see the upper and lower limits of the nose requires angulation of the beam of light, the patient's head and the speculum. The longer bladed St. Clair Thomson specula are useful for seeing the middle and posterior thirds of the nasal cavities and for lifting turbinates to expose the inferior and middle meatuses but they can only be used with local or general anaesthesia.

Examination of infants

When examining a neonate's or infant's nose, the patency of the nasal airway on quiet breathing is assessed and the presence or absence of nasal discharge is noted. The infant is best examined wrapped, with its arms included, in a shawl or blanket and held flat on its back on a bed or table with a nurse to control head movements.

Common nasal conditions requiring investigation in infancy are discharge and an inadequate airway. Slight discharge is common during the first few days of life as the nose is cleared of intrauterine and birth contaminants. Persistent 'snuffles' may be related to trauma and infection from a difficult labour. A nasal swab is taken and the nose examined to exclude a collection of infected debris or other sources of infection. Suction with a soft rubber-tipped Zöllner aural sucker is a useful technique for clearing the nasal fossae under vision.

A moderate degree of nasal obstruction may interfere with feeding and severe or complete obstruction, as seen in bilateral choanal atresia, threatens life due to the infant's inability to learn mouth-breathing. If the baby lies quietly breathing with the mouth shut, then the nasal airway is adequate. If the baby is restless and can only take a few sucks at the nipple or teat without drawing its head back and gasping for breath, then an inadequate nasal airway is probable. If mucus is seen bubbling in the nostril, or if clouding with the breath on a bright surface held beneath the nostrils can be demonstrated, then some airway must be present. Otherwise, the patency of the airway must be tested with a blunt-ended soft rubber or plastic catheter to exclude choanal atresia. It should be demonstrated that the catheter passes through into the oropharynx where it will cause gagging and can be seen through the open mouth. Suction can be used on withdrawing the catheter to remove any secretions which may have been the cause of the obstruction. Failure of the catheter to pass into the oropharynx requires x-ray examination. This may require general anaesthesia.

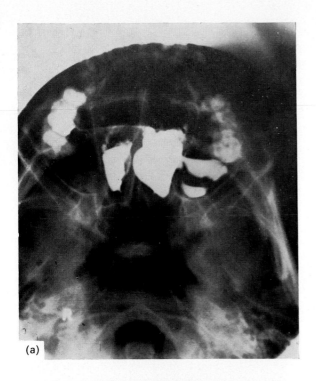

(a)

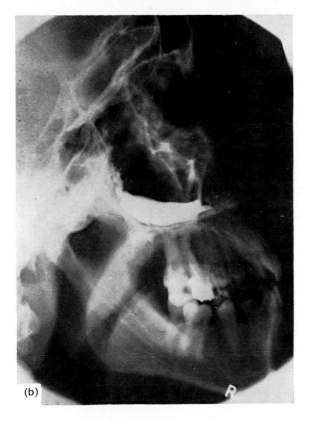

(b)

Figure 1.3 Contrast study x-rays of choanal atresia. (a) Basal view; (b) lateral view

Lateral soft-tissue x-rays must be taken first, followed by similar views taken after introducing a radio-opaque solution into each nasal cavity separately while the infant lies on its back. (*Figure 1.3* shows the appearance of bilateral choanal atresia.) Congenital nasal deformities are usually seen in conjunction with hare-lip and cleft palate and involve the alar cartilages. An abnormal fusion of the nasal processes produces a characteristic external deformity (*Plate 1a, facing page 16*).

Examination of adults

The external nose is examined by observation and palpation. Palpation permits accurate assessment of any skeletal deformity. One should note the site and relationship to the skin and underlying skeleton of any swelling or ulcer, and whether there is any defect communicating with the nasal passages, buccal cavity or antrum. Marks of recent trauma should be noted in writing in case of future legal proceedings and it is prudent to have x-rays taken if there is any likelihood of a fracture. More severe nasal injuries may have associated skull fractures. Scars which may be due to previous trauma or surgery are noted and the patient questioned as to their origin.

Many different types of swelling and cysts appear on or near the nose. Dermoids are found at the lines of fusion of the nasal processes (*Plate 1b, facing page 16*) and the philtrum of the lip and they also occur over the nasal bones and columella. A moist sinus near the bony-cartilaginous junction on the bridge of the nose is seen in dermoid cysts, with a deep extension upwards between the nasal bones which may extend to the anterior cranial fossa. A furuncle often occurs near the tip arising in hair follicles in the vestibule and presenting as a tender red external swelling. Sebaceous cysts may occur on the nose, while swellings near the alae may be dental in origin—either cysts or abscesses.

Acne rosacea with its butterfly rash over the nose and cheeks is a common condition of the nasal skin, but virtually any skin disease can affect the nose. In rhinophyma, the lower half of the nose enlarges due to hypertrophy of the skin and proliferation of the sebaceous glands. Skin neoplasms found here include epitheliomas and melanomas. Loss of tissue around the edges of the nares may be due to trauma or to healed lupus, and the surrounding skin should be examined for other evidence of disease. Superficial ulceration and inflammation of the skin surrounding the anterior nares is often secondary to discharge from the nose, especially if this is profuse or dries on the skin, producing crusts. Herpes simplex ulcers also may present in this site. They are frequently multiple and in most instances there is a history of previous attacks. Skin lesions restricted to the distribution of the maxillary division of the fifth cranial nerve are characteristic of herpes zoster and this can be complicated by superadded infection.

The shape of the nose alters with age. Loss of elasticity of the soft tissue between the columella and the caudal margin of the septal cartilage and the alar and upper lateral cartilages results in a drooping of the tip of the nose, so that the nose appears longer (Parkes and Kamer, 1973). The variations in the shape of the nose related to racial characteristics are also well recognized.

Palpation of the nasal bones and cartilages differentiates a bony deformity from a cartilaginous or soft-tissue swelling. An external deviation of the nasal bones and cartilage is probably associated with a deviated nasal septum.

Destruction of the bony septum may result from syphilis and of the cartilaginous skeleton from lupus vulgaris. Enlargement of the bony skeleton may be due to a general bone disease, such as Paget's, or to fibro-osseous dysplasia, and other bones should be examined for evidence of these conditions. Cartilaginous enlargement may be due to a chondroma or chondrosarcoma.

X-rays of the nasal bones will demonstrate recent fractures and show the degree of displacement. X-rays have a medico–legal significance but are of limited help in the management of nasal fractures.

Examination of the vestibule of the nose

The vestibule is the skin-lined anterior compartment of the nose. Its size and shape vary according to age, and from one person to another, but it is pear-shaped in adults with a narrow slit-like upper angle between the septum and ala. The skin contains hair follicles, sebaceous and sweat glands. The vibrissae become well-developed in middle-aged and elderly men. Most of the hairs arise from the lateral and medial walls. The skin lining extends further posteriorly on the lateral wall and this side is more flexible than the medial. Insertion of a speculum causes more discomfort on the medial side where the sensitive mucosal surface is nearer the front of the nose and the wall is relatively rigid. The muco-cutaneous junction is identifiable by a change of colour to pink and by the moist appearance of the mucosa, due to its surface film of mucus. The junction is also marked in some areas, usually on the lateral wall and lower half of the medial wall, by a slight ridge.

Metaplasia of the columnar mucosa to a squamous-cell lining may occur in the anterior part of the nasal passages, especially on the septum. This is usually due to frequent rubbing of these areas by the patient, through habit or to relieve irritation. The metaplasia stands out as whitish dry areas on the surrounding normal mucosa and, where these are continuous with the vestibular skin, the muco-cutaneous junction is obliterated. Frequent rubbing of the septum produces even more marked changes, sometimes progressing to ulceration and septal perforation. The anterior end of the septal cartilage may become dislocated out of its groove in the maxillary crest and protrude into one or other vestibule (*Plate 1c, facing page 16*). It causes an obvious projection into the vestibular lumen and tends to cause nasal obstruction and be subject to trauma. Various industrial dusts and fumes, notably nickel and chrome, tend to be deposited on the vestibular septum and they may cause septal perforation.

A nasal speculum may hide more of the vestibule than it reveals. Examination of this region should begin with inspection from several angles, assisted by pressing on the columella and tip of the nose to open up different areas of the vestibule. A short-bladed speculum is inserted just within the anterior nares and, deliberately, each wall and the floor are inspected. The upper angle and the upper lateral wall are particularly difficult to examine and a small mirror often gives the best view of these parts.

Staphylococcal infection of the hair follicles is common and may produce acute inflammation, or the patient may be a symptom-free carrier of bacteria. Swabbing of the nasal vestibules of hospital staff is a routine procedure when a bacteriologist is trying to trace the origin of a ward infection. A vestibular staphylococcal infection may go unnoticed by the patient while infection is transmitted to other parts of the head and neck, causing such problems as furuncles, conjunctivitis and otitis externa. Pain on examination of the vestibule suggests a furuncle or a fissure in the upper angle. The furuncle discharges into the vestibule although the main swelling is not infrequently on the external surface.

While many types of skin condition occur in the vestibule, one of the most common is a papilloma which is usually pedunculated. Malignant change in a papilloma is very rare but carcinomas and melanomas do occasionally present in the nasal vestibule.

Examination of the nasal fossae

The nasal fossae in an adult are approximately 7.5 cm long and 5 cm high. The airway through them is tortuous and its shape and size depend upon two factors:

(1) The configuration of the skeletal elements—septum, lateral wall and turbinate bones.
(2) The nasal mucous membrane, which is liable to considerable changes in thickness. These changes are particularly marked over the inferior and middle turbinates and depend upon a variety of exogenous and endogenous factors.

The nasal airway is subject, therefore, to wide variation from day to day in any one person.

The area of the nasal fossae visible on anterior rhinoscopy varies considerably but the anterior part of the septum and floor are always visible, while the area of the lateral wall that can be seen depends upon the size of the anterior end of the inferior turbinate. This is the most conspicuous feature on first inspection of the nasal fossae (*Plate 1d, facing page 16*) and patients may attend hospital for advice on this 'tumour' which they have glimpsed in the mirror. A large inferior turbinate which obstructs a satisfactory view of the middle turbinate and middle meatus can be reduced in size by the application of a vasoconstrictor solution, such as topical adrenaline.

When inspecting the nasal fossae, the following should be evaluated: the airway; the septum; the inferior turbinate and meatus; the middle turbinate and meatus; and the floor of the nose.

An examination which follows this routine avoids overlooking a particular site in the nose.

The airway

A complaint of nasal obstruction is very common and the range of individual tolerance to this symptom is wide.

For assessment of the airway, each side of the nose is examined separately, and one anterior naris is occluded without deforming the opposite side. A bright surface held beneath the nostrils to compare the area of misting may also demonstrate and compare the airways. If the obstruction is worse on inspiration, the alae nasi may be seen to collapse on to the septum. Sometimes, a previous submucous resection may cause the septum to 'flap' or impinge on inspiration against the lateral wall of the nose. If the obstruction is mainly on expiration, a 'corking' effect in the posterior choana is a possible cause and may be due either to a large posterior end of an inferior turbinate or to ethmoidal or choanal polypi. Occasionally, adhesions are seen between the septum and turbinates—usually as the result of surgical or other trauma.

The septum

The general configuration of the septum is first related to the external shape of the nose. A septal spur on one side usually means a concavity on the other but sometimes the septum is thickened and bulges into both nasal passages. This occurs as an acute condition in a septal haematoma or abscess. A chronic thickening of the septum may be due to a duplication of the cartilage or to an organized haematoma. The septum is rarely straight and small deformities are often of no clinical significance. It is also remarkable how a marked deviation of the septum found on a routine examination may be unassociated with any nasal symptoms. They should be noted, however, and a drawing is often a useful note. Examination of the septum should exclude perforation ar.1 areas of granulation.

The inferior turbinate and meatus

The inferior turbinate is the largest one and it is subject to considerable variation in size, due mainly to changes in its submucosal vascular bed. Hypertrophy of the inferior turbinate may occur when the airway is large: the concave aspect of a deviated nasal septum is usually seen to be opposed by a compensatory enlargement of the inferior turbinate. A wide airway results in drying of the mucous film and crusting. The mucosa is thick in chronic and allergic rhinitis and this is an important cause of nasal obstruction. Hypertrophy of the inferior margins of the middle and inferior turbinates and of their posterior ends is common in these conditions.

The inferior meatus is not usually visible unless the inferior turbinate is lifted upwards and inwards, and this requires anaesthesia. Sometimes, the anterior opening is very narrow and low down near the floor of the nose, making the introduction of probes and other instruments difficult. If the inferior meatus is visible, the lateral wall is seen to curve laterally in the anterior third. The nasolacrimal duct enters the meatus just below the attachment of the turbinate in this area but it is rarely visible.

The middle turbinate and meatus

The middle turbinate, like the inferior one, is subject to variations in size and shape. A large turbinate often contains an air-cell, while oedema, hypertrophy or polypoid change in the mucosa are all common. The shape is also influenced by the size of the airway, and physiological compensatory hypertrophy occurs in wide nasal fossae as with the inferior turbinate.

The middle meatus is the main drainage channel for the sinuses and the most likely place to find evidence of sinus disease. Most nasal polypi first appear in this space. While it is possible to view the area in some noses, it is often necessary to use a vasoconstrictor spray to reduce the inferior and middle turbinates for an adequate view. With the meatus exposed, the hiatus semilunaris and bulla ethmoidalis are seen anteriorly and it is possible to cannulate or probe the ostium of the maxillary antrum more posteriorly.

The floor of the nose

Foreign bodies usually lodge between the inferior turbinate and the septum and may be overlooked by failure to examine directly along the floor of the nose. A swelling in this area may extend from the teeth, the palate or the bucco–alveolar sulcus, e.g. a naso–alveolar cyst. An ulcer in the floor of the nose should be probed to exclude a communication with the oral cavity. Posteriorly, an antrochoanal polyp or a hypertrophic end of an inferior turbinate may cause obstruction.

The superior turbinate and meatus and the olfactory mucosa are not seen on routine clinical examination. Any polyp or swelling apparently arising from these areas may communicate with the cranial cavity.

The methods of viewing the post-nasal space and choanae are described in 'Methods of Examination of Mouth and Pharynx' (Volume 4).

Other examination techniques

Probing

A mucosal anaesthetic is usually needed before probing to demonstrate the consistency, mobility and site of attachment of a lesion. Ulcers are probed to detect if the underlying bone is exposed or if there is a sinus or fistula. The septum can be touched to see if the cartilage or bone is missing or to demonstrate a perforation, by passing the probe through and observing it in the other nasal fossa. The grating sensation felt on probing a rhinolith is characteristic.

X-rays

Lateral and anteroposterior x-rays and tomograms are helpful in demonstrating the nasal fossae. Soft-tissue shadows can be seen outlined against the air spaces (*Figures 1.4* and *1.5*) and the size and situation of radio-opaque foreign bodies and rhinoliths can be seen. Because the septal and nasal cartilages are radio-translucent, little information

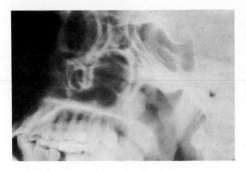

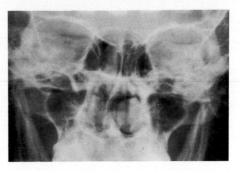

Figure 1.4 X-ray showing deviation of the bony septum and compensatory hypertrophy of the opposite inferior turbinate

Figure 1.5 X-ray demonstrating soft-tissue swelling of an enlarged posterior end of the inferior turbinate

about them, and no accurate assessment of the airways, is obtainable by x-ray examination. Xeroradiography is a relatively recent radiological technique that demonstrates the nasal bones and soft tissue particularly well (McKinney, 1974). The nasal cartilages, however, are not well delineated in these pictures.

Examination under anaesthesia

Under general or local anaesthesia, the nasal passages can be dilated with specula, such as Killian's or St. Clair Thomson's (*see Figure 1.6*) and the nasal fossae can be

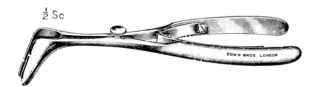

Figure 1.6 St. Clair Thomson's speculum. (Reproduced by courtesy of Down Bros. and Mayer & Phelps Ltd.)

examined to the choanae. The turbinates can be infractured and the blades of the speculum inserted beneath the inferior and middle turbinates, giving good exposure of the meatuses.

Investigation of nasal complaints

Anosmia

The cause may be intranasal or neurological.

Nasal obstruction, if severe, prevents the satisfactory circulation of odoriferous particles or vapours over the olfactory mucosa. It is more likely in such cases that the impairment will be partial and variable, whereas with neurological causes, the impairment is permanent and often total.

No easy and accurate method is available in routine clinical use for assessing olfaction. Some methods are described in Chapter 12, and Douek (1974) has described his findings in patients and control cases using an olfactometer to measure the minimal perceptible odour (MPO).

Seven primary odours are used and suggested test substances are shown in *Table 1.1*.

Table 1.1

Primary odour	Test substance
Ethereal	Ether
Camphoraceous	Camphor
Musky	Phenylacetic acid
Floral	Salicyl. aldehyde
Minty	Peppermint
Pungent	Formalin
Putrid	Thiophenol

The control cases gave reliable results. Patients with vasomotor rhinitis tended to lose the sense of smell for camphoraceous, musky and, to a lesser extent, for floral odours, while retaining the sense of smell for the other primary odours. However, these 'anosmic zones' are not yet sufficiently specific to be of use diagnostically.

In ordinary clinical practice, most cases are assessed on the history and with standard 'smell' solutions such as lemon, tar, cloves and camphor. Strong irritant odours like ammonia test the ordinary sensation of the nasal mucosa rather than the sense of smell and may help in assessing anosmia that is psychogenic or due to malingering. Any acute or chronic nasal pathology that causes marked nasal obstruction (such as a coryza or polypi) will impair the sense of smell. Not infrequently, anosmia is found with relatively mild symptoms of nasal allergy or minimal nasal obstruction. Obstruction to the smell particles is therefore only part of the explanation of anosmia. With chronic infection in the nose and sinuses also, anosmia may present with an apparently normal airway, and the cause may be chronic inflammatory change in the olfactory mucosa with degeneration of the specialized nerve endings.

Permanent anosmia can follow head injury when there is a 'shearing injury' to the fibres entering the olfactory bulb through the cribriform plate either from direct injury or a contrecoup injury. Although the more severe head injuries are associated with subsequent anosmia, relatively minor head injuries can also cause complete permanent anosmia. Anosmia may follow an attack of influenza, and impaired or absent smell sensation is not uncommon in old age. Treatment in these cases, and in most cases of anosmia without nasal symptoms, is ineffective.

Epiphora

Nasal causes of epiphora are uncommon and, although abnormalities in the inferior meatus which obstruct the naso–lacrimal duct are infrequent, they should be looked for to exclude such bony lesions as fibro–osseus dysplasia. The duct may be invaded by nasal or maxillary and ethmoidal neoplasms which can extend via the lumen to present in the medial canthus.

CSF rhinorrhoea

A cribriform plate lesion is the commonest site for a CSF leak but defects may occur in the frontal, ethmoid or sphenoid sinuses. In some cases, the leak may be from the mastoid or middle ear in which the CSF presents as a watery rhinorrhoea via the eustachian tube.

To establish whether a watery rhinorrhoea is cerebrospinal, the fluid, if sufficient, is collected in a test tube and examined for the presence of glucose. Glucose is present in lacrimal secretion so the presence of glucose is not complete proof that the fluid is cerebrospinal fluid. An excess of nasal mucus tends to cause crusting in the nose but this appearance is not seen with CSF; furthermore, mucus will dry on a handkerchief, whereas CSF does not.

Location of the CSF leak may be difficult: x-rays may show a fracture line into the frontal sinus, or the mastoid or middle ear, or in the region of the cribriform plate, ethmoid labyrinth and sphenoid sinuses. Tomograms, however, have proved particularly helpful in demonstrating sites of CSF leak. The injection of radioactive sodium into the CSF as a tracer has been used to detect the intranasal site of a CSF leak. Cotton-wool pledgets placed at the openings of the frontal and sphenoid sinuses (and along the cribriform plate) are later removed, after the injection of the sodium, and their radioactive content estimated (Crow, Keogh and Northfield, 1956). Another method described by Montgomery (1971) involves the use of fluorescein. After the intranasal application of a local anaesthetic with a vasoconstrictor, pledgets of wool are placed in the spheno–ethmoidal recess, the region of the cribriform plate and the anterosuperior angle of the nasal passage. One ml of 5 per cent fluorescein is injected intrathecally, with the patient sitting, and the nose is examined with the room darkened using an ultraviolet light source. The leak may be immediately obvious but, if not, the pledgelets are removed after 10 min and examined under ultraviolet light. If no fluorescein is seen, new pledgets are inserted into the nose and the patient is placed supine with the head dependent, and the pledgets are examined again after 10 min.

Epistaxis

This is discussed in Chapter 2.

References

Borrie, P. (1975). In *Roxburgh's Common Skin Diseases.* London; Lewis

Crow, H. J., Keogh, C. A. and Northfield, D. W. C. (1956). *Lancet,* **2,** 325

Douek, E. (1974). *The Sense of Smell and its Abnormalities.* Edinburgh; Churchill Livingstone

Lloyd, G. (1978). In *Recent Advances in Otolaryngology.* Ed. by Bull *et al.* Edinburgh; Churchill Livingston

McKinney, P. (1974). *British Journal of Plastic Surgery* **27,** 352

Montgomery, W. W. (1971). *Surgery of the Upper Respiratory System.* Vol. 1, p. 138, Philadelphia; Lea & Febiger

Parkes, M. L. and Kamer, F. M. (1973). *Laryngoscope* **83,** 157

Rees, T. A. (1972). Personal communication

2 Conditions of the external nose
T R Bull

The nose and nasal vestibules are covered with skin and may be involved in many generalized skin diseases, while a few dermatological conditions, such as acne rosacea, are especially liable to affect the nasal skin. The vestibules and surrounding skin are liable to infection because this is the main air inlet and patients frequently rub this area, causing minor abrasions and introducing infection on the finger. The hairs of the nasal vestibule are thick and strong; their follicles are a common site of both acute and chronic infection.

The normal nasal flora

Jacobson and Dick (1941) swabbed the nose in 500 consecutive patients admitted to a medical ward who had no nasal symptoms. They found the common organisms to be *Staphylococcus albus*, diphtheroid bacilli and occasionally, in apparently normal noses, they also found *Staphylococcus aureus* and *Micrococcus catarrhalis*.

The result of nasal swabs taken from staff at the Royal National Throat, Nose and Ear Hospital showed the following results (Rees, 1969). Out of 158 persons examined, 44 grew coagulase-positive staphylococci, and 38 out of the 44 organisms cultured were resistant to penicillin. Laryngectomy cases have nasal swabs taken pre-operatively as a routine and in 1969, out of a total of 25 patients, 16 grew no pathogenic organisms, five grew staphylococci, two grew beta-haemolytic streptococci, one grew pneumococci and one grew proteus.

The nose is therefore free of pathogens in the majority of normal people but it should be examined as a source of infection in institutional outbreaks. Coagulase-positive staphylococci are the most common pathogens and may cause acute or chronic infection in the vestibule.

Acute infections

The nasal vestibule is a painful site for a *furuncle* which is probably the commonest acute infection. The infecting organism is nearly always *Staph. pyogenes (aureus)*. It is important to find out the sensitivities of the particular strain of *Staphylococcus*. If the furuncle is pointing or has discharged, this information is easily obtained, but a swab from the surface of the vestibule probably reveals the type of *Staphylococcus*. The vestibule of the nose may act as a reservoir of staphylococci from which other parts of the body may become infected; alternatively, staphylococci may be transferred from other areas of the body, perhaps from ears, eyes or perianal region to the nasal vestibule, the finger nails acting as the connecting link.

Nasal furuncles are potentially dangerous because the veins of the nose drain on each side into the facial veins, which, like the ophthalmic veins, have no valves. The superior ophthalmic veins communicate directly with the facial veins and also communicate with them indirectly through the supra-orbital veins (*Figure 2.1*). The ophthalmic veins pass via the superior orbital fissure to the cavernous sinus. Severe nasal inflammatory processes may therefore extend to the venous sinuses of the brain, causing thrombophlebitis, a condition which may prove fatal despite antibiotics. Squeezing or incision of nasal furuncles is best avoided unless they are definitely pointing. The first indications of *cavernous sinus thrombophlebitis* as a complication of a

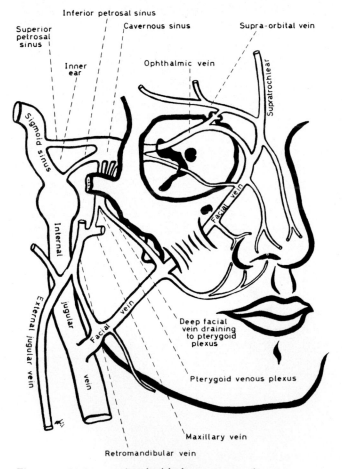

Figure 2.1 Veins associated with the cavernous sinus

nasal furuncle are those of malaise, headache and pyrexia. There may be superficial tenderness along the facial veins, with lid oedema and chemosis of the conjunctiva. Later, there is proptosis with limited eye movement. These local signs are due to the obstruction of the venous return from the ophthalmic veins.

The great majority of nasal furuncles are minor infections, however, and resolve spontaneously by discharging into the vestibule. A topical antibiotic ointment suffices as treatment for the small furuncle and vestibulitis. A severe furuncle with a general reaction, requires systemic antibiotics and, because of the potential dangers, close observation to ensure that the infection is showing an early response to treatment.

Recurrent boils suggest either local trauma, which may be self-induced, or an underlying general condition which reduces the patient's resistance to infection. Having excluded local causes, the patient's blood picture should be investigated and diabetes mellitus must be excluded.

Vestibulitis

Vestibulitis is a condition in which the skin of the nasal vestibule becomes excoriated and infected. An eczema of the vestibular skin gives a similar picture. Repeated trauma to the vestibule when the nose is rubbed or cleaned excessively by the patient is a common cause. The projection of a dislocated columellar portion of the cartilaginous septum into the vestibule is one of the commonest predisposing factors in vestibulitis. The skin overlying the projecting cartilage is thin, stretched and easily damaged with minimal trauma to the nose. Persistent infected ulceration develops. Advice to avoid unnecessary trauma, with the application of an ointment such as aureomycin, often suffices as treatment, but removal or correction of the projecting cartilage may be necessary.

Unilateral vestibulitis in a child (*Plate 2a, facing page 16*) is invariably diagnostic of a foreign body. The offensive discharge from the mucosal irritation of a foreign body causes a secondary vestibulitis. Vestibulitis affecting both nares is usually due to eczema, which may be localized to the nose or may be part of a generalized tendency to eczema. Purulent rhinorrhoea due to chronic sinusitis may also cause vestibulitis. The watery rhinorrhoea of nasal allergy or coryza may also cause an excoriation of the vestibular skin.

Impetigo

This is a contagious skin infection of the superficial layers of the epidermis caused by pyogenic staphylococcus and occasionally by a streptococcus. Pustular vesicles form and break, with yellow transparent adherent scabs. Impetigo commonly affects the face and nasal vestibules. The condition usually settles with the application of an ointment such as aureomycin.

Erysipelas

This causes an acute inflammation of the skin and subcutaneous tissues of the nose. The skin is raised and deep red in colour, with pain, heat and vesiculation, often accompanied by headache, fever and malaise. The organism is *Streptococcus*, which usually enters through a small fissure in the skin. Erysipelas in the region of the medial canthus simulates an acute frontal sinusitis, with eye closure from lid oedema (*Figure 2.2*). The diagnosis is clear, however, from the sharp margin of the reddened area of skin, the absence of intranasal symptoms and signs, and the normal sinus x-ray. Penicillin is usually curative.

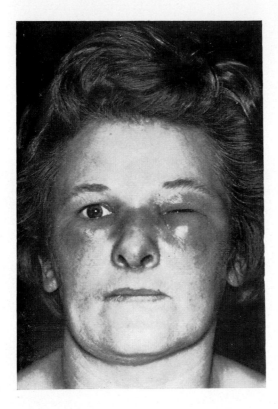

Figure 2.2 Recurrent erysipelas arising from scar of external left ethmoidectomy. Excision of scar stopped attacks

Herpes simplex

Small vesicles forming near the nostrils or lips are not uncommon with a coryza. They are painful and break down, with a watery discharge, to coalesce and form a larger irregular ulcer. The vesicles tend to recur at the same site and are caused by the herpes simplex virus. This virus may remain latent in the skin until local irritation, possibly combined with a period of lowered resistance, causes the virus to become active and the vesicles to develop. There is at present no specific cure for this condition, although antibacterial ointments such as aureomycin cream are used.

Herpes zoster

The nasal skin is affected in zoster of the maxillary division of the trigeminal nerve when vesicles involve the cheek, nose, nasal vestibule, nasal mucosa and palate. In

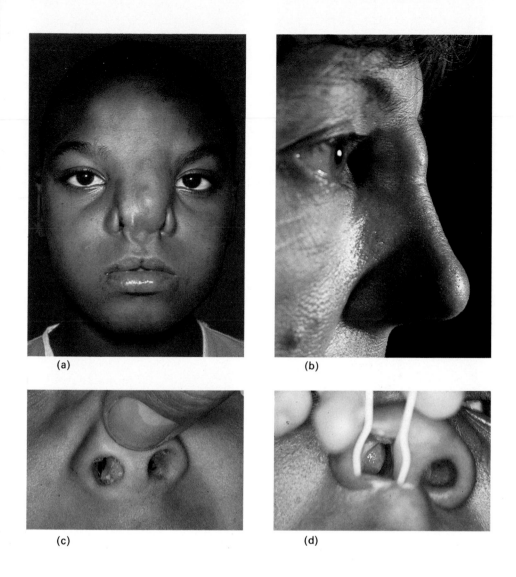

Plate 1   (a) Bifid nose; (b) nasal dermoid; (c) deviated nasal septum with vestibulitis; (d) examination of the anterior nares to demonstrate the inferior turbinate

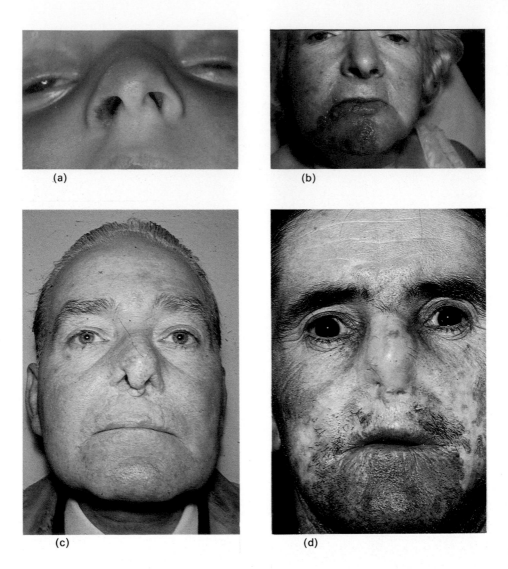

Plate 2 (a) Unilateral vestibulitis in a child with a nasal foreign body; (b) herpes zoster; (c) alar destruction from lupus vulgaris; (d) gross alar destruction from lupus vulgaris (*continued*)

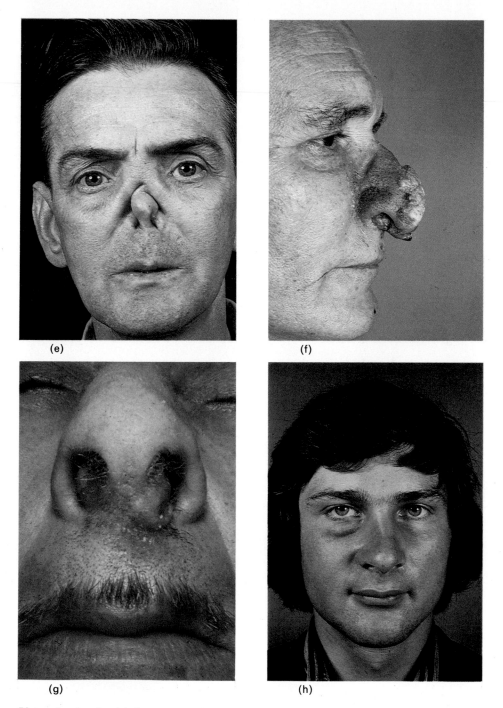

(e)　　　　　　　　　　　(f)

(g)　　　　　　　　　　　(h)

Plate 2 (continued)　(e) destruction of the external nose from tertiary syphilis (patient of Mr Charles Heanley); (f) carcinoma of the external nose; (g) carcinoma of the external nose and columella; (h) fractured nasal bones

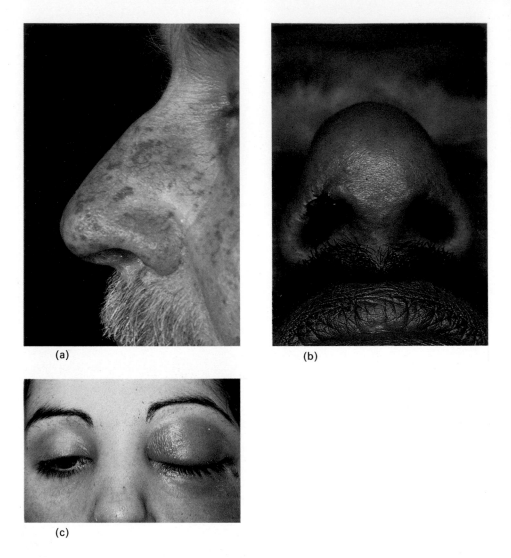

Plate 3 (a) Osler's disease (hereditary haemorrhagic telangiectasia); (b) sarcoidosis; (c) orbital cellulitis complicating acute ethmoiditis

ophthalmic herpes, the eye lesion and vesicles in the supra-trochlear and supra-orbital areas demand most attention, although vesicles also affect the nose in the distribution of the anterior and posterior ethmoidal and external nasal nerves. Pain may precede the eruption and, in the maxillary or mandibular division, may be mistaken for dental or sinus disease. Once the eruption develops, diagnosis is made by the exact limitation of the outbreak to the nerve distribution, and limitation to the midline is characteristic (*Plate 2b, facing page 16*). Secondary infection of the eruption makes diagnosis more difficult but the distribution remains unaltered. Lesions of the palate and nasal mucosa are rarely seen in the vesicular state, and they appear as discrete superficial ulcers which heal in three to four days. Treatment is restricted to the skin, with such an ointment as neomycin and hydrocortisone 1 per cent. Post-herpetic neuralgia is rare in these cases.

Chronic infections

Lupus vulgaris

Lupus vulgaris may cause skin involvement of the nose by the tubercle bacillus and occurs more frequently in women than in men. The skin invasion usually begins between the ages of 2 and 15 and occurs in someone who has already been infected by tuberculosis. Reddish-brown papules first appear on the nose, which when pressed with a glass slide, becomes white, and 'apple-jelly' nodules appear as small brown semi-translucent spots. Borrie (1975) describes two types of lupus involving the nose: (1) a slowly progressive usually non-ulcerative tuberculous infection of the skin. The disease is probably borne by the finger to the nose and the bacillus enters the deep layers of the skin from a finger scratch. The condition is characterized by miliary tubercles forming lupus nodules in the dermis. (2) An ulcerative type of infection of the skin, which may spread rapidly, and which is nearly always secondarily infected by staphylococci.

In the slowly progressive type of lupus the papules become soft, coalesce, and break down, forming shallow ulcers with undermined edges. Severe scarring and nasal deformity result with nasal obstruction of varying degree caused by contraction of the scar tissue at the vestibule. A chest x-ray is necessary and evidence of tuberculosis elsewhere in the body is to be excluded. Lupus, before adequate chemotherapy, resulted in extreme nasal deformity with virtually complete destruction of the external nose and closure of the nares (*Plate 2c, facing page 16*). Lupus is now rare, presenting with less conspicuous lesions (*Plate 2d, facing page 16*) and early treatment has eliminated such gross sequaelae.

Syphilis

Primary lesions of syphilis may present on the nose and *Treponema pallidum* is demonstrated in the exudate from the ulcer. The primary sore appears 9–90 days after exposure to infection and, if untreated, heals slowly in 3–10 weeks, leaving a thin atrophic scar.

Tertiary syphilis of the nose has the usual characteristic of the gumma. A hard, painless nodule breaks down to leave a deep ulcer with a typical punched out margin and a 'wash leather' base. A gumma heals with scarring and destruction of tissue. A painless chronic inflammatory nodule requires the exclusion of syphilis as a diagnosis.

The nasal vestibule may become involved in congenital syphilis, giving rise to 'snuffles'; and late congenital syphilis produces the classic saddle nose with occasional more severe deformity (*Plate 2e, facing page 16*). Gummatous lesions which destroy the nasal septum are in part responsible for the external deformity of the nose and cause large crusted septal perforations.

Other skin conditions

Acne rosacea

Enlarged superficial blood vessels in the skin of the nose and cheeks cause the dusky red colour and shiny surface characteristic of acne rosacea. There is usually secondary hypertrophy of sebaceous glands, and acneiform lesions may be superimposed. The disease is seen more commonly in women at the menopause. In some cases, usually males, there is enormous hypertrophy of the sebaceous glands, leading to the condition of rhinophyma (*Figure 2.3*). With gross deformity, surgical excision of the excess skin is necessary, avoiding damage to the underlying cartilage.

Lupus erythematosus

The skin lesion affects the nose and cheeks with a symmetrical butterfly distribution. There are patches of erythema and scaling which slowly become thin atrophic scars. In these areas, there is a stippling caused by filling of the orifices of the sweat glands

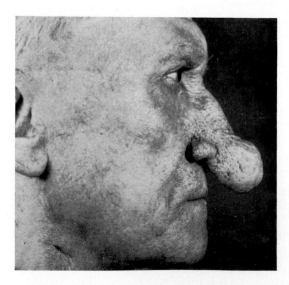

Figure 2.3 Rhinophyma

and hair follicles with horny plugs. The condition is differentiated from lupus vulgaris by the absence of apple-jelly nodules and ulceration, and the presence of stippling. In about 5 per cent of cases, the disease becomes systemic, with malaise, multiple arthritis and kidney lesions in addition to the skin changes. In these cases, blood examination will show a raised ESR and gamma globulins, leucopenia and the presence of typical LE cells—rosettes of leucocytes around nucleoprotein. Sarcoidosis, leprosy, scleroderma, yaws and rhinosporidiosis affecting the nose are described in Chapter 9.

Neoplasms of the skin of the nose and vestibules

Papillomas

Papillomas are common and may require excision on account of their appearance or irritation to the patient.

Rodent ulcers (basal-cell carcinomas)

These are common in the skin covering the nose, especially around the alae nasi. A small semi-transparent pearly nodule first appears which ulcerates and fails to heal. The ulcer *slowly* enlarges (so the history is usually long) and causes local destruction of skin, cartilage and bone but without metastasis to nodes or systemically. The diagnosis should be suspected in any long-standing ulcer on the nose and, if the diagnosis is in doubt, the lesion is biopsied. Radiotherapy or excision is curative in an early lesion.

Squamous-cell carcinoma

This may occur on the skin of the external nose or vestibule. The history is short, unlike that of rodent ulcer. A carcinoma on the external nose usually has an ulcerated centre with rolled everted edges. *Plate 2f* (*facing page 16*) illustrates a rapidly growing carcinoma of the nasal tip: *Plate 2g* (*facing page 16*) shows a carcinoma of the nasal columella. The prognosis, with treatment, for a small early lesion, before there is lymphatic metastatic spread or involvement of underlying bone and cartilage, is good. Some early neoplasms respond to radiotherapy while more advanced lesions require wide excision with radical neck dissection for cervical metastases. A painless lesion in the vestibule or on the septum is often ignored by the patient or missed by the doctor in the early stages. The prognosis with nasal carcinomas is therefore frequently not good and early metastases in the cervical nodes are seen.

Injury to the nose

Nasal fractures, with or without skin laceration, are common injuries. An external cosmetic deformity, and injury to the septum causing nasal obstruction, are the main relevant aspects of nasal fractures (*Plate 2h, facing page 16*).

Fractures of the nasal bones, like fractures elsewhere, can be simple, with or without displacement, or compound. The fractures may be associated with both skin and mucous membrane laceration, causing epistaxis as well as external bleeding. Nasal bone fractures with associated fracture of the maxillae may involve the nasal sinuses, which fill with blood. It is important to exclude associated fractures of the skull particularly those of the anterior cranial fossa or orbital margin in a case of nasal fracture. The nasal septum is frequently displaced when the nasal bones are fractured, and a septal haematoma may also form, lifting the perichondrium on one or both sides and causing marked nasal obstruction. Pain suggests secondary infection of the haematoma. Management is discussed in Chapter 3.

Reference

Borrie, P. (1975). In *Roxburgh's Common Skin Diseases.* London; Lewis

3 Injuries of the facial skeleton
R L G Dawson

The middle third of the face can be divided into the lateral middle third, which is the malar–zygomatic complex, and the central middle third, which is the maxilla and the nose. Although in many injuries all parts of the middle third of the face are affected, any part can be injured without involvement of the others. It is therefore appropriate to deal with three main sections of the middle third of the face separately, but with the understanding that, where all are injured, the individual treatment of the separate fragments must be combined and in a proper sequence, starting with the reduction and fixation of the maxilla, fitting the injured malar and nose onto the stable base of the maxilla. All of these injuries are likely to be complicated by severe haematoma and lacerations of the covering skin and other soft tissues and also by lacerations of the mucosal lining. It is therefore necessary in many cases to perform soft-tissue repair in layers following the fixation of the fractures if the covering integument is injured, or before the fixation of the fragments if the lining of the affected part is injured.

The nose

The skin, the lining, and the nasal skeleton of bone and cartilage, are all affected during injury to a greater or lesser extent. The nasal skeleton is composed of two nasal bones which are attached to the frontal bone superiorly, to the frontal processes of the maxillae laterally, to each other medially, and distally to the lateral cartilages. Deeply they are attached to the vertical plate of the ethmoid bone which continues in apposition with the vomer inferiorly and posteriorly and with the septal cartilage inferiorly and anteriorly. Posterior to the frontal processes of the maxillae lie the lacrimal bones with their attachment of the internal palpebral ligament surrounding the lacrimal sac lying in a groove in the lacrimal bone. More posteriorly still lie the ethmoid air-cells, and these also lie posterior to the upper part of the nasal bones, medial to the lacrimal bone, on each side. Injury to the lateral and alar cartilages is relatively rare compared to injury of the septum and the bony nasal skeleton, but the lateral cartilages are attached medially and are in continuity with the cartilaginous nasal septum and where an injury and displacement has occurred to the septum, the lateral cartilages themselves are likely to be displaced. Nasal injuries in children are very often confined to a green-stick type of fracture of one or other nasal bone without involvement of the rest of the skeleton, whereas in adults the whole of the bony skeleton is nearly always affected.

Mechanism of the injury

The degree of displacement and the severity of the comminution of the fracture depend upon the force and direction of the blow.

Lateral

This type of fracture occurs when the injuring force is applied to the side of the nose. There is then a displacement of the nose to the opposite side with a fracture of the nasal bones and parts of the frontal processes of the maxillae. The fragment of the ipsilateral side overrides the stable part of the frontal process, whilst the fractured fragment on the contralateral side becomes impacted beneath the stable part of the process. There is an overriding of the nasal bones in the midline and the septum, which is deflected away from the direction of the blow along the bridge-line, kicks back to occlude the ipsilateral airway along the nasal floor. Simple deviation of the nasal tip without involvement of the bony skeleton does occur when the injuring force has hit the nose below the bone. This results in a deviation of the nasal tip with a dislocation of the cartilaginous septum from the vomerine groove and the nasal spine.

Frontal

This type of nasal injury is often more severe and is due to the injuring force being applied centrally from the front. The degree of displacement and involvement of structures depends upon the degree of the injuring force. Three stages of this condition are recognized according to the severity:

Stage I   Here the nasal bones collapse centrally and spread out over the frontal processes of the maxillae, giving the appearance of an open book in an occipitomental radiograph (*Figure 3.1a*). As the dome of the nose collapses, so the septum shatters and tends to 'concertina', with overlapping of the septal fragments.

Stage II   Here there is a spreading of the nasal bones, but also impaction between the frontal processes of the maxilla, which are fractured outwards, and there is an obvious flattening in the profile of the face. The septal injury is usually greater (*Figure 3.1b*).

Stage III   This is most severe where there has been an impaction of the nasal bones between the laterally spread frontal processes, which themselves have become impacted into the antra (*Figure 3.4*). Even more serious than this is the lateral spread of the ethmoid air-cells and the lacrimal bones on each side. There is a gross disruption of the nasal septum, and a very flat profile. Lateral spread of the anterior ethmoid air-cells and lacrimal bones produces a widening of the interpalpebral distance, and pseudohypertelorism. The normal ellipsoid shape of the palpebral fissure is converted into an almond shape with a rounded inner canthal region. The incidence of

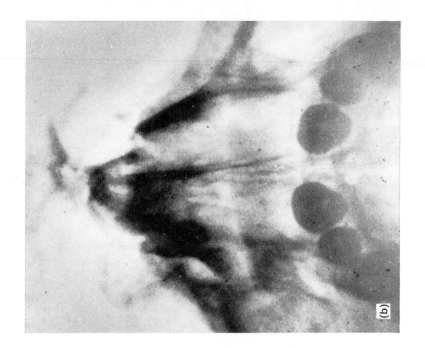

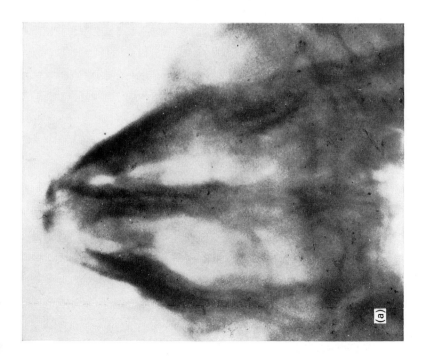

Figure 3.1 Frontal type of nasal injury: (a) Stage I, 'open-book' deformity; (b) Stage II, overriding septum. The nasal bones are depressed between the out-fractured nasomaxillary processes (frontonasal processes). (From Matthews (1967) reproduced by courtesy of Messrs. J. & A. Churchill)

cerebrospinal rhinorrhoea due to laceration of the dura in the anterior fossa is highest in this stage.

Associated injuries

Although fractures of the nose are commonly isolated injuries, they are often also associated with fractures of the malar–zygomatic complex, maxilla, frontal bone and mandible. So the treatment of a fractured nose may often represent an incident in the treatment of the whole patient, particularly in these days of multiple injuries associated with accidents at high speed.

Symptoms and signs

Besides the history of the blow on the nose, there is bleeding, usually from both nostrils, pain, and later swelling and haematoma of the nose and both lower eyelids. Nasal obstruction results both from blood clot and from the displacement of the nasal skeleton and septum. As a consequence of this nasal obstruction, or through injury to the olfactory nerves in the severe frontal types of injury, the patient may complain of inability to taste or smell.

Depending upon the type of injury the signs vary considerably. In the lateral type of injury there will be severe lateral displacement, with bruising and swelling over the nose, epistaxis from both nostrils, nasal obstruction and bilateral bruising involving both eyes and all four eyelids. Particularly there is a concentration of bruising in the lower lids. The main deformity can be felt with the overriding and instanding nasal bones and the deviation can best be assessed in minor cases by observing the nose from above, using the forehead as the horizon. In this way, even minor deviations are obvious, whereas a frontal inspection may not elicit such small deflections. The nostrils must be cleaned of blood clots and a proper inspection made of the septum. If there has been a frontal type of injury, the profile is lower than normal, the nose is wide across the bridge-line, and there tends to be more haematoma in both lower eyelids. Where a severe frontal injury has occurred as in Stage III, an increase in the intercanthal distance, and a conversion of the palpebral fissure into an almond shape, is obvious. There is usually more swelling over the nose than in the lateral type of injury and the septum can be seen to be wider than normal, causing nasal obstruction in both airways.

Radiography

Radiographs for the laterally displaced nose are not usually very helpful. The deformity is obvious and the bones can be palpated in their displaced position. Radiographs for the frontal type of injury can be more useful, but do not often add much to a careful examination, except when there is an excessive amount of swelling and the bony outline cannot be palpated. This particularly happens when the patient is examined some hours after the injury. Lateral and 30 and 60 degree occipitomental views will give all the information that is required.

Treatment

Pre-operative

If much swelling has already occurred before the patient seeks surgical help, it is best to wait for some days to allow the swelling to subside. The displaced bones are then more easily palpable, the effective surgical correction more easily determined, and any plaster fixation can be more closely applied. If a plaster fixation is put on to a nose that is badly swollen, in two or three days that plaster will be so loose that it is useless. However, children with green-stick fractures, and people with the severe Stage III of the frontal type of injury should receive early surgical treatment—the children because the fracture may be difficult to move after a few days, and the Stage III injury because the cerebrospinal rhinorrhoea often associated with this injury may cease with correction of the fracture, and the ethmoid spread can more easily be reduced at an early stage. It is justifiable in other types of injury to wait anything up to seven days so that as much swelling as possible has subsided. The patient is nursed sitting up in bed and ice applied to the eyelids in order to reduce the haematoma.

The operation

It is preferable to give a general anaesthetic with an endotracheal tube, and the pharynx must be firmly packed off. For the laterally deviated nose the displaced nasal bones are gripped with Walsham's forceps (*Figure 3.2*) and the deformity is initially increased, for disimpaction of the nasal bones, and subsequent correction of the

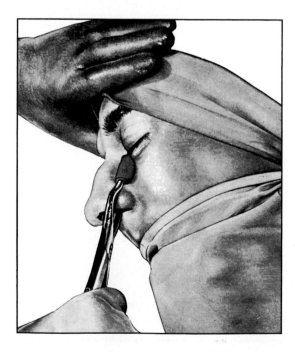

Figure 3.2 Disimpaction of nasal bones. With the aid of Walsham's forceps, the external blade of which is covered with a piece of rubber tubing, the fractured nasal bones are disimpacted on each side and re-positioned to give a smooth and rounded bridge-line

deformity. Ashe's forceps are passed on either side of the septum lifting a displaced cartilaginous septum back on to the vomerine crest, and straightening the fractured bony septum (*Figure 3.3*). The airways are inspected, cleared of blood clots and then

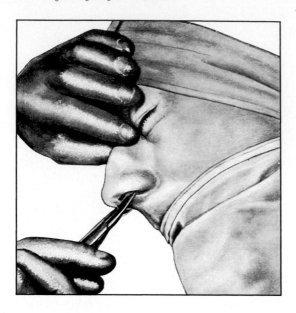

Figure 3.3 Centralizing of septum. After the nasal bones have been disimpacted and repositioned, the nasal septum is grasped on each side with Ashe's septal forceps. The septum is centralized, the fractured nasal bones being controlled

Vaseline is placed over the eyes and the eyebrows, and a plaster-of-paris splint applied composed of eight thicknesses of 7.5 cm plaster bandage. This is moulded closely to the nose, particularly in the canthal region on each side, and when it is dry it is fixed to the forehead with 2.5 cm Elastoplast and to the cheeks with 2.5 cm strapping. If there is difficulty in replacing and straightening the nasal septum, it is wise to pack each nostril with either a rubber glove finger pack or tulle gras. The plaster fixation should remain on for about 12 days. It is then removed, the airways cleaned and the patient re-examined in three months' time.

In the frontal type of injury, the nose has been spread laterally and more or less symmetrically, and at the same time the actual height of the nose has been lowered by the injury. Therefore after clearing the nostrils the septum is gripped with Ashe's forceps and these lift the nose forward and upwards away from the operating table, at the same time as the bony skeleton is pinched between the finger and thumb on each side. In this way the flattened profile is corrected and the width from the front view is narrowed. Where a Stage III frontal injury has occurred the frontal processes which have been displaced into the maxillary sinuses on each side must be lifted out either by volsellum forceps or, by a Caldwell–Luc approach, pushing the process upwards. Fixation is performed by a wiring of the medial part of the inferior orbital margin. In all types of frontal injury it is essential to maintain the forward elevation of the nasal bridge and also maintain the lateral compression which has been achieved by the finger and thumb. Therefore instead of using a plaster-of-paris fixation which is not satisfactory in this type of injury, two stainless steel wires are passed directly across the nose through the most posterior of the fracture lines and these stainless steel wires are tied over malleable lead plates on each side, while the forward elevation of the nose is maintained by the Ashe's forceps. The wires are tightened so that a good firm fixation is achieved with the lateral lead plates. In this way the wires prevent backward redisplacement of the fracture and the lateral lead plate compression maintains the corrected narrowing of the nasal bridge. In Stage III cases, where there is a tendency to redisplacement of the frontal processes into the antra, it is very often advisable to maintain a forward traction on the nose, after the lead plates have been applied, by a stainless steel frontal bar fixed to a plaster head cap (*Figure 3.4b*).

Treatment of the laterally displaced inner canthal ligament
With lateral displacement of the inner canthal ligament and widening of the intercanthal distance, it is necessary to correct the displacement by firm digital

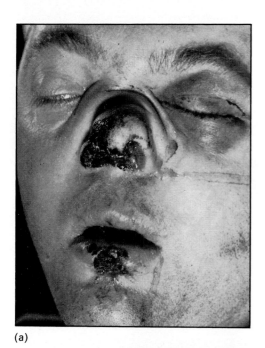

(a)

Figure 3.4 Stage III of frontal type of nasal injury: (a) complete collapse of the nasal skeleton; much of the skeleton is in the left orbit; (b) same patient showing head plates on the nose and forward traction of the fixation used for an associated fractured maxilla; (c) post-operative view of the same patient. (From Matthews (1967), reproduced by courtesy of Messrs. J. & A. Churchill)

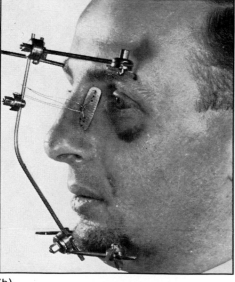

(b)

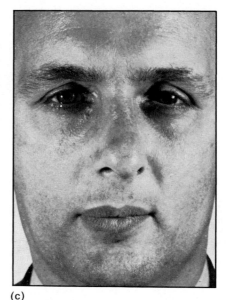

(c)

compression between finger and thumb, at the same time as the frontal nasal injury is corrected. In many cases if the upper nasal transfixion wire is placed in the actual corner of the eye, the upper part of each lead plate will maintain the canthus in its corrected position, but the lead plates must be maintained for at least three weeks, otherwise the lateral pull of the eyelid muscles in the inner canthus will displace the canthus laterally again. Recently the displaced canthal ligament with its attached lacrimal bone has been directly wired to the nasal process of the frontal bone through a midline incision over the upper nasal bridge (Stranc, 1969). This method allows a more exact reposition of the fractured bone fragment under direct vision (*Figure 3.5*). The wires are left in permanently.

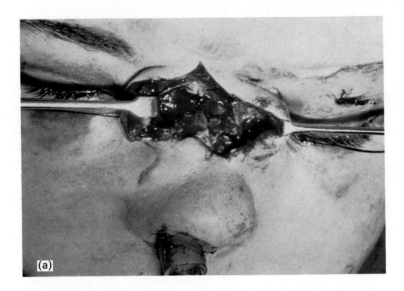

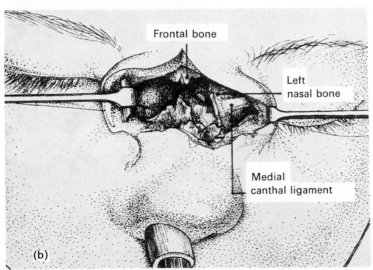

Figure 3.5 The extent of the frontal type of nasal injury in relation to the inner canthal spread (Mr. M. Stranc's case)

Post-operative treatment

The patient should sit up as soon as possible, and sleep in the sitting postion for the next two days. Icebags are applied to the eyes for the first 12 h. Any nasal packing is removed at the end of 48 h, the plaster-of-paris fixation is retained for 12 days, and the lead plate fixation with the transfixion wires is retained for three weeks. Where cerebrospinal rhinorrhoea is present penicillin and sulphadiazine are given systemically. The nostrils themselves are cleaned daily with cottonwool swabs soaked in saline and Naseptin (Hibitane) cream is applied to the nostrils twice a day. The airways become re-established after about four days when the intranasal swelling begins to subside. Pain beneath the plaster fixation is unusual and if severe it is an indication for removal of the plaster to find the cause.

Haemmorrhage   The epistaxis following immediately upon injury usually ceases reasonably soon, but in more severe injuries this haemorrhage may cease only when reduction and fixation have been achieved. Bleeding may rarely be encountered from a laceration of the anterior ethmoidal artery in the severe type of nasal injury. This will necessitate a ligation of the anterior ethmoid artery through the orbit. If the bleeding is severe, packing of the airways with adrenaline gauze or an inflatable (Simpson's) bag may be needed. Even a post-nasal pack is sometimes necessary. Only rarely is a blood transfusion required.

Haematoma of the septum   Although it is rare, if such a haematoma does develop, incision, evacuation and drainage must be performed because of the risk of infection, chondritis and subsequent saddle nose.

Cerebrospinal rhinorrhoea   This complication, although associated very frequently with high maxillary fracture incorporating a fracture at the base of the nose, is usually only met with in the pure nasal fractures when a Stage III frontal type of injury has been sustained. It is due to a fracture of the cribriform plate, or a fracture of the posterior wall of the frontal sinus, with dural laceration. Where the former type of injury has taken place, early nasal correction and fixation are indicated, penicillin and sulphadiazine are given, and the patient is nursed with the head raised. He is instructed not to blow his nose, for fear of producing a cerebral aerocoele. The rhinorrhoea seldom lasts more than ten days, but if it persists, or a cerebral aerocoele occurs, operation to close the tear in the dura with a fascial graft is indicated.

Anosmia   This can occur either as a result of obstruction of the airways, and then is not usually complete, or as a result of injury to the olfactory nerves as they pass through the cribriform plate. If it is the latter then an assessment of permanent disability must not be made for at least a year after the injury, since partial recovery quite often occurs, sometimes with unpleasant aberrations of olfactory sensation.

Lacrimal obstruction   This complication occasionally occurs in a severe type of frontal injury where the nasolacrimal duct has been crushed as it passes through the maxilla. Occasionally this can be relieved by an exploratory operation to remove the bony obstruction, but more often the patient finally has to have a dacryocystorhinostomy operation.

Later complications

Sinusitis   Frontal sinusitis may occur as a result of crushing or blockage of the frontonasal duct, and a maxillary sinusitis may occur from deviation of the nasal septum.

Atrophic rhinitis   Where there has been a loss of septum or poor septal development, very wide airways may be encountered and normal intranasal moisture is deficient. This causes crusting and rhinitis. Narrowing of the airways, at the same time as a depressed profile is built up with chip bone grafts, has a very beneficial effect on the rhinitis.

Thickened nasal bones   These may occur some months after the injury due to the deposit of periosteal new bone where much haematoma formation has occurred.

Synechiae   These are most commonly met with in the severe frontal type of injury due to the gross comminution and laceration of the septum, as well as the lateral wall of the nose, and where a lateral nasal compression with lead plates and transfixion wires has been necessary to maintain a reduced position. It is therefore always necessary to inspect the airways at the time of removal of the wire fixation and to break down any adhesions at that time.

The maxilla

'Fractured maxilla' is a term loosely applied to fractures of the central middle third of the face which, by terminology, also includes the nasomaxillary complex. In only 33 per cent of fractures of the tooth-bearing segment of the upper jaw is there no involvement of the upper part of the nasal skeleton. Therefore the upper part of the nasal skeleton is involved in 67 per cent of all fractures of the central middle third of the face which includes the fractures of the tooth-bearing segment. The central middle third of the face incorporates 13 separate bones. One can visualize the great disturbance which can occur following injury to this section, and the so-called 'fractured maxilla' frequently involves fractures of the pterygoid processes, the ethmoids, the vomer and the lacrimal bones. There is a close association also between fractures of the maxilla and fractures of the nose and nasomaxillary complex, and a close association between fractures of the malar–zygomatic complex and fractures of the maxilla.

Mechanism of the injury

The central middle third of the face is injured by direct force; the degree of comminution of the bones and to a great extent the degree of displacement of the bony fragments, is dependent upon the force and direction of the blow, or injuring object, or the speed and direction of the face when hitting a stationary object. To a certain extent the displacement following an injury is also influenced by gravity, subsequent swelling, and to a large extent by muscle spasm and muscle pull against the loose fragments of bone. The structure of the facial bones, struts of strong bone interspaced with areas of weaker bone enclosing the various sinuses, produces a cushioning effect against the force that would ultimately be directed to the cranium and the brain, and a large amount of the force is expended on injuring the 'middle third' thereby sparing the brain from serious injury. In this way many people escape fatal injury at the expense of the severely fractured face.

Various classifications to denote extent of the injury have been made, but the most useful is that of Le Fort (1901) who, working in Paris, subjected cadaver heads to varying degrees of force in varying directions and analysed the results of the injuries. As a result of his dissections he compiled three main divisions:

Le Fort I or Guerin
The fracture lines pass above the palate, fracturing the pyramidal processes of the maxilla on each side, the vomer and the lower parts of the pterygoid processes. This therefore is purely a fracture of the tooth-bearing section of the maxilla and the palate, and involves the antral floor on each side.

Le Fort II
The fracture lines pass upwards and inwards from the antral floor through the junction between the malar–zygomatic complex and the maxilla into the medial side of the orbit, across the inferior orbital margin, out again across the lacrimal bone, and upwards across the nasal bridge to meet the fracture line coming up from the opposite side. The fracture then passes backwards and downwards across the vertical plate of the ethmoids, the vomerine bone, and laterally through the pterygoid processes in their middle or upper third. The posterior wall of the antrum is also involved on each side.

Le Fort III
This injury is a craniofacial dysjunction in which the fracture lines cross the zygomatic arch, the zygomatic process of the frontal bone, the back of the orbit through the superior orbital fissure, the ethmoid, the lacrimal bone, frontal process of the maxilla, and nasal bones to meet the fracture line coming from the opposite side. Posteriorly the pterygoid processes are fractured in the upper third. In this way the whole of the middle third of the face, maxilla, nasomaxillary complex and both malar–zygomatic complexes are separated from the cranium. These are the three main divisions of the fracture, but variations and permutations can occur as can be seen in *Table 3.1*.

Table 3.1 Percentage incidence of injury type

Unilateral Le Fort I	11
Le Fort I	23
Le Fort I and II	21
Le Fort II	35
Le Fort II and III	2
Le Fort III	4
Le Fort I, II and III	2
Unilateral Le Fort II	1
Le Fort I unilateral and Le Fort II unilateral	1

The degree of displacement of the fractured bones varies according to the force and direction of the blow, gravity, swelling and muscle pull on the fractured fragments. If the blow comes from the lateral side the maxilla is pushed sideways, and a malocclusion with the mandibular teeth occurs, with a crossed bite. If the blow comes from the front, the maxilla is pushed backwards. If it comes from the front and below also, the front of the maxilla is pushed backwards and upwards whilst the posterior part of the maxilla remains down, causing a markedly open bite through premature occlusion of the teeth in the molar region. The maxilla may become impacted between the malar bones causing subsequent difficulty in reduction, but more frequently the maxilla is 'floating', easily movable from side to side, and easily brought forward into occlusion with the lower teeth. The muscles involved through spasm are those attached to the pterygoids and these tend to cause further displacement posteriorly, and trismus.

Associated facial injuries

There are frequently associated nasal, malar–zygomatic and mandibular fractures, whilst fractures of the base of the skull are also common.

Symptoms

Bilateral epistaxis, bilateral orbital haematomas, staining of both upper and lower eyelids with a greater involvement of the lower lids, a very swollen face, flattened profile, difficulty in swallowing and difficulty in breathing, are the commonest symptoms. The patients may also complain of inability to taste or smell, but pain is not a marked feature.

Signs

Shock is not common, unless the injury is associated with other injuries such as fractured long bones or thoracic or abdominal injuries, and where shock is present the examiner must look for other causes. The face is very swollen, the profile often flat, the nasal bridge wider than normal and in the Le Fort II with ethmoid injury the intercanthal distance is increased. There are bilateral orbital haematomas, and marked staining of the lower eyelids. Bilateral epistaxis has occurred, the mouth opening may be limited through trismus, and the dental occlusion is disrupted, either with a crossed bite or with a retroposed maxilla and an anterior open bite. The maxilla is usually very mobile and on tapping the teeth a 'cracked pot' sound may be elicited. This sign must be checked on several teeth because a localized alveolar fracture will give the same sign. Intra-oral inspection reveals bilateral haematomas in the soft palate and may reveal a step in the hard palate if the maxilla has been split. The number of sound teeth, both in upper and lower jaw, must be noted because these teeth will be used in the subsequent fixation after reduction. If the maxilla has fallen too far down the palpebral fissure on each side will be sloping inwards and downwards. If the posterior wall of the frontal sinus has been injured with a tear of the dura, or if the cribriform plate has been fractured, cerebrospinal rhinorrhoea will be present, the flow being increased in the head-down position and decreased on sitting up. If the olfactory nerves have been torn, anosmia will be present. If the fractured nose moves in continuity with the moving fractured maxilla, a Le Fort II fracture can be diagnosed. If, however, the fractured nose does not move when the maxilla is rocked, then there is a combination of Le Fort I and II fractures and the naso–maxillary complex has to to be treated as a separate entity at the same time as the maxilla is treated. Occasionally anaesthesia of one or other cheek may occur if the fracture line has passed through the infra-orbital canal. This can occur even without an actual fracture of the malar–zygomatic complex.

Where no teeth are present but the denture is available, this should be fitted to ascertain the degree of malocclusion. If the dentures have been broken the fragments must be preserved and reassembled by the dental laboratory. This can be done very quickly.

Radiological diagnosis

One of the accepted views for fractured maxilla is a lateral view of the face where the degree and direction of displacement of the tooth-bearing segment can be assessed and where the fractured pterygoid processes can be seen. This view may also show a gap between the nasal process of the frontal bone and the nasal bones. Also, 30 degree and 60 degree occipitomental views are used to show the state of the antra which are always cloudy if involved; the state of downward displacement of the central middle third between the malar bones is noted. A split palate can also be seen on these views, but should be confirmed with an intra-oral view of the maxilla. At the same time the films will show the state of the malar–zygomatic complexes, and posteroanterior and lateral oblique views of the mandible and a Towne's view for the condyles are usually taken. It is not necessary to have x-rays to diagnose such an injury, nor is it absolutely essential that any should be taken as a preliminary to reduction and fixation. They should really be regarded as confirmatory evidence.

Treatment

First-aid treatment
Immediately after the injury the patient can be lost unless the proper first-aid treatment is carried out. Two aims are to arrest any severe haemorrhage and to establish an airway. The haemorrhage will usually be severe only if there are associated major lacerations of the face, but the airway can be completely obstructed by the maxilla being pushed back against the posterior pharyngeal wall and falling down against the dorsum of the tongue. It is therefore necessary to roll the patient into the prone position, preferably with the head hanging over the end of a stretcher or bed, to pass the finger into the mouth behind the soft palate, and hook the maxilla forward pushing it upwards, and at the same time, if available, a nasopharyngeal tube should be passed with the other hand through one of the nostrils so that it comes to lie at the back of the soft palate in the pharynx.

One further complication, which needs urgent tracheostomy, is the involvement of the larynx with haematomatous swelling causing respiratory obstruction. Occasionally there is a fracture of the hyoid bone associated with these injuries and where there is a swelling in the neck overlying the larynx it is advisable to perform an early tracheostomy.

Definitive treatment
If the operator keeps to the following principles in the order listed, treatment will go through smoothly and quickly.

(1) The loosening of all impacted fragments until all bones can be replaced in their normal positions.
(2) The reduction and fixation of the tooth-bearing part of the maxilla.
(3) The reduction and fixation of the nasomaxillary complex.
(4) The repair of intra-oral and extra-oral lacerations, other than those on the lingual side of the dental arch, which obviously have to be repaired before the tooth-bearing segment is fixed.
(5) Removal of the throat pack and aspiration of all blood clots.
(6) The application of the intermaxillary fixation.

Mobilization and reduction   As a pre-operative measure it is wisest where possible to be prepared for a transfusion, because although these cases do not lose very much blood in the normal course of events, just occasionally, particularly in manipulation of the nose, a large haemorrhage may occur. The mouth must be cleaned, loose teeth picked out, fragments of denture removed, and where teeth cannot be accounted for, an x-ray of the chest must be ordered. A full general anaesthetic is given, a nasotracheal tube is used and a pharyngeal pack is put in by the anaesthetist. It is a possibility that the central maxillary fragment has impacted underneath the lateral elements, on one or other side, particularly along the orbital margin. Where, therefore, the malar has been also injured, it is often necessary to elevate the malars laterally through a temporal fossa approach, with a Bristow's elevator beneath the zygomatic arch on each side in order to allow the maxilla to be pulled forward. Either Walsham's nasal forceps with one blade passing along the nasal floor and the other along the palate, or Rowe and Killey's forceps can be used to grip the palate, and the maxilla can be rocked sideways and then forwards and downwards anteriorly and upwards posteriorly until it can be brought into better occlusion with the mandibular teeth. Just very occasionally it may be necessary to remove a loose fragment that has caused an impaction between a solid malar and the maxilla at the malar–maxillary buttress. Where there is a separate nasomaxillary complex, as in the combination of the Le Fort I and II fracture, it will be necessary to perform a separate nasal reduction and bring forward this complex which will not come forward when the Le Fort I fracture is reduced.

Fixation of the maxilla and the tooth-bearing segment   This can proceed following the mobilization and reduction. The method used depends very much upon how many teeth are present both in the upper and lower jaw, and on the state of the rest of the facial and cranial bones. In the past, a plaster-of-paris headcap with a German silver outrigger fixed to the front over the frontal region has been used, the cap passing well down behind the occipital protuberance. The maxilla and mandible have been fixed to the stable cranium (*Figure 3.6*). The plaster headcap has various disadvantages. It

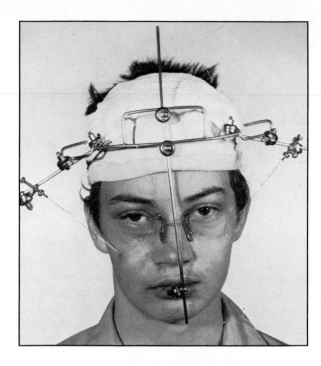

Figure 3.6 The three-point fixation for the fractured maxilla. The central frontal bar is attached to silver dental splints

is difficult to apply really well and tends to rock a little, and is therefore not a completely stable method of fixation. Very occasionally a ring of alopecia will occur and if the head cap is not fitting properly it tilts over the forehead and can cause a pressure sore. If there has been any degree of oedema of the forehead, the headcap will loosen when the swelling subsides. Therefore various operators introduced other forms of fixation, including the metal halo fixed to the skull by screws, passing through the scalp, or wires threaded through the zygomatic process of the frontal bone and emerging through the upper buccal sulcus to be fixed to the maxillary teeth posteriorly, or to the posterior mandibular teeth, these in turn being fixed to the maxillary teeth (Milton Adams). As a quick method of fixation where the malar bones are intact, a Kirschner wire can be threaded through the malar bones and across the top of the palate thereby transfixing the face. This fixation allows the face to fall, but prevents the centre bones of the face from shortening up too much. The next stage of this method was to use two Kirschner wires, each passing through a malar bone and into the hard palate with the assistant holding the maxilla in occlusion with the mandible. This two-point type of fixation prevented both lengthening and shortening of the face, but was not a very accurate procedure and depended very much upon the malar stability which so often is absent in complicated facial fractures. A better fixation, and one which gives a very stable skeletal fixation, where the bony region of the outer orbit is intact, is the box-fixation used at Mount Vernon Hospital (*Figure 3.7*). A mounted screw, either the wood screw type or preferably the Toller type, is inserted into the thickened piece of bone of the outer supra-orbital margin on each side; after intermaxillary fixation has been achieved either by interdental and intermaxillary wiring or by the application of cast silver splints, similar screws are inserted into the body of the mandible on each side, care being taken to avoid the exit of the inferior alveolar nerve. The four screws, two in the mandible and two in the

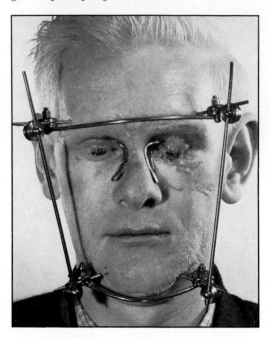

Figure 3.7 The 'Mount Vernon box' fixation following interdental and inter-maxillary wiring. The mandible is fixed to the stable cranium with intra-osseous screws and bars with universal joints

cranium, are then joined together by vertical and curved transverse bars with universal joints. In this way a very stable fixation can be achieved. The author has not used the classic head cap with the anterior frontal bar maintaining the anterior part of the maxilla forward and downwards, and the cheek wires threaded to the molar regions with screw traction to maintain the posterior part of the maxilla upward, for the last two years. The mandibular and maxillary teeth are only temporarily fixed together unless there is a large gap anteriorly with some absent teeth, through which the throat pack can be removed, because of the necessity for removing the pack and clearing out the pharynx at the termination of the operation. Therefore only temporary fixation is applied at present between the upper and lower teeth.

Reduction and fixation of the nasomaxillary elements   This can now proceed as there is a stable base and a stable upper part of the skull, and the nose can be reduced to its proper position between the two. If there has been a severe frontal injury with a Stage III displacement nasal transfixion following reduction must be performed with wires tied over lead plates on either side of the nose. The nose must then be pulled forward via the plates and fixed to a bar passing obliquely across from the upper intra-osseous screw to the lower intra-osseous screw, and fixation and forward traction must be maintained for three weeks. The box method has the disadvantage that, because it is a craniomandibular fixation, an eccentric position of the mandible may be obtained, and an eccentric position of the maxilla will follow. The craniomandibular fixation also has the disadvantage that the mandible cannot be released in order that a soft diet may be taken or a better airway achieved through the mouth if there is any respiratory complication, whereas when the craniomaxillary fixation has been made with other methods, the mandible can be released from occlusion with the maxilla at the end of a week and the patient has the advantage of being able to open the mouth fully.

Following the fixation of the maxilla and of the nasomaxillary complex, the lateral middle third or malar–zygomatic complex, can be fixed. If the antrum has to be packed it is absolutely essential that the maxilla should be immobilized first, otherwise the maxilla may be displaced by the packing. If the mandible has been fractured as well this complicates the satisfactory reduction of the maxilla because there is no fixed arch upon which the maxillary teeth can be put into proper occlusion. It is therefore necessary to restore the mandibular arch initially before immobilizing the maxilla to the mandible. If the malar bones are intact it is not necessary to form a craniomaxillary fixation by the box method. The screws can, where desirable, be drilled into the body of the malar on each side and connected to the mandibular screws in the usual way.

Special problems

The split palate   A central split of the palate is relatively common. Occasionally a split occurs laterally, producing one large fragment and a smaller one. It may demand the construction of separate silver cast cap splints for each fragment. These splints bear a hook on the palatal surface by which the split palate can be pulled together by elastic traction (*Figure 3.8*). Unless there are good mandibular teeth to which maxillary ones can be fixed in proper occlusion, the splint on each maxillary fragment should bear an extra-oral bar which is fixed to the cranial part of the suspension by stainless steel rods in the usual way.

The alveolar fragment   This is a frequent complication. If the displacement is slight, a one-piece splint can be made to incorporate the alveolar fragment. This can then be fitted and cemented into the splint and the main fragment is then cemented into the splint. If the alveolar fragment is large, then a separate cap splint is made and after

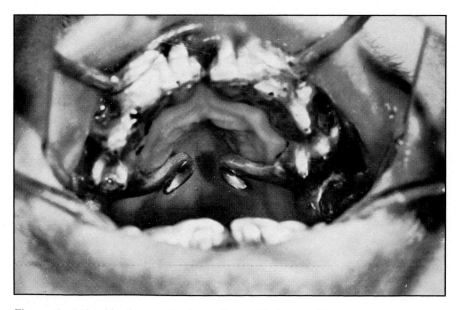

Figure 3.8   Palatal hooks to maintain a split maxilla in apposition

reduction into proper occlusion with the mandible a locking bar is made to cross between the two splints on the maxilla. Only very loose teeth should be extracted from a posterior alveolar fragment because of the risk of producing an oro-antral fistula.

The edentulous patient   Here it is not of such great importance to get an absolutely perfect correction of the maxillary displacement as dentures can always compensate minor degrees of displacement. If the original denture is available, or if a denture which is broken can be reconstituted, then obviously this is the best form of splintage. The denture is then wired to the maxilla with peralveolar wires, passing through the denture and the alveolus, and the denture can then be suspended from a plaster headcap by a frontal bar with an attachment to the front of the denture. Loops are made on each side of the posterior part of the denture, so that cheek wires can be passed through the upper buccal sulcus from the malar region. These are attached to the loops on the denture, and attached to the lateral part of the German silver outrigger on the headcap with a screw adjustment.

Delayed treatment   After two or three weeks it is usually extremely difficult to move, and disimpact by manipulation only, a fractured displaced maxilla. Therefore either an open operation is indicated with the approach through the upper buccal sulcus on each side, passing an osteotome through the fracture line and levering the maxilla free again, or slow traction can be applied to the maxilla by way of a cap splint. The traction need never be more than 1.8 kg, and passes from the front of the splint over pulleys on a Balkan beam. Three or four days is usually enough traction to bring the maxilla into reasonable occlusion with the mandible, but the operators must be on the watch constantly so that over-correction is not obtained. This is in any case only a second best procedure and first class occlusion is rarely obtained.

Cerebrospinal rhinorrhoea   This occurs in approximately 25 per cent of all patients with a central middle third fracture. It is due to a tearing of the dura at the level of the cribriform plate, or associated with a fracture of the posterior wall of the frontal sinus. Where possible it is best to nurse the patient with the head raised. This lowers the intracranial pressure. The patient must be warned not to blow his nose for at least four weeks. Penicillin and sulphadiazine are prescribed parenterally. The main initial treatment is to immobilize the maxilla and immobilize the nasomaxillary complex. Once these bones have been immobilized the tear in the dura usually heals, and it is rare that a cerebral aerocoele with increasing headache and drowsiness, or persistent rhinorrhoea occurs. If the rhinorrhoea lasts for more than four weeks there is a need for craniotomy and a fascia lata graft. Complications following a tear of the dura in this situation, manifesting as a frontal lobe abscess, aerocoele or meningitis, occurring months or years after the accident, are rare.

Post-operative treatment
The occlusion of the teeth and the stability of the fixation must be checked regularly and the entry holes of any fixation must be cleaned with 1 per cent Savlon each day. The intra-oral fixation, whether by wire or denture, or silver cap splints, must be cleaned two or three times a day, and syringed with 5 per cent sodium percarbonate solution with a Wyatt–Wingrave syringe. At the end of four weeks the craniomaxillary or craniomandibular fixation is slackened off, and the occlusion tested at the end of a

further two days. If no displacement has occurred, the fixation may be taken down, interdental wires of cap splints and dentures being removed.

Post-operative complications

Infection may occur, involving the soft tissues of the face or the entry holes of any fixation. Sinus infections are not common. Malocclusal variations happen, and if the mandible has been fixed to the maxilla in an eccentric position, quite severe pain may occur in one or other of the temporomandibular joints. Diplopia from involvement of the origin of the inferior oblique muscle in haematoma, or from collapse of the orbital floor, is usually a complication associated with fracture of the malar–zygomatic complex. Epiphora from crushing or tearing of the nasolacrimal duct may be a temporary phenomenon, but occasionally the duct has to be relieved of its pressure at a secondary operation in about four weeks, with an incision along the lateral side of the nose. If, following decompression, the epiphora persists, dacryocystorrhinostomy is needed. Pressure sores and areas of alopecia may occur from a badly fitting plaster headcap; cheek wires may break or screws come loose. Electrolytic ulceration of the entry holes of the screws is occasionally seen if an insulator is not incorporated in the fixation, when a bar is attached to a cap splint and then attached to an intra-osseous screw in the process of fixation. The ulceration is due to a minute electrolytic discharge formed between dissimilar metals and the effect of this is manifested in the ulceration at the site of entry of the screw.

Anosmia

This results through injury to the olfactory nerves as they come through the cribriform plate. It is therefore associated with Le Fort II and Le Fort III fractures. It has an uncertain prognosis; about half of all cases of anosmia fail to recover at all. At least a year should elapse before a final assessment is made. Other cases show a partial recovery. Some of the sensations of smell and taste are normal whilst others are completely abnormal, showing aberrations sometimes of a most unpleasant kind.

Fractures of the malar–zygomatic complex

This complex represents the lateral part of the central middle third of the face and consists of the malar (zygomatic) bone itself which forms the orbital rim; the orbital floor; and the posterior wall, the floor, the anterior wall and the lateral wall of the maxillary antrum. It is attached to the maxilla at the malar–maxillary process, to the frontal bone at the external angular process and to the zygomatic process of the temporal bone by its own zygomatic process.

This complex is fractured by a direct blow, except in the rare cases of orbital floor 'blow-out' where pressure is transmitted to the thin orbital floor by a sudden impact on the globe. The extent of comminution, the degree of displacement and the direction of displacement, depend upon the force, direction and size of the injuring object, or the force with which the face hits a stationary object. If, however, the area of impact is small, such as from a high velocity bullet, a localized compound injury is suffered, and the majority of the complex is preserved intact. Local depressed fractures of the zygomatic arch are another type of fracture often caused by rings or some other narrow objects.

Symptoms

The patient usually provides a good history. He complains of swelling of the cheek, unilateral epistaxis, flattening of the cheek, numbness of the cheek and the side of the nose, the upper lip and the upper teeth and gums on the side of the injury. The patient may also complain of inability to open his mouth properly, and of double vision.

Signs

There is gross swelling of the eyelids with haematoma, particularly of the lower lid, a certain amount of proptosis due to haematoma in the orbit, and peripherally a subconjunctival haemorrhage in the inferior and outer part of the bulbar conjunctiva (*Figure 3.9*). Later when the swelling has gone down there may be enophthalmos to quite a severe degree. This is often associated with herniation of the lower orbital

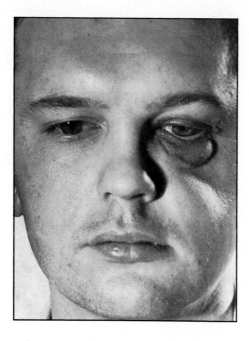

Figure 3.9   Fracture of the malar–zygomatic complex: note flat cheek, orbital haematoma and conjunctival haemorrhage

contents through the fractured orbital floor into the antrum. The enophthalmos combined with the inferiorly displaced malar will produce an eye which is appreciably lower than the normal one. Diplopia is frequent, and is usually due to involvement of the inferior oblique muscle in haematoma, and to prolapse of its origin into the antrum. The site of the diplopia is usually found in the upper and outer field of vision on the affected side. There is a sensory loss in the area supplied by the maxillary part of the trigeminal nerve, viz. the cheek, the side of the nose, the upper lip, the upper teeth and the buccal sulcus. With involvement of the masseter muscle in the fracture there is a degree of trismus, and this may be much worse if a localized depressed fracture of the zygomatic arch has occurred, which prevents a free forward running of the coronoid process of the mandible on mouth opening, and may virtually block this movement. A localized depression of the zygomatic arch may be associated also with a transverse fracture of the coronoid processes of the mandible, thereby involving the temporalis muscle and providing a contributory cause of the trismus. Intra-orally the haematoma can be seen in the cheek on the affected side and the bone can be palpated in the displaced position through the upper buccal sulcus. Some days after the injury, when the swelling has gone down, a marked flattening of the cheek is obvious. It is essential first of all in the examination for a fractured malar that the eye level should be noted and swelling of the cheek and other signs listed above should be observed when viewing the patient from the front. The patient must then be examined from the back with the fingers palpating the malars on both sides to compare the normal and the abnormal one. The fingers should be run along the infra-orbital margin to note any obvious depression, and backward displacement may be assessed by comparing the two sides with a finger placed on each malar prominence.

Radiological examination

Occipitomental views, 30 degree and 60 degree, should be taken to show the antra and the orbital margins, whilst a submentovertical view can be taken to outline the zygomatic arch. They are useful particularly when the face is very swollen, but are by no means essential. Stereoscopic radiographs are more useful because the total displacement can be visualized.

Treatment

If a patient with a fracture of this complex seeks very early treatment it is possible to correct the deformity before very much swelling has arisen. If, however, a large swelling of the cheek is present when the patient first seeks surgical help, it is very often wise to leave the patient for four or five days until the majority of the swelling has gone down and then the full deformity can be noted.

One severe contraindication to reduction of the fracture must be mentioned, and that is when there is a blind eye on the opposite side. Very occasionally manipulation of a fracture of the malar–zygomatic complex has resulted in a spicule of bone injuring the optic nerve on the side of the injury, causing blindness of that eye.

The reduction of the fracture is performed under general anaesthesia with an endotracheal tube. The pharynx is packed off. An initial approach is made by the Gillies incision high up in the temporal fossa where a small strip of the scalp is shaved (*Figure 3.10*) The incision is oblique and well away from the zygomatic arch, avoiding both the transverse and the vertical branches of the superficial temporal artery. The incision passes down to the temporal fascia which is then incised and a Bristow's elevator is passed down beneath the temporal fascia and therefore beneath the zygomatic arch. It is hooked round the inferior border of the arch, at the junction of the arch and the malar bone. Then, with the full pressure on the wrist of the operator and not on the middle fossa of the skull, the malar bone is elevated into place. In approximately 45 per cent of all cases this procedure is effective and there is no need for any fixation. The malar sits on the malar–maxillary buttress and remains stable in the reduced position. The cheek is marked with ink to warn the nurses that the patient

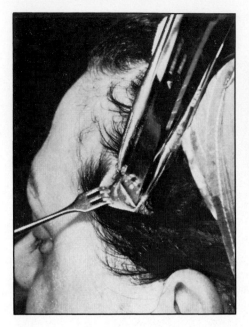

Figure 3.10 The straight lift of Gillies, the Bristow's elevator passes deep to the temporal fascia. The incision must be high in the hair, never over the arch

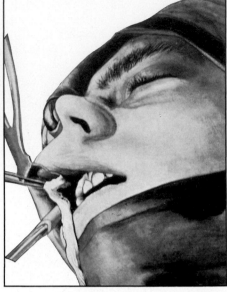

Figure 3.11 The anterior wall is packed up through a buccal sulcus incision

should not be allowed to lie upon that side of the face. The wound in the temporal fossa is closed with interrupted silk. When the malar is not stable the external angular process must be exposed through a small incision, and the bone ends found and wired with 0.5 mm stainless steel wire. It is possible that a wire may also have to be inserted into the infra-orbital margin at the junction with the maxilla if this area is not stable. This is done through a transverse lower eyelid approach. Where the anterior wall of the antrum has been grossly comminuted and flattened, and where there is a collapse of the orbital floor, the antrum must be packed through a Caldwell–Luc approach, and the bone fragments having been moulded into place with a finger in the antrum, are held up with an elevator, whilst 2.5 cm ribbon gauze, soaked in paraffin–flavine emulsion, is packed into the antrum, until a good firm contour has been achieved (*Figure 3.11*). The antral pack is finally removed at the end of 14 days through the buccal sulcus incision which then heals up completely as long as the ostium is kept open with 1 per cent ephedrine nose drops. The antrum is washed out through the buccal sulcus incision with normal saline twice a day for three days after the pack has been removed. Any persistence of an oro-antral fistula in this site indicates a sequestrum present in the antrum.

Where there a good anterior wall of the antrum, and therefore good cheek contour, but where there is still a depressed eyeball, it means that there has been a collapse of the orbital floor with probable herniation of contents of the orbit into the antrum. This can be corrected by a transverse lower lid incision along the malar line and a subperiosteal dissection, replacing the contents of the orbit from the antrum back into the orbit again. A polythene or Silastic plate, suitably shaped to cover the gap, is then inserted so that herniation does not recur (*Figure 3.12*). These foreign bodies stay in this position extremely well and it is very rare to get an extrusion, in spite of the fact that they appear to be in direct contact with the torn antral mucous membrane.

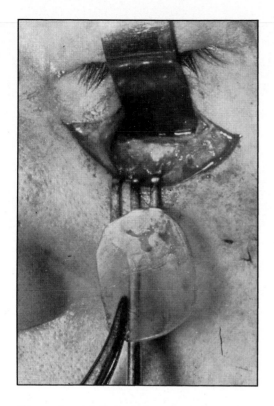

Figure 3.12 Polythene plate being inserted along the collapsed and fractured orbital floor to maintain eye elevation and prevent herniation of the orbital contents into the antrum

Correction of diplopia can be achieved in this way, and the use of polythene and Silastic in this situation has largely superseded the use of shavings of iliac bone graft.

Other methods of fixation which can be used are:

(1) Skeletal fixation, using two mounted screws, one into the malar body and one into the frontal bone at the superior orbital rim, and joining them together with a stainless steel bar and universal joints.
(2) Silver cap splints and an extra-oral bar to a mounted screw into the malar body, again joined by a bar and universal joints (*Figure 3.13*)
(3) A mounted screw into the malar body, attached to a plaster headcap (*Figure 3.14*). This is an unstable type of fixation and has been largely superseded.
(4) A Kirschner wire, getting stability on the normal malar, through the normal maxilla and normal septum into the unstable malar—in other words, transfixing the face (*Figure 3.15*).

All these methods have two objects in view—to restore contour and restore function. External fixations can be dismantled at the end of three weeks.

A local displaced fracture of the zygomatic arch is almost always capable of quick and permanent correction through the lift and oral temporal approach. The bones have angulated in and are still in contact; when levered out they 'click' out and stay

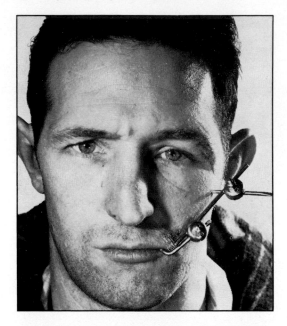

Figure 3.13 The malar supported through a mounted screw attached to a silver cast splint to the upper teeth

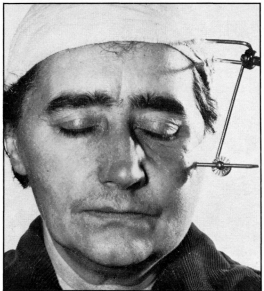

Figure 3.14 The malar supported by a mounted wood screw attached to a plaster headcap

out. An old fracture has to be broken down, and it is sometimes advisable to splint the arch by three circumferential wires tied over a wooden spatula along the arch, one wire passing anterior to the fracture, another posterior to the fracture to stabilize the wooden spatula, and the third wire passing around the fracture site. These wires are tied tight, and thereby keep the bones reduced in the outward direction.

Late treatment
If the patient presents any time up to four weeks after the accident, unless he is a child manipulation is usually successful in reducing the fracture. Almost always in late

attendances, an additional form of fixation to the straight temporal lift must be used. After that time an osteotome is usually needed to break down the fracture lines, and a polythene or Silastic plate, or iliac bone graft is very often needed for the collapsed orbital floor. For very old cases of displacement with a marked flattening, iliac onlay bone grafts can be used also to build up the malar prominence and the anterior wall.

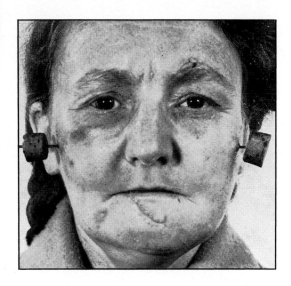

Figure 3.15 The malar supported by a Kirschner wire drilled through the normal malar and across the nose into the fractured malar

Post-operative complications
Infection of the antrum is uncommon. It is most likely to occur when the antrum has been packed, and persistent infection after removal of the packing, with an oro-antral fistula, indicates a sequestrum and the necessity for further exploration and intranasal antrostomy for drainage.

An *orbital haematoma* may be an extremely alarming phenomenon. If exophthalmos persists with the risk of exposure of the cornea it is necessary to make an incision through the lower lid into the floor of the orbit, and to drain this area. It sometimes happens in association with antral packing, and the pack must immediately be removed.

Surgical emphysema, particularly on blowing the nose, may occur through leakage from the ruptured antrum. This does not need treatment except the avoidance of blowing the nose.

Recovery of the sensation in the damaged maxillary division of the trigeminal nerve usually occurs by the end of three months. Sometimes it never recovers and the patient suffers a permanently numb cheek, nose, upper lip and upper teeth. Parts of the nerve may recover and other parts may produce unpleasant forms of parasthesiae, or formication. Persistent pains in the distribution rarely occur, but on occasion it can be so severe that avulsion of the nerve may be necessary.

Persistent diplopia is not infrequent to a minor degree. After six months it is sometimes possible for the ophthalmic surgeon to perform a muscle adjustment. A slight degree of diplopia even then is a very common final result, but does not seem to inconvenience patients very much. They become well adjusted to it.

References

Le Fort. (1901). Translated by W. W. James and
    B. W. F. Fickling. (1941). *British dental Journal*
    21, 85
Mathews, D. N. (1967). *Recent Advances in the
    Surgery of Trauma.* London; Churchill

4 Cosmetic surgery of the nose
R L G Dawson

Plastic surgery

Plastic surgery is concerned with the preservation or restoration of the function of the nose, and the preservation or restoration of the appearance. The treatment of the various forms of nasal obstruction usually lies in the realm of the ear, nose and throat surgeon, but the exterior of the nose and its appearance is frequently the subject of consultation between him and the plastic surgeon. The latter may be called in to deal with severe airway stenoses, or conversely where the airways are so large that atrophic rhinitis develops.

The nasal conditions that come to the plastic surgeon can be either congenital or acquired. The acquired ones are usually the result of old injuries, chronic infections and new growths, and occasionally damage from irradiation. It is necessary when dealing surgically with the nose to ensure that the three principal layers of the nose, the skin, the bones and the lining, all receive adequate attention.

Congenital abnormalities

The commonest is the familial hump nose which is too long, and which so often is a fearful anxiety to the patient. He has a sense of ugliness and inferiority which can affect his working and social life. The ideal nose should be one-third of the length of the face. There should be a 'stop' between the nasal process of the frontal bone and the nasal bones, and the nose should come out at an angle of 35 degrees from the face. The angle between the columella and the lip varies, and in women should be about 100 degrees, whilst in men it can usually be 90 degrees. The actual length and shape of nose depends not only upon the sex of the individual, but also upon the facial configuration; a lady with a long oval face would look stupid with a small turned-up nose, and such a patient should have a longer nose with a less obtuse nasolabial angle, whereas a round-faced woman can take a small turned-up nose, with a more obtuse nasolabial angle.

The presenting nose must therefore be examined in relation to the patient. One must note the general configuration of the face, the presence or absence of a nasal hump, the nasofacial angle and the nasolabial angle, the width of the present nasal bones and frontonasal processes, the state of the lateral cartilages (which are usually relatively unobtrusive but can be quite ugly), and the extent and size of the alar cartilages, particularly at the tip. Irregularity of the nostrils may be due to a twisted anterior septum presenting in one or other nostril. There may be a 'hanging tip' to the nose, that tip being very prominent furthest away from the lip. The actual width of the nostril on each side must be noted because, if the tip is to be lowered and there is already a wide nostril, it will become so wide that wedges must be removed from the alar base on each side. The presence or absence of valvular nostrils is also important, for if the patient already has this condition and the cartilages are trimmed, the condition may be made worse.

A number of patients fix their disappointments and failures in life upon what they consider to be a deformed nose, and one must be careful of these people; it is usually advisable to obtain a psychiatric opinion before subjecting them to a rhinoplasty, and they may very frequently have to go back to the psychiatrist after the operation has been done. There are, of course, other people who are so psychologically disturbed that it is frankly dangerous to take them on for surgery.

The operation for cosmetic rhinoplasty (*Figure 4.1*)

Pre-operative photographs are necessary, principally as a safeguard for the surgeon. The patient is starved for 4 h and has a usual premedication. The writer recommends a general anaesthetic with an endotracheal tube through the mouth, the tube lying straight down over the chin and not coming out of the corner of the mouth. The anaesthetist packs the pharynx firmly and puts three swabs of cotton wool on orange sticks soaked in a solution of 10 per cent cocaine and 1:1000 adrenaline up each nostril. He leaves them there for 10 min. The patient is operated upon lying at an angle of 30 degrees with the head up. Some surgeons use hypotension and then there is no need to use adrenaline and cocaine. Being opposed to this form of anaesthesia, the author prefers to inject 1.25 per cent Xylocaine with 1:100 000 adrenaline, 1 ml into the subcutaneous tissues on either side of the nose, 1 ml into the columella and 1 ml along the nasal bridge-line. It is of advantage then to wait for about 10 min until the cocaine, and the adrenaline–Xylocaine have taken effect.

The future shape of the nose is marked out in profile with Bonney's blue ink, and excess intranasal hairs are removed, as these not only get in the way of surgery of the nasal tip, but also tend to cake with blood clot afterwards and become painful. A Joseph's double-edged, curved-on-the-flat, pointed knife, is inserted at the junction between the alar and lateral cartilages and, passing superficial to the lateral cartilage and superficial to the nasal bones and the frontal process of the maxilla, separates the skin from the nasal skeleton as high as the frontal bone on each side. A blunt-ended bistoury knife is then inserted over the bridge-line to free the skin, and is then slipped down through the nasal tip just posterior to the columella between the columella and the septum, to the base of the septum. In this way all the skin is lifted off the nasal skeleton and the lateral cartilages and the septal and alar cartilages are separated from each other. Small curved scissors are then passed up over the bridge-line, to cut the procerus and corrugator muscles off the skin over the nasion. This is followed by the use of a Howarth elevator to scrape the muscle off the nasion downwards, and the muscle is then removed with a curved haemostat. An Aufricht nasal retractor is then inserted beneath the skin, and the lateral cartilages are separated from the septum on each side as far as the nasal bones. The estimated amount of lateral cartilage to be removed is then cut in strips attached to the nasal bone, from each side, along the bridge. The height of the septal cartilage that has to be removed along the bridge-line is cut from below upwards with a pair of cartilage scissors in line with the nasion. There are now three pieces of cartilage, two lateral strips and one central strip, lying free except where they are attached at their upper ends. A McIndoe nasal chisel is then inserted, with the bevel down towards the nose, beneath these three free strips until it impinges against the nasal bones that have to be removed. The bony hump is then chiselled off in line with the lowest part of the nasion. The free bony hump with its three attached strips of cartilage is then removed and the future bridge profile can be seen. The lower end of the septum is then shortened to the appropriate amount, and one must be warned not to take too much away, as it is extremely difficult to correct a nose that is turned up too much. It is therefore safer to take too little off the septum than too much. The nasal tip then sits back against the trimmed lower end of the septum and on the new height of the nose. The pointed lower end of the septal cartilage is then rounded off a little. Where there is a very prominent tip and the upper lip tends to be drawn up towards the tip of the nose, the anterior nasal spine must be chiselled away when the lower part of the septum is removed, so that the nasolabial angle becomes more acute. As the tip of the nose is set back, so the upper lip tends to lengthen a fraction. This is usually an advantage as many of these patients have a particularly short upper lip which tends to disappear behind the tip of the nose when they smile.

The new profile of the nose having now been achieved, it is necessary to narrow the nose by lateral saw cuts, or lateral osteotome cuts using a 5 mm osteotome, separating the nasal lining from the bone with a Joseph's elevator. The alar margin on each side must be pulled out a little, an incision made over the lower end of the frontal process of the maxilla and a Joseph's periosteal elevator passed up to separate the periosteum. A nasal saw is then passed into the incision as high as the frontal bone and just anterior to the medial canthal ligament. The nasal bones and frontal processes are then cut with the blade of the saw in the coronal plane, the handle of the saw being depressed towards the face. In this way the saw cut is made as far back as possible. The chisel is then passed up alongside the septum on each side and the attachment of the nasal bone and the frontal process to the frontal bone is chiselled off. The bones now being loose are depressed in, thereby narrowing the bridge-line. The columella is now re-attached to the lower end of the septum in its new position by catgut sutures passing through the septum and then back through the columella and tied. Three are usually sufficient. The tip of the nose can be depressed or lifted according to the direction of the suture. The tip of the nose always tends to fall after the operation to conform with the new height of the septum. As the nose has now been shortened there is an overlap of the lower border of the lateral cartilage on each side into the nasal cavity, and this overlapping portion is cut off with the scissors.

Finally the nasal tip itself is reduced by everting the tip of the nose with a finger on the skin pushing downwards and with a rake retractor pulling the edge of the ala upwards, so that the alar cartilage at the tip presents. An incision is made at the new level of the septum through the upper part of the medial crus of the alar cartilage, but

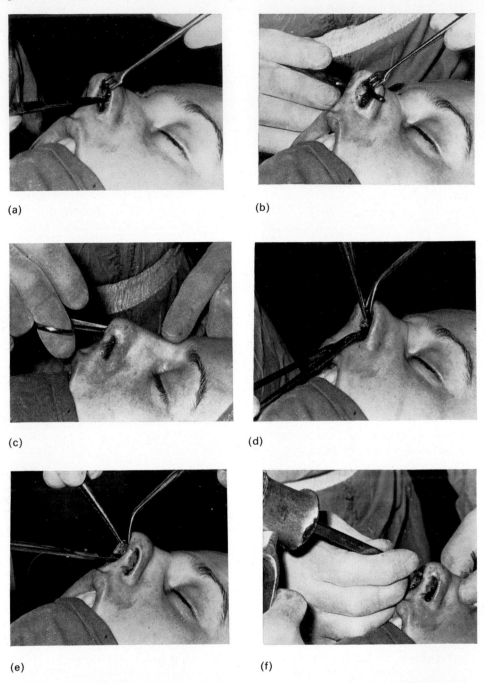

(a)

(b)

(c)

(d)

(e)

(f)

Figure 4.1 (a) Introduction of Joseph's double-edged, curved-on-the-flat knife between alar and lateral cartilages; (b) Joseph's blunt-ended bistoury has cut down over the dorsum of the septum and is now separating septum from columella; (c) fine curved scissors now separate the procerus muscle from the skin. It is then removed from the nasal bones with a Howarth elevator; (d) the lateral cartilages are separated from the septum and the necessary amount removed in line with the septum; (e) the excess septal prominence is cut up to the bony hump with cartilage scissors; (f) the bony hump is removed with a McIndoe chisel

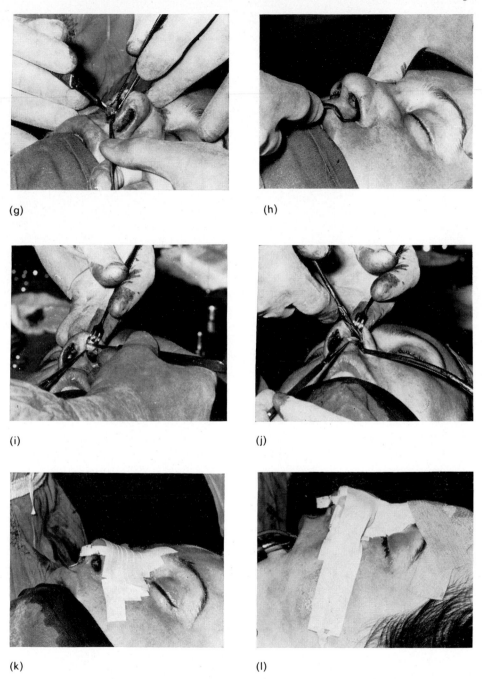

(g)   (h)

(i)   (j)

(k)   (l)

Figure 4.1 (cont.)   (g) The lower end of the septum is removed to lift the nasal tip and shorten the nose; (h) the lateral saw cut, in the coronal plane, through a separate alar incision; (i) the alar cartilage dome, having been undermined, and turned inside out, is reduced in size by removal of a determined amount from the upper edge; (j) the upper edge of the alar cartilage dome is finally removed with scissors; (k) strapping (1.25 cm) moulds the nose into its new shape; (l) the final plaster-of-paris splint is applied and held in place by Elastoplast. Note the really close fit in the canthal region

this incision must not go completely through the whole width of the cartilage. There must always be a small rim left intact. A hook then pulls the upper edge of the alar cartilage out and dissection with small curved scissors further loosens it. The upper portion of the dome can then be removed, which often includes both the lining and the dome cartilage, but in very large tips where much cartilage has to be removed it is advisable to dissect the lining off the cartilage first. Where the lining has to be dissected away from the cartilage it will tend to fall down unless it is lightly packed up into the dome of the nose with a little tulle gras at the end of the operation. If the tip of the nose is fat there is quite an excess of subcutaneous tissue. When the portion of the alar cartilage is removed equally on both sides the fat can be removed by everting the skin and removing it with small curved scissors.

The operation is now complete, the saw cuts and cartilage removal have been entirely symmetrical and the nose must now be fixed in its new position. A length of 1.25-cm zinc oxide strapping is split into two 0.6-cm tails, intact at the upper end. The upper end of the strapping is laid along the bridge-line of the nose and each of the tails is passed round the tip, to adhere with that of the opposite side. This performs a compression to mould the new tip. Strapping (1.25 cm) is then put in layers crosswise from the tip of the nose down the alar cartilage on each side. These pieces of strapping gradually get smaller as they go up the nose till the final piece is put across the nasion. This strapping moulds the nose, allows the operator to see the final shape the nose will take up and prevents to a large extent the formation of haematoma. A rigid fixation is then applied in the form of a plaster-of-paris splint of eight layers of 7.5 cm plaster-of-paris bandage after Vaseline has been applied to the eyelids and the eyebrows. The plaster of paris is then moulded and fixed to the face with Elastoplast and 2.5 cm-wide zinc oxide strapping.

Post-operative treatment
The patient will lose blood and blood-stained serum for two days post-operatively and therefore a small bolus of gauze is attached beneath the nose on the upper lip. Ice is applied to the eyelids to prevent haematoma from forming and the patient is nursed in the sitting-up position as soon as he is conscious. Any packs are removed on the second day. Erythromycin 250 mg four times a day for five days and Naseptin cream to the nostrils, are given routinely to prevent infection of the columella with *Staphylococcus*. The patient remains in hospital for three days and returns to the hospital for removal of the fixation and cleaning of the nose two weeks after the operation. If the plaster is removed earlier the nose tends to swell too much and the writer has lengthened the time of the nasal fixation from 7 to 14 days with more satisfactory results. There will still be a little swelling over the glabellar region and nasal tip. This swelling will gradually go down over the next three months. The full benefit of the operation is often not seen for at least six months.

Various special points need to be mentioned:

The treatment of the hanging tip   This is a difficult problem where the actual anterior part of the nasal tip hangs well down below the rest of the columella. It can be tackled by a greater amount of septal shortening immediately behind the hanging tip, so suturing the tip back to a higher level. Where the lower rim of the medial crus of the alar cartilage is particularly prominent it is usually best to remove this rim locally through a small incision on either side of the upper part of the columella, directly over the prominent portion of the medial crus. Symmetrical removal of this portion can be achieved. Closure is by small sutures of 5/0 silk which leave no permanent marking.

The very large bulbous tip   In some noses even when a satisfactory reduction of the hump of the nose has been achieved, the actual tip of the nose stands up in a most ugly way. This can be tackled by a fairly large cartilage dome removal with preservation of the lining combined with removal transversely of a portion of the columella. The portion to be removed lies almost at the base of the columella and the size of it depends upon the estimate of how much the tip must be brought down. When repairing this area the sides of the columellar excision are sutured together with 5/0 silk. This is an efficient way of reducing the excessive prominence and leaves a virtually invisible scar. The alternative is to perform a *Lipsett operation* on the alar cartilages. In this procedure the normal intercartilage incision which is always made to elevate the skin from the nasal skeleton is combined with a marginal incision just inside the actual margin of the ala, extending from the alar base to the dome and then down on the inner side of the columella. It then passes transversely at the base of the columella to meet the incision that has separated the columella from the lower border of the septum. The alar cartilage is then dissected out from the nose, covered with its lining skin, the medial crus being dissected first, then the dome, then the lateral crus. The attachment is only on the base of the ala and it is through this base that the blood supply to the cartilage and to the lining is maintained. The cartilage can then be brought out on a hook on each side of the nose and a new dome can be made by multiple small transverse cuts across the alar cartilage, in a predetermined position. The cartilage can then be bent to form its new dome, and the actual height of the nose can be reduced by a removal of a predetermined amount from the lower end of the medial crus. Each alar cartilage with its newly formed dome is put back into position, and four or five catgut sutures inserted along the intermarginal incision, in the dome, and in the columella. These are of 4/0 catgut quite loosely tied, otherwise the alar margin will be notched. They maintain the cartilage in its new position. The normal alar strapping fixation is then applied, and the nostrils packed for two days post-operatively. This method has the one advantage that the whole of the alar cartilage can be brought out, based on its lateral attachment only, and can be trimmed so that not only the upper border of the dome can be removed, but also the new dome can be made, under direct vision.

Alar base excision   In negroid noses, or where the tip of the nose has had to be lowered so much that a negroid type of nostril has been achieved, a wedge can be removed from each alar base. In Europeans the wedge is seldom more than 0.6cm and more skin should be removed than lining. Obviously a wedge excision of the alar base cannot be used when the Lipsett approach to the alar tip has been performed, otherwise the whole blood supply to the alar cartilage and lining would be cut off. The incision for removal of the wedge which is marked out in exact measurements on each side, should be just 1 mm in front of the actual alar groove. It must never be put into the alar groove, otherwise an ugly depressed scar will be obtained. Once the wedge is removed the small alar artery is ligated, and the lining repaired with 4/0 catgut and the skin with 5/0 silk. These sutures are removed at the end of five days. It is important not to remove too much, or too small a nostril with difficult airways will result.

The bifid nasal tip   This is usually a square tip and therefore the upper border of the alar cartilage dome has to be removed. It is then sometimes possible to remove the soft tissue from between the medial crura in the upper part and pass a catgut suture between the two cartilages to bring them close together. If it is a widely bifid tip it is best to remove an ellipse of skin and subcutaneous tissue from between the two cartilages from the exterior, suture the cartilage together under direct vision after removal of the soft tissue between them, and then suture the skin with 5/0 silk. The resulting scar is minimal.

The crooked nasal tip   This is due to a bend in the septal cartilage at the tip, the tip of the nose passing over to one or the other side. During the cosmetic rhinoplasty after the central bridge-line and the lower end of the septum have been freed the displaced septum is separated from the nasal floor and the shortened lateral cartilage is sutured to the septum on the contralateral side. In this way the septum is held over in an over-corrected position away from the side to which it has bent. The suture used should be a 4/0 chromic catgut and subsequent external fixation must over-correct the deformity; suturing the shortened lateral cartilage back to the septum acts in the same way as the guy-rope of a tent.

Valvular nostrils   In this common condition the nostrils flap against the septum on inspiration, thereby causing obstruction to the intake of air. This is due to lack of rigidity of the alar and lateral cartilages and the most satisfactory procedure is to perform an intercartilagenous incision, and dissect the skin off the lateral cartilage thereby making a pocket on either side. A portion of the lining of the nose overlying the upper border of the lateral crura of the alar cartilages is then removed. The denuded alar cartilage is passed over the lower border of the lateral cartilage and held in place by fine catgut mattress sutures passing through both the alar and lateral cartilages and tied into the lining of the nose. A fine catgut suture can also be used to close the gap between the lining attached to the alar cartilage and the lining attached to the lateral cartilage. In this way a double layer of nasal cartilage is formed on either side and produces the required rigidity with a very slight flaring of the nostrils.

The nose of a person suffering from cleft lip and palate (*Figure 4.2*)

The extent of the deformity of the cleft lip determines the amount of deformity of the nose, but all grades of cleft lip, even the smallest notching of the vermilion border show, to a greater or lesser extent, the classic deformities of the nose that are associated with the maldevelopment of this area. The columella is deflected towards the normal side. The dome of the cartilage on the abnormal side is lower in the vertical dimension, and retroposed. It is less well developed. The medial crus lies slightly lower in the vertical dimension than on the normal side. The lateral crus of the ala is much flatter than normal and the alar base is displaced downwards and backwards because there is underdevelopment on the affected side of the maxilla. It is also displaced further laterally than normal. The lateral cartilage follows this outward displacement and lies on a flatter plane than on the normal side and the nasal bones and the frontal process of maxilla on the abnormal side tend to be wider and flat with a deviation of the nose as a whole to the normal side.

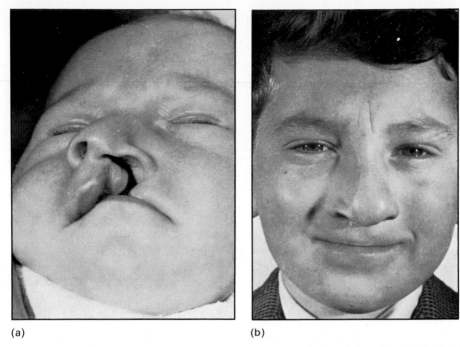

(a)   (b)

Figure 4.2   (a) The cleft lip nose showing flat, wide, recessed ala and the columella deviated to the normal side; (b) same patient showing the residual nasal deformities

The operative procedures that can be performed to correct these deformities concentrate on the bony skeleton and on the nasal tip. It is justifiable to perform a definitive operation upon the nasal tip at about 13 years old, whereas a correction of the bony skeleton must wait until the nose has finished its growth, at about 17 years old.

Operations upon the nasal tip
The displaced alar base can be brought in towards the columella by lifting a wedge based on the upper lip from the abnormally wide nasal floor and transposing that wedge into the defect created by incision of the alar base, transferring the alar base medially to fill up the gap left when the wedge of tissue has been transferred from the nasal floor. In other words, a Z-plasty is performed, using the alar base as one limb of the Z and the nasal floor as the other limb. In this way the base of the ala can be approximated to the columella. If the columella is grossly displaced towards the normal side a similar Z-plasty can be performed using the columella as one limb of the Z and a portion from the nasal floor on the abnormal side as the other limb.

The flat low alar dome can be reformed by reversing the Lipsett flap, basing it on the medial crus, using marginal and intercartilaginous incisions which tail off towards the alar base and meet. In between these incisions lies the dome of the alar cartilage and the lateral crus which is mobilized with its lining skin attached. It is then brought to the exterior still attached at the columella and a new dome created by transverse riberation of the cartilage. The lateral crus is then advanced up and sutured to the normal dome on the opposite side with fine chromic catgut and the defect so created by the advancement of the lateral cartilage medially, that is left on the inner side of the alar base, is closed by direct approximation of the skin edges. In this way the alar base is lifted upwards from its downwardly displaced position, and the new dome created on the abnormal side. The marginal incision is closed with two or three loosely tied fine catgut sutures and the nostril packed lightly with tulle gras. It is often advisable to perform a reduction of the dome on the normal side also, as this assists in the matching of the two sides of the nasal tip. Adhesive strapping surrounding the nasal tip, passing up over the nasal bridge-line, is held by transverse strips of similar strapping, and it is kept in place for seven days. The nostril pack is removed at the end of two days. It is not advisable to perform the alar base shift medially at the same time as the lateral crus is advanced, two separate operations being necessary. The writer does not advise inrolling of the displaced lower edge of the abnormal alar cartilage dome, which usually results in a rather ugly notch.

The bony skeleton

This is corrected at about 17 years of age, and is centralized by the normal lateral saw cuts, but a wedge must be removed from the nasal bone and frontal process of maxilla on the flattened abnormal side to allow the nose to be moved across to the straight position. The nasal bones are separated from the septum by a chisel passing up on either side and cutting across at the top of the junction of the nasal bone and frontal process. Strapping fixation covered by a plaster-of-paris splint is maintained for 12 days. Where a severe nasal deformity has occurred (and nowadays with the modern surgical approach to cleft lip and palate defect, the nose is the most lasting stigma of the condition) there is very often a severely twisted septum with the vomer running almost horizontally from the normal palatal side. When the palate has been closed this vomer presents a severe obstruction. It is therefore often necessary, in the severe cases, to perform a submucous resection.

Cleft of naso-lacrimal groove (*Figure 4.3*)

In this condition there has been a failure of the tissues from the lateral part of the face to meet the tissues of the nasal complex. This leaves a gutter of mucous membrane showing between the lower lid and area of the caruncle of the orbit, and the nasal cavity, with a failure of the alar base to develop properly and a failure of attachment of the alar base to the cheek. There is also a failure of the bone and superficial tissues to close over the gutter to form a proper naso-lacrimal duct and lacrimal sac. There is therefore a coloboma of the lower lid, and a gutter on the side of the nose, with a gap where the alar base should meet the cheek. These patients require an attachment of the alar base to the cheek with a transposition naso-labial flap to fill the defect on the lateral side of the nose, surgical closure after excision of the mucosal gutter, a conjunctivorhinostomy and correction of the coloboma of the lower eyelid.

Nasal dermoid cysts (*Figure 4.4*)

These cysts are formed by the inclusion, within the developing septum, of a portion of epithelium. Where the primary cartilage has been replaced by bone epithelial

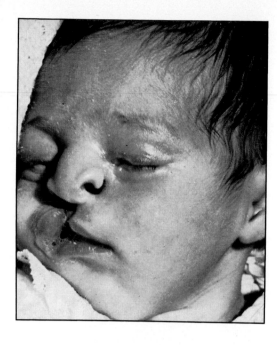

Figure 4.3 A naso-lacrimal cleft on both sides and a cleft lip on the right

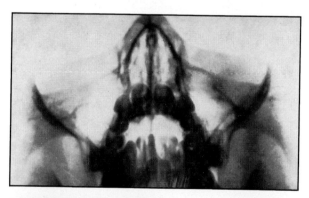

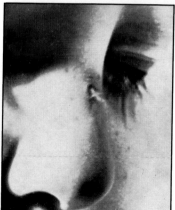
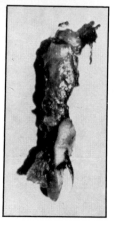

Figure 4.4 The nasal dermoid. The x-ray shows the cystic cavity in the septum

remnants may be left which gradually grow, causing a widening of the nasal septum, or even a double septum to develop in its upper part. The lower part of the nasal septum always appears to be single. There is widening of the septum associated with a widening of the nasal bridge, and with a small pit which is usually in the midline, but can be displaced to one or other side. It is usually about halfway down the nasal bridge-line but can be at the tip of the nose or up at the base of the nose. This little pit has a few hairs sprouting out of it. A 60 degree occipitomental view of the nose will sometimes show a cystic cavity.

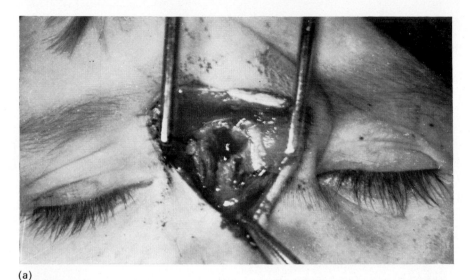

(a)

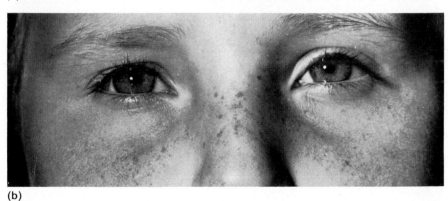

(b)

Figure 4.5   (a) The operation for nasal dermoid. The cavity has been unroofed and the cyst removed; (b) the ultimate scar is small

The eradication of this cyst can be difficult (*Figure 4.5*). The nose has to be split from just distal to the pit to approximately the glabella. The pit is circumcized and the sinus is traced between the nasal bones. The nasal bones surrounding the sinus are nibbled away and the cyst is found lying between the two leaves of the nasal septum. It is sometimes necessary to outfracture the nasal bones and frontonasal processes on each side using a small chisel to take the bones off the frontal process. A more direct and extensive view can then be obtained if the sinus passes backwards towards the sphenoidal sinus. Occasionally these dermoid sinuses have to be traced up to and into the base of the skull. When the cyst and its sinus have been removed the outfractured nasal bones, with the frontal processes of the maxillae attached, are brought together and held in the narrowed position with trans-nasal stainless steel wires tied over lead plates. These plates must remain on for three weeks. Where an extensive operation has been performed, it is advisable to prescribe sulphadiazine and penicillin for at least five days post-operatively.

The frontonasal glioma

This is a midline swelling over the bridge of the nose, causing a wide nasal bridge, splayed out nasal bones and frontonasal processes, composed of gliomatous tissue. It is often from the frontal lobe and in continuity with it. The glioma has a stalk and it must be removed with its stalk, through an external nasal approach. The outfractured nasal bones are subsequently brought together and held in the narrowed position with lead plates.

Acquired abnormalities

Deformities resulting from an old trauma

The laterally displaced nose (Figure 4.6)
Lateral displacement can be confined only to the cartilaginous portion, the bony bridge being intact, and this is probably the hardest type to correct. There is usually a gross angulation of the lower part of the septum taking the tip over, with a 'kick back' into the airway on the side of the injury. The lower end of the septum presents in the contralateral nostril. In this type of case the 'swinging door' operation is indicated.

   The usual intercartilaginous incision is made on each side, extending over the septum and then down between the septum and the columella separating these two structures. The lateral cartilages are detached after the covering skin of the nose has been mobilized up over the dorsum of the bony skeleton, and the lateral cartilage on the ipsilateral side is shortened in its coronal or vertical plane. This lateral cartilage will then be reattached to the nasal septum when it has been straightened, thereby holding it in its proper position. After the dorsum of the septum has been freed the mucoperichondrium on the concave side of the bent septum is stripped off the cartilage from the columellar incision backwards beyond the bend in the septum. At the bend, the cartilaginous septum is divided, but still remains attached to the perichondrium on the opposite side through the whole of its extent at the actual bend. The skin and mucosa of the nasal floor is then lifted on each side of the septum, the nasal spine is chiselled away, and the vomerine crest is removed as far back as the hinge of the septum that has just been made. A new bed in the proper position is thereby made, and the bent part of the septum is swung into place. The septum now is free completely except for the hinge of the mucoperichondrium on the convex side of the bend and it is attached to the columella after a groove has been made between the two medial crura with dissecting scissors to receive its lower end. The suture, which passes through the columella, through the septal cartilage and then back through the columella again, is tied over a small piece of tulle gras. The lateral cartilage on the convex side of the septal bend is then attached to hold the septum over in its proper position. Trans-columellar and trans-septal catgut sutures are then passed in the usual way to fix back the columella to the lower end of the septum. Both nostrils are packed for two days, the nasal skin being held down against the skeleton with 2.5 cm Elastoplast or zinc oxide strapping for one week.

This operation may have to be combined with a formal infracture for displaced nasal bones where there is a combination of both bony and cartilaginous skeletal deformity. After lifting the nasal skin through the usual incision and freeing the columella and the lateral cartilages from the septum, the surgeon makes lateral saw cuts, and a chisel is passed up on either side of the septum to separate the nasal bones, cutting outwards at their junction with the nasal process of the frontal bone. It may be necessary to shorten the lateral cartilage on one side and tether the tip over into its new position. The nasal skeleton is then fixed with zinc oxide strapping and plaster of paris for 12 days. More usually, however, it is advisable to straighten the nose but to delay a submucous resection for a subsequent operation because of the risk of synechiae if the submucous resection and the nasal straightening are performed at the same time.

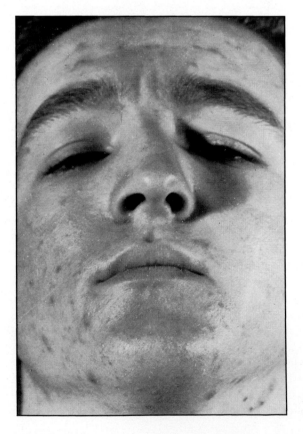

Figure 4.6 The laterally displaced nose. Post trauma

For the long-neglected 'frontal type' of nasal injury with overlapping nasal bones, it is necessary to perform a lateral saw cut at the site of the old fracture on both sides, separate the nasal bones from each other with a chisel, and then transfix the nose with wires tied over lead plates, to be kept on for three weeks.

Loss of septal support

This is a very common deformity, following on severe untreated trauma to the septum, or haematoma and subsequent infection of the cartilaginous septum, with complete loss. The tip of the nose is kept up to a certain extent by the alar cartilages but the nostrils are splayed out, the tip is flatter than normal and the maximum deformity can be seen just above the alar cartilage domes where there is usually an obvious saddle. This injury may or may not be associated with a fracture and displacement of the nasal bones. Where the septal loss has occurred in childhood the nasal bones grow in a divergent way, spreading out laterally, and sometimes causing flattening of the profile. It is therefore necessary to perform corrective surgery in two stages.

The first stage narrows the nose and straightens the bony skeleton so that a good base can be obtained upon which a bone graft can be put later to raise the whole profile of the nose. At the same time it may be justifiable to remove any severely displaced septal remnants, so that there is virtually no septum left at all. After the usual plaster-of-paris fixation the patient is discharged for future operation in about four months' time, when the tissues have softened down enough to allow for a bone graft.

Some surgeons use rib cartilage instead of bone, but the writer prefers bone from the iliac crest. Other surgeons use implants and in the past have used ivory, ivalon, polythene and now use Silastic, but these implants tend to be extruded, particularly if any injury is sustained, and in the writer's view the only indication for using Silastic is in a child, where there is a badly collapsed nose which is to be temporarily supported in order to stimulate the forward growth of the central part of the face. The Silastic can then be removed when growth is finished, at about 16 or 17 years, and can be replaced with a bone graft.

The decision to use a bone graft depends upon the actual deformity of the nose. Where there is a reasonable bony bridge of good elevation it may only be necessary to support the nasal tip as far as the bony bridge. If a total loss of septum has been sustained there is very often a retracted columella, which cannot be seen from the lateral view, and is an extremely ugly deformity. In such cases a bone graft is used to support the lower part of the nasal bridge combined with a bone graft to bring down and maintain the columella in a more satisfactory position. This is usually a thin graft shaped like a boomerang, one end of the graft resting on the nasal spine, the other end in apposition to the lower edge of the nasal bones. Where there is a flat bony bridge-line with a flattened tip but still with a columella visible from the side, and very little columellar retraction a cantilever type of bone graft is used of one strip hollowed out on the surface which fits over the nasal bones thinning down to a blunt point where the graft will come up against the alar cartilage domes. The bone graft must never lie between the alar cartilages, as this produces a nasal tip which is much too wide. It must always be behind the alar cartilage domes. Where there is a combination of retracted columella, a flattened bony bridge-line, and a flattened nasal tip, the graft is bigger and must extend along the whole length of the nose down into the columella.

The nose is infiltrated with normal saline only. No adrenaline is used, because the operator must be able to see if the skin is pale when the graft is inserted. The saline is used in order to define the tissue planes for easier dissection. The incision is made vertically down the centre of the columella, the gap between the two medial crura is defined, then the dissection passes between the alar domes, between the two leaves of the septal mucoperichondrium and over the bony bridge-line. The operator will find that the difficult part of doing this dissection, done usually with McIndoe scissors, is at the lower edge of the nasal bones. The dissection must pass laterally over each side of the nose, in order to free the nasal skin extensively, and should not be made subperiosteally. The bone graft must lie on top of the nasal periosteum and no special cut need be made into the nasal processes of the frontal bone in order to receive the bone graft. Ideally this bone graft should be lying relatively free and symmetrically upon the nasal bridge; thus if the tip of the nose is hit a fracture of the graft will not occur since the bone graft is not united to any part of the nasal skeleton. If extensive lateral dissection of the skin from the side of the nose is not made, too much tension will occur when the bone graft has been inserted, with the risk of skin necrosis. If a boomerang bone graft has been used with the nasal tip supported by the columella it is not necessary to dissect up over the nasal bridge, but just as far as the nasal bones allow, separating the two leaves of the mucoperichondrium from the septum. The cavity thus formed is now packed with a little gauze and the operator changes his gloves and takes a bone graft from the iliac crest. This second part of the operation is performed at this time and not as the first part of the operation, because sometimes the nasal lining is torn during the dissection to form the cavity into which the bone graft is to be put, in which case, if there is a severe tear, the operation should be abandoned and repeated again in three months' time. This bone is removed from a lateral hip wound over the iliac crest, care being taken not to detach the anterior superior iliac spine. When the bone graft is removed the periosteum is stripped from both plates and from the crest and usually it is wisest to remove a small block of bone from the whole width of the iliac crest, of the right length and about 2.5 cm deep. The edges of the crest where the graft has been removed are bevelled off, the muscle is sutured together across the gap, and a corrugated drain is used for two days. Subcutaneous catgut and medium silk close the skin wound, and with a wad of gauze is bound into the slight depression and a firm spica bandage applied. The bone is now taken and shaped according to the desired type and dimension, is sprayed with Polybactrin powder and inserted into the cavity along the nasal bridge-line and into the columella. The cantilever graft must sit up on the nasal bridge against the nasal process of the frontal bone where it is bevelled to fit, and the marked tension of the skin on this part of the graft, if it has been properly shaped on the cantilever principle, maintains the tip of the nose in its elevated position. There is no need for a further graft in the columella. Where the boomerang graft is used, care must be taken that there is no projection of the end of the graft as it lies against the lower end of the nasal bones. The alar dome cartilages are then sutured across the end of the bone graft with fine catgut and the columella incision closed with fine silk. Elastoplast (2.5 cm) fixation is used; the Elastoplast divided to surround the nasal tip and then pass over the bridge-line. Further layers of Elastoplast are placed across the nose. A plaster-of-paris splint must never be applied because of the risk of necrosis of the skin where it is sandwiched between solid bone graft and rigid plaster. The Elastoplast fixation is kept on for seven days and the sutures are removed from the columella after that time.

Loss of septal support and a flat central part of the face

This deformity occurs following a severe injury to the nasal skeleton and particularly to the anterior nasal spine region during childhood, and a flat central part of the face results. The dental arch is perfect, but just above the dental arch the bone has not developed properly and the upper lip turns back towards the nose, rather like a monkey. There is a small nose with a slightly retracted columella, a loss of all tip support because the catilaginous septum has gone, a deformed nose with wide divaricating nasal bones, and a flat profile (*Figure·4.7*).

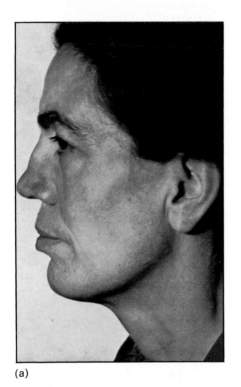 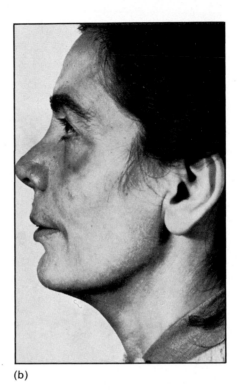

(a)   (b)

Figure 4.7 (a) Old injury to nose in childhood showing a low saddle deformity, a retracted columella and lack of anterior nasal spine development, with a flat central part of the face; (b) same patient after an L-shaped bone graft and an inlay bone graft beneath both alar bases and across the top of the upper lip

After preliminary infracture and narrowing of the bridge-line the second stage of the operation usually consists of a boomerang type of bone graft. Access to the nose is made with a vertical columellar incision with two limbs branching out from the lower end of this incision slightly across the nostril entrance at the junction with the upper lip on both sides, as an inverted Y. The two leaves of the mucoperichondrium are separated and a cavity is made to receive the boomerang bone graft. Further cavities are made beneath each alar base and across the upper lip at the junction with the nose, so that the whole of the upper lip and both alar bases are brought forward by packing with bone chips removed at the same time as the boomerang graft was taken. In this

way the saddle nose, the retracted columella, the flat middle part of the face with the
retroposed alar bases, and the flattened upper lip, are all corrected. Elastoplast
(2.5 cm) is applied across the upper lip and across the nose and is removed after seven
days. These patients usually suffer quite a large amount of swelling of the central part
of the face, but this quickly goes down over the week following the operation.

So far, definitive treatment for congenital disfigurement and post-traumatic
disfigurement with loss of nasal tip support has been described; equally important is
the loss of lining of the nasal airways.

The loss of lining may be caused by the use of sclerosing solutions in mistake for
adrenaline when severe epistaxis is to be controlled. There is severe fibrosis between
the septum and the lateral walls. It is necessary to divide all the adhesions and to make
gutta percha moulds of the opened nasal passages, upon which are draped split skin
grafts removed from the hairless inner side of the upper arm. The grafts are draped
raw side outwards, and stuck to the moulds with Mastisol. The moulds bearing the
skin grafts are then inserted into the nasal passages and a piece of adhesive strapping
passed round the nostrils to maintain them in place. Usually two moulds are made for
each side, and suitably marked, the spares then being sent to a dental laboratory
where they are converted into clear acrylic moulds with a hole bored through the
centre. At the end of three weeks the moulds are changed, the clear acrylic ones
replacing those of gutta percha, and the patient must wear these for six months. If they
are permanently removed earlier a contracture of the skin graft will occur, and
stenosis will become severe again.

Loss of lining also occurs as a result of syphilis and leprosy and following irradiation
treatment of eosinophilic granuloma. In these conditions one meets with a very severe
collapse of the distal half of the nose, the cartilages and lining having been destroyed.

These are cases for the *classic post-nasal inlay.* An incision is made in the upper buccal
sulcus and all soft tissues of the central middle third of the face are cut off the bones.
The periosteum must be left attached to the bone. The septal remnants are divided,
the division of the soft tissue from the skeleton being continued up to the dorsum and
to the nasal bones. In this way, all the soft tissues can be lifted off the face and restored
to their original shape again. Overcorrection must be performed before the gutta
percha mould is made to lie inside the cavity so created, to force the soft tissues of the
nose into an overcorrected position. The skin graft is taken from the inner side of the
thigh, and draped as a sheet over the gutta percha mould, to adhere to the mould with
Mastisol. The mould rests on the upper part of the front of the maxilla and the skin
and soft tissues covering the mould and the lining skin graft are pressed down upon the
mould with layers of 2.5 cm Elastoplast dressed over the nose and over the lower lip.
The mould is removed under general anaesthesia three weeks after the operation, the
cavity cleaned out and the mould re-inserted. The patient is then instructed how to
take the mould out, syringe out the cavity and then re-insert the mould rapidly once
a week. If a mould is left out during the early days post-operatively for more than
2 min, contracture of the skin graft will occur which will necessitate re-operation, but
as the months go by the mould can be taken out for longer intervals. At the end of six
months the potentiality of the skin graft to contract is finished, and the patient is then
fitted with an acrylic intranasal support which he wears permanently. In some cases
it is possible to put a thin bone graft between the covering nasal skin and the split skin
graft lining and to close the opening in the buccal sulcus, thereby avoiding the
necessity to wear an acrylic support.

Loss of cover of the nose

This can occur as a result of trauma, and in rare accidents over half the nose can be lost. It is much more usual however, to lose an alar margin, frequently as a result of a dog bite. If the loss has been a large one and is not suitable for repairing with local flaps, or with a composite graft from the ear, it is best to suture the lining to the skin edge to avoid contracture and then to perform a reconstructive operation later. Tissue loss can occur also as a result of burns, frost-bite or therapeutic irradiation for new growths. Chondritis is particularly liable to occur when therapeutic irradiation is used on the nasal tip.

The benign lesions that involve the covering of the nose are:

(1) Capillary haemangiomas of the port-wine stain variety which remain flat and of good texture until middle age when they tend to become very lumpy.
(2) A mixture between capillary and cavernous haemangiomas where there is involvement of the subcutaneous tissues as well.
    Besides the necessity to resurface the nose, there is the need to reduce its size as well. In the latter type of haemangiomas a combination of surgery and sclerotic fluids such as saturated saline injections (30 per cent) or selective diathermy coagulation deep in the cavernous haemangioma is used.
(3) A pigmented naevus also requires removal and resurfacing.
(4) A molluscum sebaceum, diagnosed by its rounded and umbilicated appearance with dilated vessels upon it and the rapidity of its growth, very often requires removal, and restoration of nasal cover.

Rather on its own in this section there is the rhinophyma (*Figure 4.8a*), one type coming on in relatively young people, associated with a thickening and acne-like infection of the cheeks as well, and a close association with Roseacea and achlorhydria. The other type of rhinophyma which tends to be a more irregular lumpy condition, comes on in middle age, getting progressively worse. This is a relatively simple but bloody condition to treat, and it is advisable to infiltrate the area with 1:200 000 adrenaline solution before surgery.

Surgery consists of shaving down the grossly enlarged sebaceous element until a satisfactory shape is achieved. When this has been done the raw area is covered with a layer of tulle gras, gauze and some wool. These dressings are held in place with Elastoplast across the nose and obliquely from cheeks to forehead. At the end of ten days the remnants of the sebaceous glands which have been left have produced a complete re-epithelialization of the nasal skin (*Figure 4.8b*).

Haemangiomas and the pigmented naevi must be removed and the raw areas resurfaced with post-auricular Wolfe graft skin (*Figure 4.9*), which is a very good colour match. If the area is too big three-quarter thickness free skin grafts taken from the abdomen, or a Wolfe graft taken from the supraclavicular region can be used. Where possible the defect should be made symmetrical; in this way the graft is not so noticeable. Tie-over sutures are used with a pressure dressing which is not disturbed for ten days.

A basal-celled carcinoma ultimately results in a loss of nasal cover. It is commonest in the inner region and at the alar base. In the inner canthal region the recurrence rate

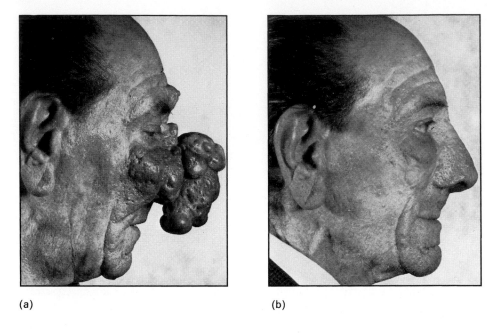

(a)   (b)

Figure 4.8   (a) A rhinophyma of 20 years' duration; (b) post-operative appearance of same patient. This has been achieved by simple shaving of the rhinophyma only

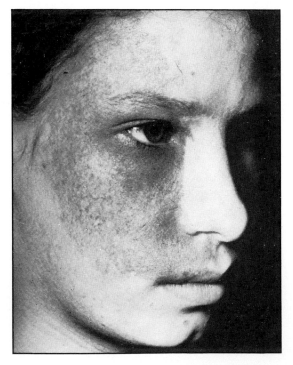

Figure 4.9   A post-auricular Wolfe graft has been used to replace a capillary haemangioma on the side of the nose

after radiotherapy is relatively high, and the growth is in close proximity to the lacrimal sac, the nasolacrimal duct, and the ethmoids, which are not infrequently invaded (*Figure 4.10a*). If the growth is not deeply involved, removal and a post-auricular Wolfe graft is the treatment of choice. If, however, a very large depth of

(a)

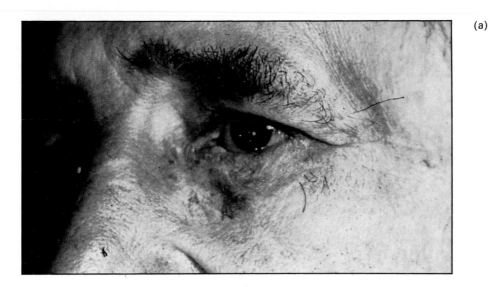

(b)

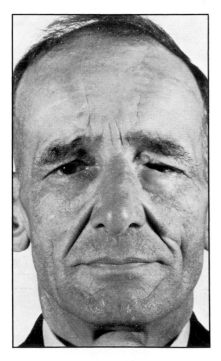

Figure 4.10 (a) A recurrent basal cell carcinoma invading the lacrimal sac, and upper and lower eyelids, and caruncle, and ethmoids; (b) same patient after excision of the basal cell carcinoma and repair by a forehead flap

tissue has to be taken, down to the nasal bone and the frontal process of the maxilla, a Wolfe graft is not an acceptable repair, first because the contour is bad and secondly because there may be bare bone upon which a free skin graft will not survive. Therefore a glabellar flap is frequently used, the donor area of the flap being sutured by direct approximation. For larger defects which may involve the removal of the inner third of both eyelids, the ethmoids, and the nasolacrimal apparatus, a forehead flap (*Figure 4.10b*) based on the opposite supra-orbital arteries, or a midline forehead flap can be used, the lining being achieved by a reflection of the bulbar conjunctiva as far as the limbus of the cornea. It is not necessary to close a hole into the nasal cavity of the size of a thumbnail if the forehead flap is being inset into a fairly wide area around that hole.

Basal-celled carcinomas of the alar base also have a rather sinister outlook because they tend to invade the maxilla, and post-irradiation recurrence in this area is relatively frequent. A wide excision of the localized rodent ulcer is performed with preservation of the uninvaded lining. A large nasolabial flap is brought up, based upwards from the nasolabial fold to be sutured into place, and the defect from the donor area is closed by direct approximation. If there is involvement of the nasal lining and involvement of the peripheral area adjacent to the cheek it is safest to excise widely, to suture to nasal lining, and to use a skin graft as a temporary measure to achieve healing on the cheek. The area should then be watched for nine months, and if at the end of this time there is no evidence of any recurrence, a reconstruction can be achieved by a cheek rotation flap to the defect abutting the nose. Either a composite graft, for a small defect, or a central forehead flap for a large defect, can be used to restore the contour of the nose.

Epitheliomas of the nose are commonest on the dorsum and here there is usually a slight ulceration and roughening of the skin. A biopsy confirms the diagnosis, and the whole of the dorsal skin of the nose should be removed and replaced with a split-skin graft. If there is no recurrence of the growth in nine months the dorsum of the nose can be repaired with a forehead flap which gives the best contour and colour match.

Melanoma of the nose is a rare condition with a severe prognosis. When on the ala, a wide excision and suture of skin to mucous membrane should be performed but early repair by forehead flap should be delayed until it is obvious that there will be no local recurrence. It is usually wisest to wait a year and in the meantime to provide the patient with a prosthesis to wear on a spectacle frame.

Operations to restore the cover to the nose
A *split-skin graft* has already been mentioned. After haemostasis the three-quarter thickness graft is sutured into place with long tie-over sutures, used to fix the flavine wool pack; 2.5 cm Elastoplast strips are used for further fixation. The graft is not dressed for ten days.

The post-auricular Wolfe graft is particularly useful for the side of the nose and inner canthal region. A pattern of the defect is marked out on the back of the ear, and the post-auricular sulcus is distended up with normal saline giving a flat area to excise. The Wolfe graft is taken half from the back of the ear and half from the mastoid area, and the wound closed by direct approximation with a subcuticular catgut suture. All fat is trimmed off the undersurface of the graft and it is then sutured into place using long tie-over sutures, and a continuous fine silk everting mattress suture. The pressure dressing is not disturbed for ten days.

The composite graft: if there is a small notch in an alar margin, a portion of the lobe of the ear matching the size of the notch is removed, and the lobe defect sutured directly. The edges of the defect to be grafted are trimmed and the composite graft sutured into place using 4/0 catgut for the lining and fine silk for the exterior. It is then best to pack the nostril with ribbon gauze and penicillin cream. The graft will go through various colour changes, first of all white, then blue, and where successful it will finally become slowly pink. This is a graft of skin and fat and skin again on the deep surface. Where the whole of the nasal rim has been lost it is reasonable to remove the rim of the helix, from the junction of the upper part of the helix to the scalp. The donor wound is closed by direct approximation of the two layers of skin over the cartilage, and the composite graft which now contains a small element of cartilage and skin on both sides, is sutured into place and packed in the usual way.

Nasolabial flaps are very useful for small but deep defects on the side of the nose. The flap can be reasonably long in relation to its width and a 4:1 ratio is safe on the face. It is based upwards on the side of the nose, and it is taken from the nasolabial fold, the donor areas closed by direct approximation. The flap can be rotated through 90 degrees to lie in the defect on the ala. There is often a small 'dog ear' at the point of rotation of the flap, which can be trimmed off three months later as a minor operation under local anaesthesia.

Glabellar flaps are based downwards, usually on the opposite side of the glabella to that of the defect which they have to fill. They can be quite long because of the good blood supply. They descend and are rotated through 90 degrees to fill the defect which is usually in the canthal region. A small adjustment of the 'dog ear' may be necessary some three months later. The donor area is closed by direct approximation.

The forehead flap (Figure 4.11) is by far the best for extensive nasal reconstruction. For a total reconstruction of the lower half of the nose, which has been lost through accident or through surgery for new growth, the lining has to be provided by turning down the remaining nasal skin based on the edge of the defect, so that the nasal skin is then turned to look inwards with the raw surface uppermost. In this way a lining for the alar margin on each side can be obtained and also a lining for the future columella. The nasal skin in the centre is sutured to a small flap turned up from the centre of the upper lip. In this way lining skin is obtained and the forehead is used to cover the whole area, from the nasion down to and including the nasal tip. It is now best to make a pattern of the approximate size of the proposed nose in tinfoil which can be moulded so that it stands up in its proposed position. This pattern is then placed on one side of the forehead with the edge for the columella and alar margins lying just above the eyebrow, and what will be the skin of the nasion area just below the hairline. The pattern is marked out and then a line is drawn across the scalp over the top of the frontal area in the hairline down to the temporal area on the opposite side. The pattern reaches to the midline and an incision along this edge of the pattern can be prolonged upwards a little way so that a greater length of flap can be achieved. The lower incision, along the future alar margins and the columella is made through the skin only and then just in the subcutaneous tissues the dissection is carried up for a distance of 0.8 cm before taking the full thickness of the scalp down to the pericranium. This thin distal 0.8 cm is turned in when the flap is pulled down to make the new nose, and sutured to the down-turned nasal skin that is being used as a lining. In this way a rounded margin is achieved for both alae.

The flap is then dissected up, and an incision made along the margins of the flap and

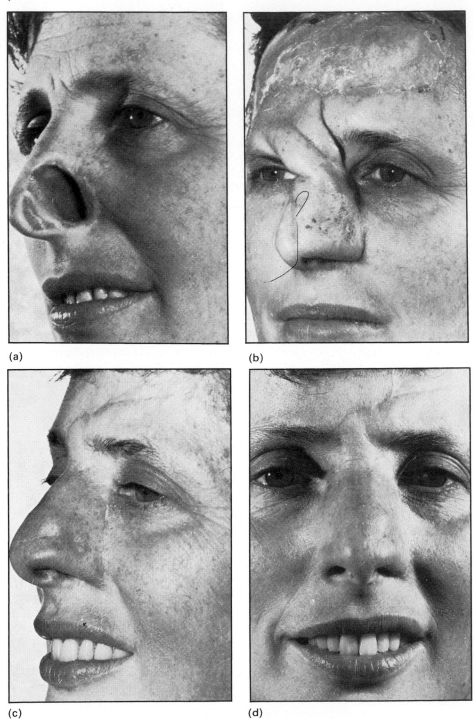

(a)

(b)

(c)

(d)

Figure 4.11 (a) The forehead flap rhinoplasty. The defect following removal of a carcinoma; (b) the forehead flap in position. The donor area grafted with split skin; (c) the forehead flap now forms the whole of the left side of the nose; (d) the flap has covered the whole left side of the nose

prolonged over the upper part of the frontal area in the hairline, whilst the vertical midline incision is prolonged a little upwards. The whole flap is then turned down based on the superficial temporal and supra-orbital arteries of the opposite side. Haemostasis is achieved on the donor area by gripping the aponeurosis with haemostats, and turning them back over the scalp. It is important to take all bleeding vessels on the flap edge and ligate them, otherwise bleeding may occur to such an extent that the distal part of the flap does not get enough blood supply. The flap is sutured into place, feeding it distally all the time, beginning with the suturing of the columella and of the alar margins and then pushing down the flap so that an excess of tissue lies at the tip. Suturing is proceeded with as high as possible with medium silk but there is a bridge across the normal tissue at the bend of the flap and on this bridge a piece of tulle gras is placed. A split-skin graft is taken from the thigh and sutured into place on the forehead and these sutures not only fix the graft but also act as haemostatic sutures. A firm pressure dressing is applied and there is always a very good survival of skin, as the pericranium is very vascular and is a firm and smooth bed. The skin grafts also extend onto the undersurface of the down-turned pedicle.

A double figure-of-eight suture is now used to mould the nasal tip, tied over two dental rolls, one on each side of the nasal tip, on the surface, and two small tulle gras rolls in the nostrils. These are tied firmly but not too tightly, otherwise necrosis of the tip of the flap will occur. All sutures are removed at the end of seven days. The dressing of the forehead skin graft is taken down at the end of ten days. Three weeks after the first operation the pedicle that bears the flap for the reconstruction is divided, and that part that is not needed for the nose is replaced on the forehead and scalp, after removal of the appropriate amount of the skin graft. The remnants of the forehead flap attached to the nose are then sutured into place in the glabellar region.

It will be necessary to make some small adjustment to this forehead rhinoplasty about six months to one year after the initial operation, and at this time it is usual to excise an ellipse of skin along the dorsum and two ellipses, one on either side, just above the alar margin. This produces a narrowing of the rather redundant dorsum, and produces a groove in the normal position just above the alar margin.

The Italian rhinoplasty, using the inner side of the upper arm, is indicated when the forehead skin is not in a good enough condition to be used. It is, however, a difficult flap to use—difficult for the patient. The positioning of the patient puts him to a lot of discomfort and inconvenience, with the hand on the top of the head, and the nose against the upper arm. The flap is initially inset on the glabellar region and not to the tip, and therefore it is much more difficult to get an excess of tissue in the tip where it is always needed. Finally, the colour match is not as good as the forehead provides.

Tubed pedicles can be used. This procedure has been described using skin from the neck, but the available skin is only enough for a small defect; from the acromio–thoracic region, where the colour match is not good and the inset is initially on the glabellar region with the same difficulty of putting excess into the tip; and from the abdomen, brought up on the wrist as a conveyor with the same disadvantages of the initial glabellar inset and poor colour match. They all have their indications, however, but the forehead rhinoplasty is by far and away the best method.

5 Congenital diseases of the nose
R Pracy

The nose is such an important and such a neglected organ that severe congenital abnormality, unless recognized, may be incompatible with life. It is probably for this reason that severe congenital abnormalities of the nose are very rare. For the purposes of this chapter structural abnormalities will exclude those whose effect is purely cosmetic.

Anatomy and embryology

In order to understand the various congenital abnormalities which may occur in the region it is necessary to keep certain important aspects of developmental anatomy in mind.

The nose is formed between two and 28 days of intrauterine life by the sinking in of olfactory pits of ectoderm. Above these lie the forebrain and below them the primitive oral cavity (*Figure 5.1*).

The olfactory pits are invaginated from the area of the olfactory placodes, which are thickenings of the ectoderm on either side of the face. The mesoderm between the olfactory cavity and the buccal cavity becomes thinned out between the 35th and 38th

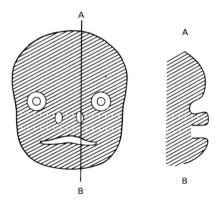

Figure 5.1 Embryology of development of choanae (schematic). Sagittal section through nasal pit of 28-day embryo

73

day of intrauterine life. The two layers of epithelium rupture, leaving a primitive choanal opening posterior to the premaxilla. At this stage the horizontal processes of the maxilla and the palatine bones develop from masses of mesoderm lying laterally. This gives rise to the formation of the secondary palate. This mesoderm too becomes invaded by the olfactory pit which grows caudally to meet the foregut growing anteriorly. Where the two epithelial surfaces meet they rupture giving rise to the secondary or definitive posterior choanae.

The external nose is developed mainly from the fronto–nasal process, but lateral contributions are also derived from the lateral nasal processes. Most of this development takes place in the second month of intra-uterine life and fusion of the fronto–nasal process, comprising elements of the septum and the dorsum of the nose and the lateral nasal process, should be complete by the end of the second month. Above this lies the metopic suture which closes at a variable time after birth.

Malformations

Complete absence

This is an extremely rare abnormality but cases have been reported by Wakely (1904), Denis (1919) and Walker (1961). Gifford and McCollum (1972) reported two cases associated with complete absence of the nasopharynx. The children learned to mouth-breathe, but feeding presented problems.

Partial absence of the nose

This is also a rare abnormality but cases of failed development of one nasal cavity are reported and the author has known a case of unilateral choanal atresia. Notching of the nasal cartilage is sometimes seen and this may be associated with hypertelorism.

Cleft tip

Hypertelorism may be associated with partial or complete cleft of the tip of the nose and in some of these patients the premaxilla is missing. The repair of such abnormalities should be carried out by the otolaryngologist and plastic surgeon working as a team. No precise advice can be given which will cover all cases, but in general some kind of primary soft-tissue repair should be carried out in infancy once the full extent of the abnormality in the deeper tissues has been determined. Correction of bony abnormalities should not be attempted until growth has stopped.

Proboscis lateralis

This consists of a tube of skin arising from the region of the inner canthus of the eye and is associated with hypoplasia of the nose on the affected side. The nasolacrimal duct does not open into the inferior meatus and the abnormality appears to be associated with imperfect fusion of the fronto–nasal and lateral maxillary components.

Repair consists of some form of dachryocystorhinostomy associated with the use of the tubular process to feed into the hypoplastic area.

Cysts

Dermoid cyst formation due to imperfect fusion may be seen in the nose, in the nasal cavity or in the post-nasal space. It has been suggested that small areas of epithelium sequestrate and form cysts. Occasionally these sequestrated areas retain a minute communication with the surface epithelium and a sinus results.

Clinical picture
The patient presents with a swelling in the midline, on the dorsum of the nose, which may be associated with splaying of the nasal bones. The swelling does not increase in size on coughing or crying. Occasionally the swelling presents at the nostril, giving rise to nasal obstruction, or a finger-like projection appears below the posterior end of the soft palate and interferes with feeding. In one case seen the projection came out of the mouth on crying and gave rise to laryngeal irritation and choking. Posterior cysts arise from the roof of the naso-pharynx, laterally in the fossa of Rosenmuller. They can usually be removed in the neonatal period by means of a snare. The snare should be guided into the posterior nasal space through a nostril, fed round the cyst and the wire closed gradually. This helps to reduce the post-operative bleeding.

Dermoids in the nasal cavities should be removed as soon as it is certain that there is no intracranial communication. Dermoids on the dorsum of the nose should be removed at about the age of 3–4 months before they have had the opportunity to produce severe distortion of the nasal architecture.

Nasal glioma

This is a solid tumour, usually present at birth, which increases steadily in size causing nasal obstruction and deformity of the nasal skeleton. The tumour does not contain brain tissue and may be connected intracranially by a stalk, from which the tumour derives its blood supply. It does not increase in size on straining or crying.

Diagnosis
It is vital to distinguish nasal glioma from nasal encephalocoele. Nasal glioma should be removed by the otolaryngologist using an external operation. Nasal encephalocoele communicates with the subarachnoid space and must therefore be treated by the neurosurgeon.

Nasal gliomas are solid, they do not increase in size on coughing or crying, and they are not associated with a large defect in the floor of the anterior fossa. They should be removed by a modified lateral rhinotomy incision.

Encephalocoeles

Encephalocoeles may present in the nasal cavity or they may present over the glabella. The management of intranasal encephalocoeles lies within the province of the neurosurgeon.

Frontal encephalocoele is rare but it is important to recognize it as it may be confused with a frontal dermoid. Frontal encephalocoele like nasal encephalocoele communicates intracranially. It increases in size on straining, coughing or crying, and it is an abnormality which is more commonly seen in Asia and is possibly associated with a widening of the intercanthal space. It appears to be associated with failed closure of the frontal neuropore. Sometimes pressure over the swelling may give rise to somnolence in the baby.

If the bony defect is small and is demonstrated radiologically and the encephalocoele protrudes only on straining or crying, it can be approached most conveniently and safely by external operation. The defect in the bone should be carefully closed. If, however, the encephalocoele is large, it will have to be treated by craniotomy and the patient should therefore be treated by the neurosurgeon.

Posterior choanal atresia

This rare abnormality is probably the commonest congenital disease of the nose. The incidence is approximately 1 : 60 000 of live births and unilateral atresia makes up 60 per cent of all cases seen. The condition is seen in girls twice as commonly as it is in boys.

Pathological anatomy
The essential features of the developmental anatomy of the nose are outlined at the beginning of the chapter. Posterior choanal atresia occurs when the olfactory pits do not extend backwards completely and a barrier results between the nasal and post-nasal spaces. The extent of the failure determines whether this is a membranous or a bony atresia. Furthermore bony choanal stenosis may be found which may cause symptoms, particularly when the infant develops upper respiratory tract infection. The shape of the nasal cavity in these cases is important because only when this is appreciated will it be obvious that it is impossible to cover bare bone with mucosa, as has been advocated by certain authors.

The nasal cavity tapers to a point posteriorly in bony atresia and this narrowing may be seen as far anteriorly as the posterior end of the premaxilla. It is important to realize that this tapering is circumferential and thus, it is at the level of the bony obstruction that the area of mucosa available is minimal (*Figures 5.2* and *5.3*).

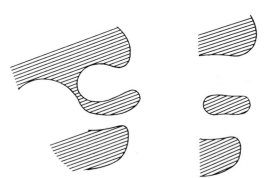

Figure 5.2   Embryology of development of choanae (schematic). Later stage with differentiation of primary palate and bucco-nasal membrane

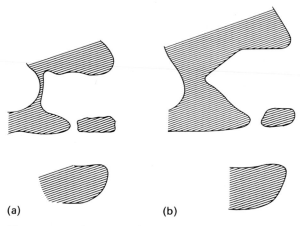

Figure 5.3 Embryology of development of choanae (schematic). (a) Secondary palate invasion of mesoderm and formation of naso-pharyngeal membrane. (b) Incomplete development leading to atretic pit

Clinical picture

By instinct the neonate breathes through its nose. If for any reason this is not possible it will asphyxiate. If the mouth is opened and an airway is inserted then the child will immediately breathe easily. However mouth-breathing without the help of an airway is a function which is only acquired slowly and with difficulty.

The symptoms of bilateral choanal atresia may fall into two categories:

(1) Breathing only when the mouth is held open.
   In such patients violent efforts to nose-breathe are made. Lips and cheeks are indrawn and the colour deteriorates. There is also indrawing of the soft tissues of the neck and thoracic cage. Opening the mouth leads to an immediate improvement in the situation.
(2) Feeding difficulties.
   These are due to the impossibility of sucking when the mouth is closed because this makes breathing impossible. Such children have to be fed by tube, pipette or by McGovern's nipple. This is a modified top of a breast pump. Three holes are cut in it. Milk can then be dripped through one of the laterally placed holes while air is taken in through the central hole.

Patients with unilateral atresia have symptoms which are less easily defined. The condition is unlikely to be recognized in the neonatal period and it must be suspected in a baby who is breast-fed and who experiences difficulty in sucking when one particular nostril is occluded by contact with the mother's breast. This difficulty will of course be accentuated during periods of upper respiratory tract inflammation.

Snoring is *not* a sign of choanal atresia, either bilateral or unilateral.

Management

The essential step which must be taken if cerebral hypoxia is to be avoided is the protection of the airway. This can be achieved either by an indwelling endotracheal tube or by a Waters airway strapped in position over the mouth. The baby should not be fed unless it is intended to delay possible surgical treatment. If this delay is anticipated then the baby should be fed by a tube.

Examination

Once the airway has been secured the infant should be examined by the otolaryngologist, radiologist and neonatologist. The otolaryngologist passes catheters into the nostril but they do not pass into the post-nasal space. The radiologist outlines the obstruction with a watery solution of Dionosyl. The neonatologist looks for associated developmental abnormalities such as blindness or heart disease which are known to be associated with choanal atresia. The plan of treatment is based upon the prognosis offered by the neonatologist and the radiological demonstration of the nature and extent of the obstruction. If surgical relief of the obstruction is proposed it should be carried out *early* in order to avoid possible complications commonly associated with the setting up of an artificial airway.

There is no contraindication, in the absence of other demonstrable abnormality, to operation within a few hours of birth.

Possible treatment

The aim of treatment is to establish permanent patent posterior choanae. This may be achieved by either transnasal or transpalatal approaches.

Membranous atresia   Where the atretic membrane is thin and removal of bone is not anticipated a transnasal approach is to be preferred. Under endotracheal general anaesthesia with a hypopharyngeal pack, a small Hagar's dilator is passed through the membrane. The hole thus made is then dilated using dilators of increasing diameter until 14/16 French Gauge is felt to pass easily. A Portex tube is now passed through the nasal cavity from the post-nasal space and secured in position by sutures. Usually a tube of 3.5 mm will be passed without difficulty. Pure membranous atresia accounts for approximately 10 per cent of all cases.

Transpalatal operation for bony atresia   Where it is anticipated that bone will have to be removed, a transpalatal operation should be carried out. This was first proposed by Brunk in 1909, modified by Blair in 1931 and by Ruddy in 1945. It is essential to have endotracheal general anaesthesia and packing of the hypopharynx. The surgeon sits at the head of the table looking down on the operative field. A small rolled towel is placed under the shoulders. The mouth is held open by means of Killian's mouth gag. The tongue plate helps to keep the endotracheal tube out of the operative field. The baby's eyes are protected with Vaseline gauze before the towels are applied.

The area of the incision is infiltrated with 1:300 000 adrenaline solution. A 'U'-shaped incision with the convexity of the U facing towards the surgeon is made on the hard palate, and is carried as far forward as can be sewn up efficiently and comfortably. This allows for the closure to be made over a bony support. The straight limbs of the U follow the margins of the hard palate posteriorly and pass lateral to the greater palatine artery and over the posterior 0.5 cm of the alveolas (*Figure 5.4*).

A mucoperiosteal flap is raised by means of a sharp elevator which presses principally on the bone of the palate. In this way tearing of the flap is avoided. An assistant retracts the flap and the elevation is continued posteriorly until the posterior border of the hard palate is identified.

Beginning in the midline the bone of the palate is drilled away from posterior to anterior until the base of the septum, the atretic plates and the unopened mucosa of the

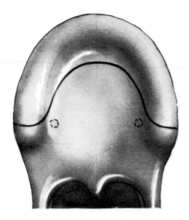

Figure 5.4   The incision. (From *Operative Surgery*, 3rd edn. *Nose and Throat*. Ed. by Rob, C. and Smith, R. London; Butterworths)

nasal cavities are exposed. Very careful measurements must now be made, and the greatest care taken not to damage what mucosa there is. The posterior end of the septum and atretic plate are drilled away, again leaving the mucosa intact. The superior and lateral limits must be defined. Superiorly the removal stops when the atresia reaches the level of the roof of the nasopharynx. The lateral limit is the canal of the greater palatine artery and these limits must be sought and confirmed repeatedly by the passage of a blunt probe. This ensures that the largest possible choanae are constructed. The mucosa of the superior surface of the soft palate and of the nasal cavities is now divided and tubes are passed into the nasal cavities from the post-nasal space. (In bilateral atresia these tubes may be connected posteriorly and should be sewn together at the anterior nares. They should be maintained in position for a minimum of two weeks and can be left for up to 28 days.) The flap is then sutured back into position. A $\frac{5}{8}$ circle Denis Brown artery needle will be found to be ideal for this suturing (*Figures 5.5* and *5.6*).

Post-operative treatment
Tubes have been left in nasal cavities. Such tubes are foreign bodies, furthermore they interfere with the humidification of the nose. Therefore the patient is covered with prophylactic antibiotics while the tubes are *in situ* and humidity is supplied.

Stitches are removed after seven days. Tubes are removed after 14–21 days and following removal of the tubes the choanae are kept patent by the passage daily of gum elastic bougies of appropriate diameter. The parents should be instructed in the use of the bougies and this routine should be maintained until it is certain that post-operative stenosis will not occur.

Complications
(1) Infection   Bacterial rhinitis may follow the operation. This is because the tube acts as a foreign body and it may be that the prophylactic antibiotic does not cover the organism causing the rhinitis. If this is suspected nasal swabs or post-nasal swabs should be sent for culture and sensitivity tests and the more appropriate antibiotic given.

(2) Fistula formation   If a great deal of bone has had to be removed a fistula may form. However, this usually closes once the tube is removed. If it does not close a form of closure has to be undertaken using a flap based on the greater palatine artery.

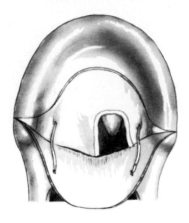

Figure 5.5   Exposure of the atresia. (From *Operative Surgery*, 3rd edn. *Nose and Throat*. Ed. by Rob, C. and Smith, R. London; Butterworths)

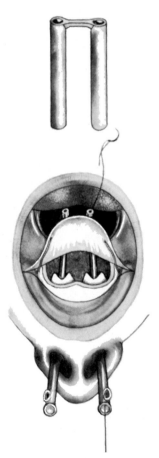

Figure 5.6   Splinting. (From *Operative Surgery*, 3rd edn. Nose and Throat. Ed. by Rob, C. and Smith, R. London; Butterworths)

(3) Closure of the choanae   Undue optimism on the part of the surgeon or unwilling parents may lead to the formation of a dense membranous stenosis formed of scar tissue due to lack of daily bouginage. Where this is extreme it may be necessary to reopen the transpalatal incision.

References

Gifford, G. H. and McCollum, D. W. (1972). *Pediatric Otolaryngology*, p. 932. Ed. by Ferguson and Kendig. New York; Saunders

Ruddy, L. W. (1945). 'A transpalatine operation for congenital atresia of the choanae in the small child or infant', *Archives of Otolaryngology*, **41**, 432

Walker, D. G. (1961). *Malformations of the Face*, p. 191. Edinburgh; E. & S. Livingstone

6 The nasal septum
David Brain

Injuries of the septum

The anterior part of the nasal septum projects in front of the plane of the piriform aperture and is frequently damaged when the nose is injured. The severer injuries may result in a haematoma formation and/or septal deviations.

Septal haematoma

When the septum is subjected to a sharp buckling stress, submucosal blood vessels are often torn and if the mucosa remains intact, this will result in the formation of a haematoma. If the injury is severe enough to fracture the septal cartilage, the blood will often pass through to the other side and produce a bilateral haematoma. The blood mainly accumulates in the subperichondrial layer and this will usually interfere with the vitality of the cartilage which is avascular, and which depends on the perichondrium for its nutrition. Avascular cartilage can probably remain viable for three days, but afterwards the chondrocytes die, and absorption of the cartilage follows. Cartilage absorption can occur with alarming rapidity and Fry (1969) has suggested that the process is hastened by enzyme action, probably in the form of one of the tissue collagenases. Small haematomas will not cause this necrosis of cartilage, but may slowly absorb leading to permanent thickening of the septum with gross fibrosis.

Symptoms and signs

The dominant symptom is nasal obstruction, and initially there may be some discomfort. Examination is best made without a speculum, and there is a smooth rounded bilateral septal swelling which often extends to the lateral nasal walls causing complete obstruction (*see Figure 6.1*).

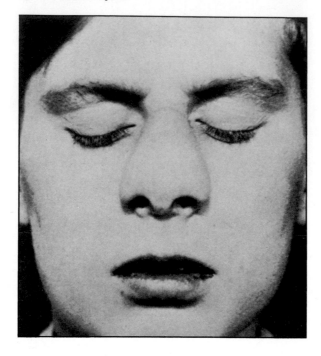

Figure 6.1 A large septal haematoma (Mr. C. A. Keogh)

Treatment

Fry (1969) has shown that early surgical drainage of the haematoma reduces the risk
of cartilage necrosis, and is therefore the treatment of choice. A long incision should
be made at the most dependent part of the haematoma as soon as possible. If the
cartilage is still intact, bilateral incisions are necessary. The mucoperichondrium is
then replaced against the underlying cartilage and is held in this position by intranasal
packs. A broad-spectrum antibiotic should also be given to reduce the risk of secondary
infection.

Complications

External deformity of the nose
The cartilaginous dorsum of the nose is supported by the septal cartilage and if this
support is lost, dorsal saddling in the supra-tip area will result. If this type of injury
occurs during childhood, it may also affect the development of the whole of the mid-
third of the face with resulting maxillary hypoplasia.

Septal abscess
A haematoma may easily become infected and this will frequently lead to abscess
formation. This complication is usually associated with an increase in the severity of
the pain, together with the usual manifestations of toxaemia such as pyrexia and a
raised pulse rate. The advent of secondary infection makes extensive cartilage necrosis
virtually inevitable, and is an even more pressing indication for surgical drainage.

Septal deviation

Septal deviations are extremely common but are usually not severe enough to affect nasal function. The incidence of these deformities is much higher in the leptorrhine type of nose found in the Caucasian races.

Aetiology

Direct trauma
Many septal deviations are due to direct trauma and this is frequently associated with damage to other parts of the nose such as fractures of the nasal bone.

The birth moulding theory
In many patients with septal deviations there is no obvious history of trauma. Gray (1972) explains these cases by means of his birth moulding theory (*see Figure 6.2 and 6.3*). Abnormal intrauterine posture may result in compression forces acting on the nose and upper jaws (the widest part of the face). Displacement of the septum can result and the nose can be exposed to further torsion forces during parturition. Jeppesen and Windfeld (1972) found 29 cases of septal dislocation in 907 newborn infants (3.19 per cent). Dislocations were more common in primipara and where the

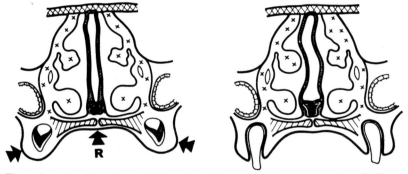

Figure 6.2 Combined septal deformity. Diagrammatic representation of effect of equal pressures on septal growth, producing deviation deformity and splaying out of vomer-cartilage junction. Note irregular hypertrophy of lateral nasal wall. (From *Modern Trends in Diseases of Ear, Nose and Throat* (1972). London, Butterworths. Reproduced by permission of Mr. Lindsay Gray)

second stage of labour lasted more than 15 min. Dislocations were generally to the right in the case of LOA presentations and to the left with ROA presentations. Subsequent growth of the nose accentuates these asymmetries.

Pathological anatomy

Deformities of the nasal septum can be classified as:

(1) Spurs
These are sharp angulations which may occur at the junction of the vomer below, with the septal cartilage and/or ethmoid bone above. This type of deformity is usually due

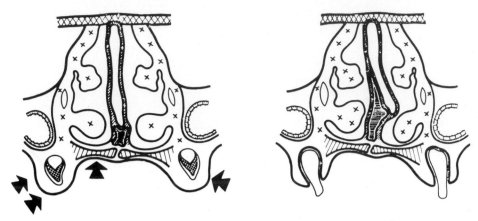

Figure 6.3   Combined septal deformity. Diagrammatic representation of effect of unequal pressure on septal growth producing spur deformity. Note elevation of palate, with tilting of vomer to the opposite side, unequal growth of the vomer, irregular hypertrophy of the lateral nasal wall and changed alignment of teeth. (From *Modern Trends in Diseases of Ear, Nose and Throat* (1972). London; Butterworths. Reproduced by permission of Mr. Lindsay Gray)

to vertical compression forces. Fractures through the septal cartilage may also produce sharp angulations. These fractures heal by fibrous union and the fibrosis extends to the adjacent mucoperichondrium. This increases the difficulty of the flap elevation in this area (*see Figure 6.4*).

(2) Deviations
These lesions are characterized by a more generalized bulge. 'C'- or 'S'- shaped deviations occur which can be either in the vertical or horizontal plane, and they usually involve both the cartilage and the bone.

(3) Dislocations
Here the lower border of the septal cartilage is usually displaced from its medial position and projects into one of the nostrils (*see Figure 6.5*).

Septal deviations are also often frequently associated with anatomical abnormalities in adjacent areas including:

(1) The lateral nasal wall
A compensatory hypertrophy of the turbinates and ethmoidal bulla usually occurs on the side of the septal concavity.

(2) Maxilla
The compression forces which are responsible for the septal deviations are often asymmetrical and may also involve the maxilla, producing flattening of the cheek, elevation of the floor of the affected nasal cavity, distortion of the palate and associated orthodontic abnormalities. The maxillary sinus is usually slightly smaller on the affected side.

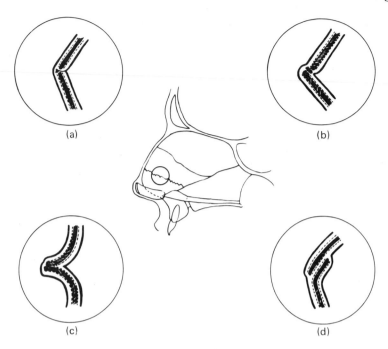

Figure 6.4 Some of the commoner septal cartilaginous fractures. (a) Edge-
to-edge angulation; (b) Angulation with overlap; (c) Bowing of both edges
at the fracture line; (d) Duplication. If a fracture–dislocation occurs during
the growth period, the displaced edges continue to grow and usually increase
the deformity. (From Bernstein, 1973. Reproduced by permission of W. B.
Saunders & Co.)

(3) The external nasal pyramid

Anterior septal deviations are often associated with deviations in the external nasal
pyramid. Deviations may affect any of the three vertical components of the nose and
there are three common types which are in order of severity:

(a) Cartilaginous deviations   In these cases, the upper bony septum and the bony
pyramid are central but there is a deviation of the cartilaginous septum and vault (*see
Figure 6.6*)

(b) The 'C' deviation   In this lesion, there is displacement of the upper bony septum
and the pyramid to one side and the whole of the cartilaginous septum and vault to the
opposite side.

(c) The 'S' deviation   Here the deviation of the middle third (the upper cartilaginous
vault and associated septum) is opposite to that of the upper and lower thirds.

With deviations of the nose, the dominant factor is the position of the septum.
Beekhuis (1973) has succinctly summarized this principle with the dictum 'as the
septum goes, so goes the nose'. The first step therefore in treating the twisted nose, is
to straighten the septum, and if this objective is not achieved, there is no hope of
successfully straightening the external pyramid.

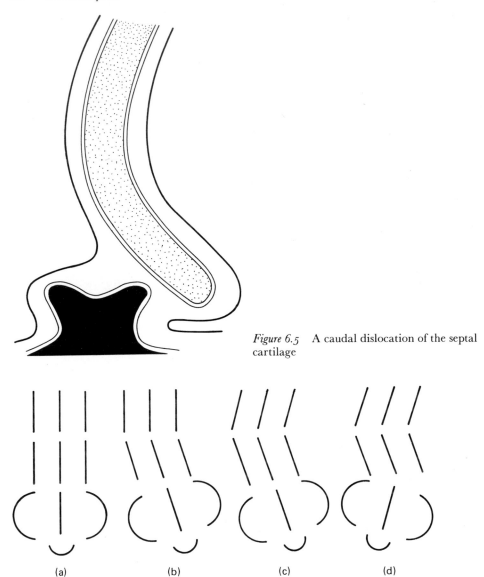

Figure 6.5   A caudal dislocation of the septal cartilage

Figure 6.6   (a) Normal nose; (b) A straight bony pyramid with a deviation of the cartilaginous pyramid; (c) 'C'-shaped deviations of both bony and cartilaginous pyramids; (d) 'S'-shaped deviations of both bony and cartilaginous pyramids

There is therefore a sound pathological basis to the concept of straightening a twisted nose by means of a one-stage septo–rhinoplasty procedure.

The effects of septal deviations

Only the more severe deviations affect nasal function and therefore require treatment. In these cases there may be:

(1) Nasal obstruction
This is always found on the side of the deviation and is also often present on the opposite side due to the hypertrophic changes in the turbinates.

(2) Mucosal changes
The inspiratory air currents are often abnormally displaced and frequently become concentrated on small areas of nasal mucosa, producing an excessive drying effect. Crusting will then occur, and the separation of the crusts often produces ulceration and bleeding. The protective mucous layer is often lost and resistance to infection reduced. The mucosa around a septal deviation may become oedematous as a result of Bernouilli's phenomenon, which states 'that when there is a flow of gas through a constriction, it produces a negative pressure'. This negative pressure will in turn predispose to mucosal oedema in the affected area thus further increasing the obstruction.

(3) Neurological changes
It is possible that the pressure exerted by septal deviations on adjacent sensory nerves can produce pain. This concept was first elaborated by Sluder (1927) and the resultant condition has been called by Shalom (1963), 'the anterior ethmoidal nerve syndrome'. In addition to their direct neurological effects, reflex changes perhaps may result from septal deformities which affect the naso–pulmonary and nasal reflexes.

Symptoms

The symptoms caused by septal deviations are entirely due to their effects on nasal function. As seen from the last paragraph the dominant symptom is nasal obstruction but this is rarely severe enough to cause anosmia. Douek (1974) has investigated many patients who were suffering from anosmia and this symptom was never due to an uncomplicated septal deviation.

Signs

Septal deviations are usually quite obvious on anterior rhinoscopy. It is important to first inspect the nasal vestibules without using a speculum because the blade of this instrument can easily straighten the septum and thus hide a caudal deviation. Cocainization may facilitate the inspection of some of the more posterior deviations. The septum cannot be considered in isolation and it is therefore necessary to perform a careful inspection of the lateral nasal wall to determine the size of the turbinates. Examination must also include the external nasal pyramid, the palate and the teeth as these structures are often also involved to some degree with septal deformities. Whenever sinus complications are suspected, x-rays of the paranasal sinuses are indicated.

Typically, septal dislocations in the newborn are associated with asymmetry of the nostrils, an oblique columella and a tip which points in a direction which is opposite to the dislocation. The nostril on the affected side looks distinctly flattened. These characteristic features are not always present and it is therefore necessary to perform an anterior rhinoscopy and the compression test. In this latter test, the nasal tip is pushed backwards and if there is a septal dislocation, it will collapse against the philtrum of the upper lip.

Indications for submucous operations on the nasal septum

Septal deviations

Minor septal deviations are extremely common and do not as a rule require surgery, which should be reserved for the more severe deviations which interfere with nasal function. The anterior lesions are usually best treated by a septoplasty technique. They are also often associated with deformities of the nasal pyramid, and a septo–rhinoplasty will then be indicated. The more posterior deviations are usually quite effectively treated by the classic submucous resection technique. The conventional reduction rhinoplasty usually produces some narrowing of the nose and this may well result in minor septal deviations which had been symptom free pre-operatively, afterwards causing troublesome nasal obstruction. The septum should therefore be examined much more critically when any surgery of this type is contemplated.

Closure of septal perforations

Most techniques which have been described for the closure of septal perforations involve the submucous elevation of the flaps for this purpose.

Source of grafting material

Submucous resection of nasal cartilage and less commonly vomerine bone, is sometimes required to obtain graft material for other operations such as tympanoplasties.

To obtain surgical access

Submucous resection of the septum has been advocated as giving the necessary access for the following surgical operations to be performed:

   (a) Hypophysectomy (Hirsch, 1952).
   (b) Vidian neurectomy (Minnis and Morrison, 1971).

The development of septal surgery

The study of the history of septal surgery is both interesting and instructive. It clarifies the basic problems encountered in treating septal deviations, and demonstrates the limitations of the various techniques which have been evolved to solve them. During the nineteenth century, surgeons started tackling these problems by a variety of techniques which have now been completely abandoned. Acute spurs and angulations were removed either by shaving down the convexities (Langenbech, 1843; Diefenbach, 1845; Chassaignac, 1851), or by performing a complete removal of the deviation by punch forceps (Rubrecht, 1868). The usual result of these operations was to exchange a septal deviation for a perforation. These techniques are only of historical interest, and there is little doubt that the first major breakthrough in surgical therapy occurred about the turn of the century with the development of the SMR (submucosal removal) operation.

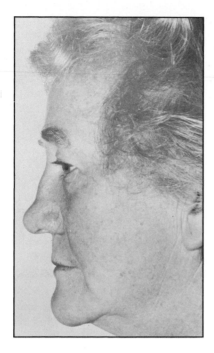 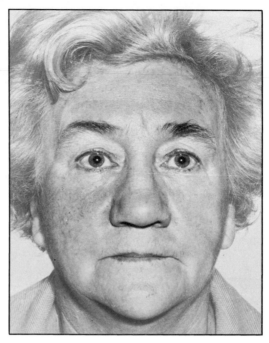

Figure 6.7 Gross supra tap saddling and retraction of the columella following an SMR

Figure 6.8 Widening and bulbosity of the nasal tip following an SMR

As so often happens, the idea of effecting a submucosal removal of the deviation, occurred to several surgeons working independently at the same time. Probably the earliest was Ingalls in 1881 but the names of Killian and Freer are usually associated with the refinement and popularization of the actual procedure. It was Killian (1904) who described the technique which is most commonly practised today, with a retention of both dorsal and caudal struts of cartilage to prevent any subsequent change in the external shape of the nose. Freer (1902) adopted a much more radical approach as, in his view, the septal cartilage did not contribute to the support of the nasal pyramid and could be completely removed if necessitated by the extent of the pathology. He admitted that 'saddling' of the dorsum did sometimes occur in the supra-tip region, but said that this was always due to rough surgery, which had damaged or partly removed the upper lateral cartilages.

The SMR was undoubtedly a great advance and was widely adopted throughout the world. With subsequent experience, it was evident that there were certain problems associated with this operation. For surgical purposes, the septum can be divided into anterior and posterior parts, by a vertical line drawn from the frontal nasal spine, to the maxillary nasal spine. Deviations posterior to this line can be easily and effectively treated by the SMR technique. The problems occur when using this technique in the anterior part of the septum. All too frequently, the operation was followed by a supra-tip depression and columellar retraction (*see Figure 6.7 and 6.8*). To minimize these complications, most surgeons adopted the conservative Killian technique, but retention of dorsal and caudal struts does not ensure complete immunity, and also the deviations may be found in the region of the dorsal and caudal struts, and would therefore not be cured by this operation. These complications occur much more frequently than is generally realized because it often takes many months to develop. Immediate saddling is rare; usually it occurs as a result of scar contraction in the septum (*see Figure 6.9*). Some surgeons have attempted to solve the problem of scar contraction by replacing all or part of the excised cartilage, while others have avoided producing a large defect in the cartilaginous septum, by mobilizing and re-positioning the septum in the central position, so that the bulk of the cartilage is retained, and is still attached to its mucoperichondrium as part of a compound flap. The first significant improvement was made by Metzenbaum (1929) of Chicago, using the latter concept. The operation was only applicable to caudal dislocations of the septum without fragmentation of the cartilage and gross fibrosis (*see Figures 6.10, 6.11, and 6.12*). He likened the principle to that of a swinging door but late failures were fairly common. A swinging door has a hinge on one side and free edges on the other three borders. In the Metzenbaum operation, the hinge was effectively produced by the incision at the level of the deviation. There was an existing free border inferiorly and one was produced posteriorly by separation of the cartilage from the vomer. There was not however a free border anteriorly where the septum was often tethered to displaced upper lateral cartilages (*see Figure 6.13*) and the traction from this source, and also sometimes from the mucoperichondrium which was liberated only on one side above the incision, produced increased tension on the unfreed side during healing, which was prone to cause a recurrence of the deflections. To overcome these problems Peer, in 1937, completely excised the deviated caudal segment of the cartilage. If possible, he reinserted it as a free graft, but if the tissue was either unsuitable or inadequate, he obtained a similar sized graft resecting cartilage from the central or more posterior part of the quadrilateral cartilage (*see Figure 6.14*). This operation developed the concept of cartilage excision followed by cartilage replacement. The original Peer operation was extended to include removal of the entire cartilaginous

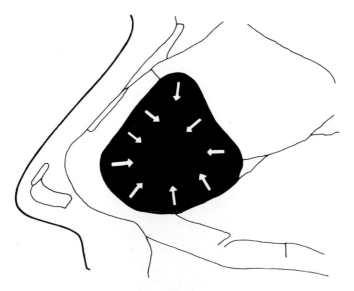

Figure 6.9   The contracting scar which develops after an SMR

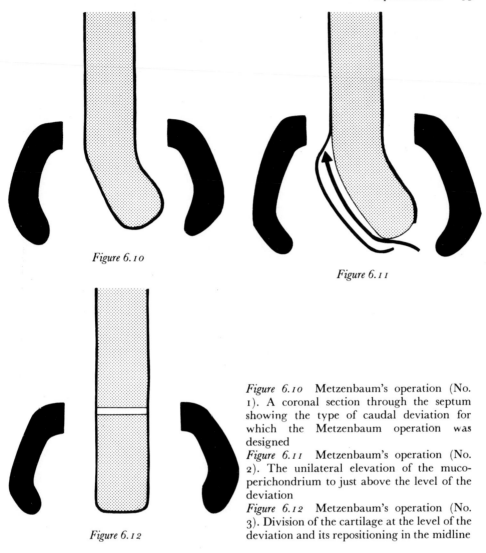

Figure 6.10

Figure 6.11

Figure 6.12

Figure 6.10 Metzenbaum's operation (No. 1). A coronal section through the septum showing the type of caudal deviation for which the Metzenbaum operation was designed

Figure 6.11 Metzenbaum's operation (No. 2). The unilateral elevation of the muco-perichondrium to just above the level of the deviation

Figure 6.12 Metzenbaum's operation (No. 3). Division of the cartilage at the level of the deviation and its repositioning in the midline

septum. This concept reached its logical conclusion in the Galloway operation of 1946. Galloway removed the entire nasal cartilage, and replaced the anterior septum with a single free autograft cut from the excised cartilage. Galloway also described a useful detail of operative technique, in the manner in which he facilitated the placing of the graft with traction sutures (*see Figure 6.15*).

Afterwards, the graft was held in place with mattress sutures, and the traction sutures were removed. Subsequent experience with this operation showed that it was by no means always successful because:

(1) Unequal scar contraction between the two septal flaps sometimes led to a recurrence of the deviation.
(2) Absorption of the autograft sometimes occurred leading to saddling of the supra-tip region.

(3) The lower end of the graft sometimes immobilized the membranous septum and
gave it a rather peculiar and unnatural appearance.

In 1948, Fomon endeavoured to solve the first and third of these problems by the use
of small autografts. The whole principle of septal removal, followed by septal
replacement, has some inherent drawbacks and consequently the alternative solution
of mobilization and re-positioning of septal cartilage has been revived and further
developed. This septoplasty concept has in particular been popularized by Cottle and
his associates.

The principles of septal surgery

From the experience over the last 90 years, it is evident that from a surgical point of
view, the septum can be divided into anterior and posterior segments by a vertical line

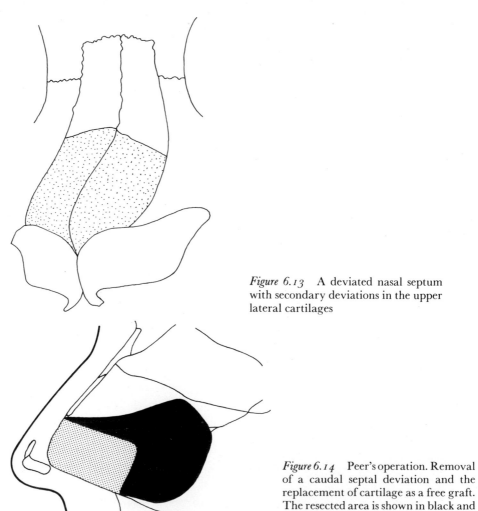

Figure 6.13   A deviated nasal septum
with secondary deviations in the upper
lateral cartilages

Figure 6.14   Peer's operation. Removal
of a caudal septal deviation and the
replacement of cartilage as a free graft.
The resected area is shown in black and
the graft is shown as a dotted area

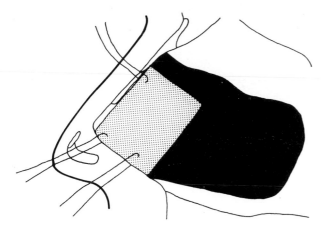

Figure 6.15   The Galloway operation

drawn between the nasal processes of the frontal and maxillary bones (*see Figure 6.16*). Deviations in the posterior segment can be easily and effectively treated by the classic Killian SMR operation, whereas those in the anterior segments should be treated by a more conservative septoplasty technique.

Anaesthesia for septal operations

Septal surgery can be satisfactorily performed under either local or general anaesthesia. The high quality, and ready availability of anaesthetists, has resulted in a preference for general anaesthesia in the UK. A general anaesthetic is also invariably required for children and nervous adults. It is necessary to pack the nose about 15–20 min before the operation with ½-inch ribbon gauze which has been soaked in cocaine and adrenaline. This will greatly diminish the amount of bleeding at operation. The postural nerve block technique described by Curtiss (1952) is easily the best of the local anaesthetic methods. It was evolved from the earlier technique of Moffett (1941) but is much simpler and quicker, and is quite as effective. The patient is placed in the Proetz position with the chin and external auditory meatus in the same vertical plane. Then 2 ml of a 4 per cent cocaine solution is introduced into each nostril using a special angulated needle. The cocaine gravitates into the superior meatus where it blocks both the ethmoidal and sphenopalatine nerves. The patient is kept in this position for 10 min. A little 2 per cent lignocaine is finally injected into the columella. This method gives far better results than the older technique of using cocaine and adrenaline packs as it is often difficult to get these packs beyond the septal deviations.

Septoplasty

The basic steps of a septoplasty are:
(1) Incision.
(2) Exposure.

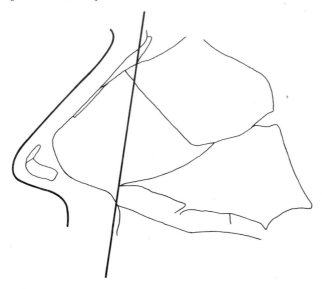

Figure 6.16   Surgically the septum is divided into anterior and posterior segments by a vertical line passing between the nasal processes of the frontal and maxillary bones

The cartilaginous and bony septum is exposed by the complete elevation of a mucosal flap on one side only. Contact between the cartilaginous septum and the mucoperichondrial flap on the other side is maintained as much as possible because in addition to ensuring the viability of cartilage, it also greatly reduces the risks of such complications as haematoma and abscess formation, perforation and over-riding of the different segments of the cartilages.

(3) Mobilization and straightening.

The septal cartilage is then freed from all its attachments apart from the mucosal flap on the convex side. Many deviations are maintained by extrinsic factors such as the caudal dislocation of the cartilage from the vomerine groove (*see Figure 6.5*). Mobilization alone will often correct this type of problem. When deviations are due to intrinsic causes as for example healed fractures, it is necessary to combine mobilization with some direct surgery on the cartilage such as a strip excision of the fracture line.

Bony deviations are treated either by fracture and re-positioning, or by submucous resection of the deviation.

(4) Fixation.

The septum is then maintained in its straightened position during the healing phase by sutures and splints.

Incision

The incision is best made at the lower border of the septal cartilage as was originally advocated by Freer. A unilateral (hemi-transfixation) incision is adequate for a septoplasty, and for the right-handed surgeon, this is usually most conveniently made on the left side. The advantages of this incision have been tabulated by Bernstein (1973b) in the following fashion:

(1) The incision is placed in a relatively avascular plane.
(2) The mucosal edges here are both thick and tough, thus reducing the risk of tears. If tears do occur here, a satisfactory repair is normally quite easily performed.
(3) It provides easy access to the whole of the septum, including the caudal septal border, and the region of the anterior nasal spine with its associated pre-maxillary crest.
(4) If the septoplasty is to be combined with a rhinoplasty, it is easy to extend the incision through to the opposite side and thus produce a full transfixation incision. It is important to make the incision as high as possible because a low incision through the membranous septum may be followed by a retraction of the columella (*see Figures 6.17* and *6.18*). The first step is therefore to displace the columella downwards and to the opposite side by means of traction, exerted with dissecting forceps or a Cottle columellar clamp. The lower border of the septal cartilage will then be plainly visible and the incision then made down to the perichondrium, which is incised and the sub-perichondrial flap elevation then commenced.

Exposure

It is usually best to expose the cartilaginous and bony septum by elevating the mucosal flap on the concave side. The difficulties of the flap elevation are partly due to the anatomy of the various tissue layers and can also be often greatly increased by fibrosis and scarring in these layers following previous trauma. The surgical anatomy of this

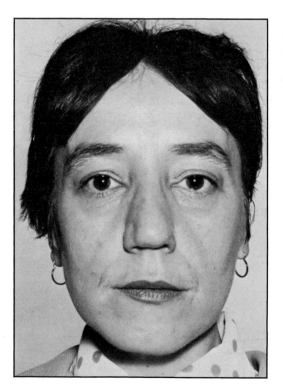 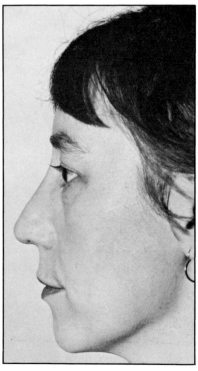

Figure 6.17 Retraction of the columella following an SMR (front view)

Figure 6.18 Retraction of the columella following an SMR (side view)

region is of extreme importance and must be clearly understood if mucosal tears are to be avoided. It is easy to elevate the mucosal flaps across both the ethmoid–vomerine suture and the ethmoid–septal cartilage suture, because very few periosteal or perichondrial fibres pass into either of these suture lines (*see Figure 6.19*). The difficulties of flap elevation mainly occur at the junction of the septal cartilage above, with the anterior nasal spine, pre-maxillary crest and vomer below. This is due to the fact that the perichondrium encloses the cartilage in a complete envelope which does not fuse with the periosteum. The periosteum forms another inferior envelope over the

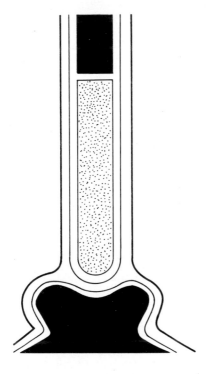

Figure 6.19   Muco-perichondrial and muco-periosteal layers in the septum. Septal cartilage—dotted area; ethmoid and vomer—black

adjacent bony septum and here one gets a sort of joint capsule which can permit a side-to-side movement of the septal cartilage (*see Figure 6.19*). The sub-perichondrial plane over the septal cartilage is therefore not continuous with the sub-periostial plane below and the difficulty in uniting these two planes can easily lead to tears. For this reason most iatrogenic perforations occur along the chondro–vomerine suture, particularly anteriorly because the bony groove is widest here, and the problems are greatest.

As a general principle of flap elevation, it is usually best to leave the most difficult areas to the last, since they can be approached then from several directions and under direct vision. A suitable technique for dealing with these problems has been evolved by Cottle *et al.* (1958) who started the elevation over the septal cartilage and worked upwards and backwards always keeping above the chondrovomerine junction. This step in the operation was called the production of the 'anterior tunnel'. Once this had been accomplished, attention was then directed to the posterior end of the incision and the periosteum over the anterior nasal spine was incised and then elevated backwards on both sides over the pre-maxillary crest, then the vomer; again keeping below the chondrovomerine suture. These were the so-called 'inferior tunnels' (*see Figure 6.20*). Finally, the most difficult elevation was performed which involved uniting the anterior and inferior tunnels under direct vision using a sharp dissector or knife. This is the so-called 'Maxilla–Pre-maxilla' approach of Cottle.

Mobilization and straightening

The first step is to separate the lower border of the septal cartilage from its osseous base. In many cases, this lower border has been dislocated from its osseous groove and

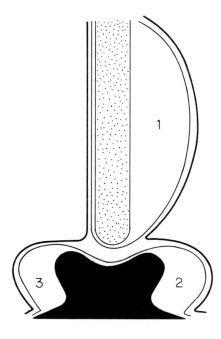

Figure 6.20 Cottle's maxilla–pre-maxilla approach to extensive nasal septum surgery. (1) Left anterior tunnel; (2) Left inferior tunnel; (3) Right inferior tunnel

there is also a considerable amount of fibrosis which can greatly distort the anatomy. A sharp dissector or knife is always required. The lower border of the septal cartilage is encased in a perichondrial envelope, and it is usually possible to continue the sub-perichondrial elevation downwards over the concave side of the septum, then around its lower border and upwards for a few millimetres in the convex side. When the cartilage has been freed, an attempt is made to re-position it back into the midline where it should rest in its osseous groove. Usually this is impossible due to the excess height of the septal cartilage and it is then necessary to remove a strip of cartilage about 3–4 mm wide from its lower border (*see Figure 6.21*). This excised cartilage is part of the quadrilateral plate and may be up to 4 cm long. It can make an ideal autograft, should one be required at a later stage in the operation. It should therefore be kept in some sterile saline during the rest of the operation in case this need arises. It is usually also necessary to straighten and lower the vomerine crest in order to make a suitable bed to accommodate the septal cartilage. The anterior nasal spine must not be removed. When deviated it can be fractured and re-positioned in the midline. The next step is to separate the septal cartilage from the perpendicular plate of the ethmoid. A Cottle elevator is inserted under the mucoperichondrial flap on the concave side and the chondro–ethmoid suture is exposed. Firm pressure is exerted on

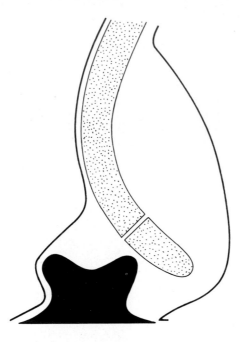

Figure 6.21   Removal of a strip of cartilage from the lower border of the septum thus enabling the dislocation to be reduced

the septal cartilage posteriorly with the elevator, and the cartilage will readily be separated from the ethmoid. The elevator is then moved backwards and it slips easily through the disarticulated chondro–ethmoid suture to start elevating the periosteum on the convex side of the ethmoid plate. This plane of dissection is extended downwards to the vomer and then forwards up to the dorsum.

Large vomerine spurs are best treated by classic submucous resection. More generalized bony deviations can frequently be re-positioned in the midline after preliminary fracture. The final complete separation of the septal cartilage is achieved by removal of any residual adjacent part of the vomer and the perpendicular plate of the ethmoid. There should be a gap of about 1 cm in all areas except the anterior nasal spine (*see Figure 6.22*).

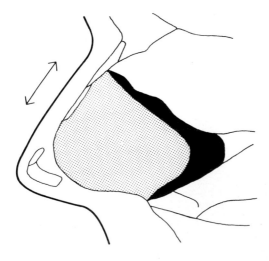

Figure 6.22   Septoplasty. In order to mobilize the septal cartilage it is always necessary to free it completely from the ethmoid and vomer posteriorly and also sometimes from the upper lateral cartilages

If the external nasal pyramid is twisted, it is important to separate the skin and subcutaneous tissue off the underlying upper lateral cartilages. This will allow the skin afterwards to be draped easily over the straightened cartilaginous dorsum without the risk of cutaneous traction on the upper lateral cartilages producing a recurrence of the deviation.

This uncovering of the cartilaginous dorsum is easily performed through the classic intercartilaginous incisions (*see Figure 6.23*). Usually a 15 blade Bard Parker knife is used to make the incision at the level of the internal nares. Anteriorly, each cartilaginous incision is united with a transfixation incision. A series of opening and closing movements with a pair of Knapp scissors will enable the elevation of the subcutaneous tissues off the cartilaginous dorsum to be easily effected (*see Figure 6.24*).

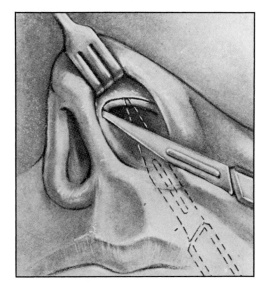 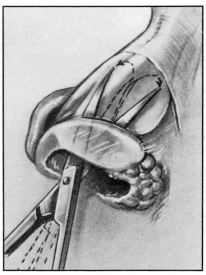

Figure 6.23 Inter-cartilaginous incision at the level of the internal nares. (From Seltzer and reproduced by kind permission of J. B. Lippincott & Co.)

Figure 6.24 Elevation of the soft tissues off the upper lateral cartilages. (From Seltzer and reproduced by kind permission of J. B. Lippincott & Co.)

The plane of dissection should be directly above the perichondrium, as most of the blood vessels are found in the more superficial layers. The upper lateral cartilages are firmly united to the cartilaginous septum. There are often secondary changes in the upper lateral cartilages associated with a twisted nose. When this occurs, it is necessary to separate the upper lateral cartilages from the septum and this is best done submucosally. By now the septal cartilage has been fully mobilized and in the absence of intrinsic deviations, should be easily re-positioned in the midline. A careful examination should be made at this stage and the mobility of the septum checked by moving it from side to side with a septal elevator. If there is any reduced mobility, its exact site should be noted and further trimming at this point may be necessary. Possible other factors include a large turbinate, which may have to be fractured laterally or actually reduced in size by partial turbinectomy, submucosal resection of the bony turbinate or submucosal diathermy. I favour the latter technique as the worst secondary haemorrhage which I have ever experienced following a septo–rhinoplasty occurred from the lateral nasal wall after a partial turbinectomy has been performed. At times, the mucosa on the narrow side of the nose is too short to allow the septum to return to the midline. This problem can be solved by cutting through the mucosa at the junction of the nasal floor and the septum. There will be a residual dehiscence on the floor of the nose after the septum has been re-positioned into the midline, but this will re-epithelialize quite rapidly afterwards. Any residual obstruction is usually due to intrinsic deviations in the septal cartilage. Old fractures in the cartilage often heal by fibrous union and this often results in severe angulations which are best treated by the removal of a narrow strip of cartilage along the line of the deviation. This will break the spring of cartilage and can then be usually re-positioned into the midline (*see Figure 6.25*).

Sometimes the septal lesion is so severe either due to previous disease (for example, a septal haematoma), or where extremely radical surgery is necessary to correct the deviation, that one is left with too little supporting cartilage anteriorly to maintain the normal shape of the nasal pyramid and the columella. This is the type of problem that is not infrequently found in the professional boxer. In such a nose, the anterior residual septal cartilage can be supported with a free bone graft, taken preferably from the thinner part of the perpendicular plate of the ethmoid, or if this is impossible, from the rather thicker vomer. A suitable piece of bone can be obtained with a pair of heavy angled Fomon scissors and chisel. It can then be cut to the shape of the dorso-caudal septum, and two holes then drilled in it to accommodate the fixation sutures. The bone graft is placed alongside the residual septal cartilage and sutured in position. Bernstein (1973b) has shown that bone is much more satisfactory when used in this supporting role than cartilage, which frequently absorbs (*see Figure 6.26*).

Fixation

At the end of the operation, the septum should be lying freely in the midline and if this objective has not been achieved, no suturing or splinting will prevent subsequent failure. If it has been necessary to make multiple incisions in the cartilage, over-riding of the segments can be a problem and this is best corrected by a Wright suture (*see Figure 6.25*). Here, a through-and-through mattress suture is used, with one arm passing between the segments of the cartilage and the other through all three layers of the septum. A figure-of-eight suture, immobilizing the lower border of the septum to the anterior nasal spine, is then inserted. Finally, the septo–columellar incision is closed with a few sutures. Silastic splints are then inserted into the nose. The nose is packed with $\frac{1}{2}$-inch ribbon gauze impregnated with BIPP.

The classic submucous resection operation

The incision and exposure stages are the same as for septoplasty. Afterwards, an incision is made through the septal cartilage about 1 cm above and parallel to its lower border. The incision should be made through the cartilage, but not through the opposite perichondrium. The mucoperichondrium can then be elevated off the far side of the cartilage through this incision. A pair of angled scissors can then be introduced and used to cut through the septal cartilage in a direction which is parallel to and at least 1 cm posterior to the nasal dorsum. It is then possible to remove the

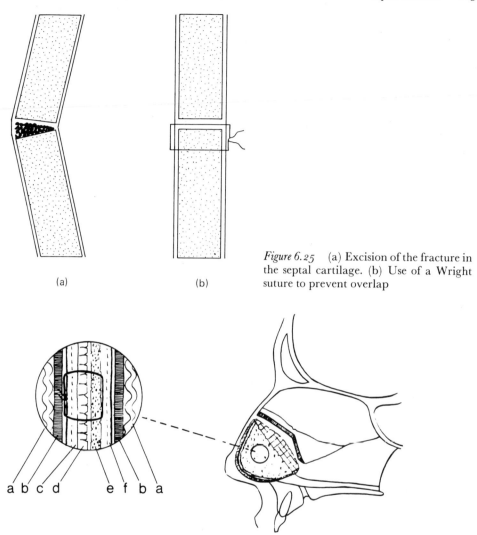

Figure 6.25 (a) Excision of the fracture in the septal cartilage. (b) Use of a Wright suture to prevent overlap

(a)   (b)

a b c d   e f b a

Figure 6.26 Bernstein's technique of supporting a deficient septal cartilage with a bone graft from either the ethmoid or the vomer. (a) Nasal packing, (b) Silastic splint, (c) muco-perichondrium attached to (d) cross-hatched cartilage, (e) bone graft, (f) freed perichondrium. (Reproduced by kind permission of W. B. Saunders)

obstructing cartilage and bone leaving these dorsal and caudal struts of cartilage to maintain the support of the nasal dorsum and columella. The cartilage is removed with Luc's forceps or a Ballenger's swivel knife. Any deviated bone in the region of the vertical plate of the ethmoid is then removed. The next step is to elevate the flaps off the maxillary crest and vomer. The periosteum covering this is not in the same plane of cleavage as the cartilaginous dissection. A separate breakthrough has to be made with a knife or dissector on to the bone to elevate the periosteum. The crest is finally removed with a hammer and gouge or with a Jansen–Middleton bone forceps.

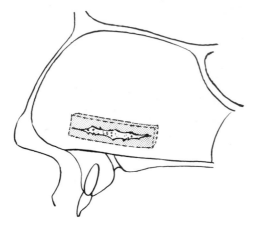

Figure 6.27   The support of mucosal tears with a free cartilage or bone graft prior to suture of the tear. (From Bernstein, 1973. Reproduced by kind permission of W. B. Saunders)

If the flap is torn, this does not matter unless there is another tear on the other side exactly opposite, when a septal perforation will inevitably result unless a satisfactory repair is effected. The site of the tears is first reinforced by the introduction of a small autograft of septal cartilage or bone between the flaps and the lacerations are then sutured (*see Figure 6.27*). Some surgeons routinely replace septal cartilage and bone after performing the classic Killian technique. The almost universal use of central heating in North America tends to produce atrophic changes in the nasal mucosa and Briant (1977) considers there is a very definite risk that this tendency is increased following the loss of support of the septal cartilage and bone, and that septal perforations for this reason are by no means uncommon following a perfectly performed Killian-type operation. For this reason, he advocates that the excised cartilage and bone be straightened in a Cottle's crusher and then re-inserted between the flaps.

Post-operative care
Packs are removed after 24 h and splints after seven days. Chemotherapy is not usually required.

Septal surgery in the growing nose

Since the turn of the century, it has been widely believed that the nasal septum plays an important role in the development of the facial skeleton and in particular, the nose. For this reason most surgeons have avoided performing surgical operations on the growing septum due to the fear of producing some retardation of growth.

Some of the earliest work was done by Hayton (1948), who made a careful study of 31 patients aged between 6 and 14 who had been treated in Logan Turner's clinic in Edinburgh by the classic Killian operation. In ten of the patients, there was some broadening of the nose, which was associated with a supra-tip depression. As a consequence of this work, it became the established conventional practice to avoid all septal surgery on patients under about 16 years of age and it is only recently that this concept has been challenged.

Animal experimental work over the years has in many ways clarified the position.

Sarnat and Wexler (1966) produced moderate-sized septal perforations in young rabbits, and noticed that this invariably led to the subsequent depression of the corresponding segment of the nasal dorsum, and also an under-development of the maxilla, with a type-3 dental malocclusion. Hartenstrom (1970) repeated these experiments on puppies and got similar results. Fuschs (1969) removed the mucoperichondrium from the nasal septum in young rabbits leaving the cartilage intact. This was followed by a septal deviation to the operated side and the retarded development of the nasal pyramid. More recently, Bernstein (1973a) has resected the septal cartilage in young puppies through a dorsal incision, which left the mucoperichondrium intact on both sides. Afterwards, none of the dogs showed any retarded growth of the nose or of the maxilla, and there was no tendency to dental malocclusion. Microscopically, the excised cartilage was usually replaced by fibrous tissue. In several of the dogs, the excised cartilage was replaced between the flaps as an autograft. All these grafts survived, but some marginal absorption did occur at times. Afterwards, the autografts continued to grow proportionately with the rest of the septum. Fractures in cartilages usually healed by fibrous union, but in several specimens it was found that the two surfaces of cartilage fused together by means of new cartilage growth. From this experimental work, it would appear that the mucoperichondrium plays a much more important role in septal growth than the cartilage, and that a conservative septoplasty in children does not lead to any stunting of growth.

Reduction of septal dislocation in the newborn

This should usually be done as soon as possible and at any rate within three weeks of birth. The method of reducing these dislocations was described by Metzenbaum (1936). A little 4 per cent lignocaine gel is usually inserted into the nostrils and the cartilaginous part of the nasal pyramid is then firmly held between the thumb and first finger of the surgeon. It is then lifted upwards and at the same time, an elevator is inserted under the lower edge of dislocated cartilage which is manipulated back into the midline. A faint click can usually be heard when it has returned to its corrected position.

Septo–rhinoplasty

The external nasal pyramid and the septum are both anatomically closely connected, and functionally interrelated, and are best considered as a single unit. Many traumatic and other clinical problems affect both parts of the nose, neither of which can be satisfactorily considered in isolation. The best solution for many of these lesions is a one-stage septo–rhinoplasty operation which has many advantages over the main therapeutic alternative which involves a preliminary Killian submucous resection, followed by a subsequent rhinoplasty performed several months later. These advantages include the following:

(1) The Killian operation does not straighten dorsal or caudal struts, and as straightening the septum is a key to straightening the nose, these two-stage operations give much poorer results.

(2) The Killian operation involves the sacrifice of much cartilage and bone which often provides the best grafting material for the rhinoplasty and which would under these circumstances normally be lost.

(3) The patient is saved two operations and two hospital admissions.

(4) It is much more dangerous to lower the nasal hump in a patient who has previously been subjected to a submucous resection as there may not be a wide enough dorsal septal strut to allow this to be done with safety.

(5) The contracting scar after a Killian submucous resection takes at least a year to mature, and it is undesirable to perform a second operation until this has occurred as it is likely to prejudice the result of the rhinoplasty.

Although major reconstructive rhinoplasties are rightly the province of the plastic surgeon, the basic corrective rhinoplasty which is involved in the treatment of the traumatic nose, together with its associated functional problems, should fall within the province of the suitably trained ear, nose and throat surgeon. Many of the problems involved in these cases are similar to those encountered in the cosmetic corrective rhinoplasty and it is impossible to separate these two subjects completely. I will however be concentrating on the more functional type of septo–rhinoplasty and the more purely cosmetic aspects of the subject are dealt with in Chapter 4.

Functional aspects of the nasal pyramid

The structure of the external nasal pyramid has some bearing on the function of the nose and is another reason why it is of importance to the ear, nose and throat surgeon. Examples of this include the fact that:

(1) Some noses are so twisted that it is impossible to restore a satisfactory airway by septal surgery alone. Here a septo–rhinoplasty is absolutely necessary if one is to produce a good nasal airway (*Figures 6.28* and *6.29*).

(2) The position of the nasal tip has an important bearing on the respiratory air currents. A drooping tip with an acute naso-labial angle results in the air currents being displaced upwards into the narrower part of the nasal cavity and this can result in obstruction (*Figure 6.30* and *6.31*). A simple digital elevation of the tip will clear the obstruction in such a patient and this constitutes a simple and useful clinical test (*Figure 6.32*).

Functional examination

This is partly covered in a previous section on septal deviations. An assessment of nasal respiration is usually made on the basis of simple clinical tests together with a subjective history and the careful inspection of the nasal anatomy.

An idea of the inspiratory air currents can be obtained by holding a metal tongue depressor or a mirror under the nostrils and observing the pattern of the frosting produced. Alar collapse is usually maximal during the negative inspiratory pressure phase and if present, can easily be seen during deep inspiration. The effect of occluding each nostril in turn on the breathing should be observed but it is important, in

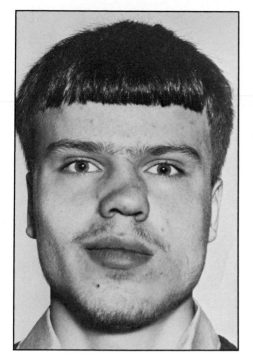

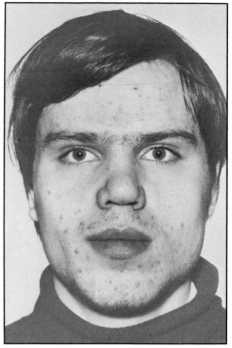

Figure 6.28 Severe nasal injury with 'S' deviation

Figure 6.29 Appearance after a one-stage septo–rhinoplasty

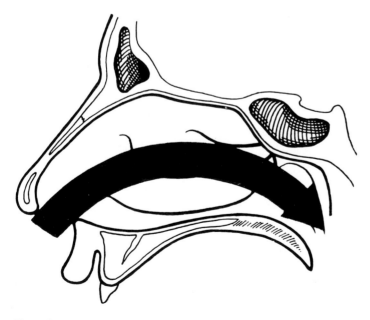

Figure 6.30 Normal inspiratory air currents. (From Denecke and Meyer, 1967. Reproduced by kind permission of Springer-Verlag (New York) Inc.)

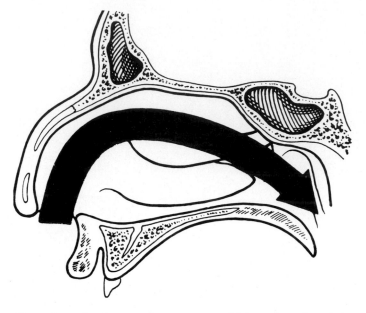

Figure 6.31 Inspiratory air currents are higher when there is an acute naso–labial angle. (From Denecke and Meyer, 1967. Reproduced by kind permission of Springer-Verlag (New York) Inc.)

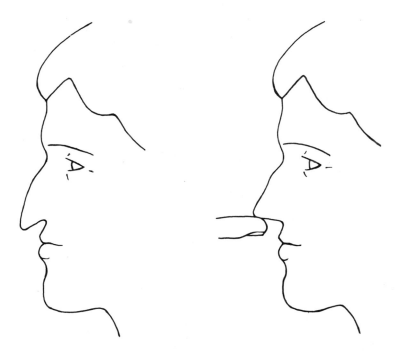

Figure 6.32 Simple digital test to show whether elevation of the tip will improve the nasal airway

carrying out this test, that there is no distortion of the nasal vestibule or any change in the naso–labial angle. Additional help can be obtained by carefully listening to the nasal breath sounds which should be quiet and regular. Obstruction produces noisy and laboured breathing. Undoubtedly some form of simple and reliable rhinometry would be of considerable value but no ideal technique exists at the moment. Probably the best of the available methods was introduced by Cottle (1968) who evolved a rhinometer with an electronic writer and this is available commercially.

Assessment of the external nasal pyramid

Before being able to analyse this problem, it is necessary to decide what a good nose should look like and here of course aesthetic values vary, not only from continent to continent, but also from country to country, and in some cases from one ethnic group to another. In this chapter however, I shall be considering only the Caucasian nose. Although some particularly gifted individuals have an intuitive artistic flair it is important to express the problems mathematically.

The enormous impact that quantitative audiometry has made on ear surgery is familiar to all of us. Rhinology has rather tended to lag behind in this quantitative approach but satisfactory techniques are now available in the assessment of the nasal pyramid and are a pre-requisite if good results are to be obtained.

When considering a patient for a septo–rhinoplasty, there are four questions which one needs to answer:

First What is wrong with this particular patient's nose? This is, of course, a diagnostic exercise.

Second What basic changes do I need to effect in this nose, in order to correct the defects? This involves planning the objectives of the operation.

Third Which operative techniques are available which are most likely to enable me to achieve these objectives? Here it is important to emphasize there are certain problems which are not capable of correction by our present known methods.

Fourth Are there any physical or psychological contraindications to the operation on this particular patient?

Most of the literature on septo–rhinoplasty is obsessed with the question of operative technique. This is very unfortunate because unless the first two questions have been correctly answered, no compensatory skills in surgical technique will save one from failure. A septo–rhinoplasty should be like a well-tailored bespoke suit. It should be planned, cut and fitted to suit the requirements and needs of each individual patient. The operation must be made to fit the patient and not the patient to fit the operation.

A full assessment will of course involve both a functional examination of the nose and a cosmetic analysis of the nasal pyramid. In making observations on the shape of the nose and face, it is important that they are integrated into numerical form. This is the basis of the so-called 'biometric analysis' which has been elaborated by Fomon (1970). Firstly, it is important to describe the various integumental points used.

(1) *Frontale (F)*—The most prominent part of the forehead.
(2) *Glabella (Gl)*—The point in the midline of the forehead at the level of the superciliary arches.

(3) *Nasion* (N)—The deepest part of the fronto–nasal angle.
(4) *The sub-nasion* (Sn)—The deepest part of the naso–labial angle.
(5) *Mental point* (M)—The most prominent part of the centre of the chin.
(6) *Gnathion* (Gn)—The lowest point of the chin. (*See Figure 6.33*).

These observations are best made from standardized photographs of the individual. On the frontal photographs, one should draw four horizontal lines:

(a) through the hairline;
(b) through the eyebrow;
(c) through the naso–labial junction;
(d) at the lower border of the chin.

Ideally, these spaces should be of equal height. The uppermost space is the most variable, and probably the least important from the standpoint of disfigurement. The nasal index can also be calculated from the frontal photographs. This necessitates measuring the width and height of the nose. The nasal index is calculated by dividing the width by the height, then multiplying by 100. The range of normality is 42–47 in the narrow or leptorrhine type of nose found in the Caucasian races, and between 53 and 58 in the platyrrhine type of nose found in Negroes.
The lateral photograph enables one to measure certain important angles:

Naso–frontal angle: This is an obtuse angle approximately 120 degrees, formed between the forehead and the bony nasal dorsum (*Figure 6.34*).
Naso–labial angle: This is located between the base of the nose and the upper lip with its apex at the sub-nasion. Ideally this angle is approximately 90 degrees in men and up to 110 degrees in women (*Figure 6.35*).
This is one of the main differences between the male and female nose.
The angle of nasal projection: This was formerly measured between a line drawn from the nasion to the mental point, and the line of the axis of the nasal dorsum. Because of great variation in the projection of the mental point, the lower landmark which is now used, is a point which lies midway between the sub-nasion and the alar–facial junction. This angle varies within normal limits between 23 and 38 degrees (*Figure 6.36*)

The initial examination is started by inspecting the nose carefully from both sides, in front and below, and also from above. The shape of the dorsum should be observed carefully for humps, depressions or lateral deviations. If there is extensive saddling of the dorsum, serological tests for syphilis should be performed. Deviations can, of course, involve the bony pyramid, the upper cartilaginous vault and/or the lower cartilaginous vault. Lateral deviations are probably most easily seen by looking down the nasal dorsum, from a position above and in front of the nose. It is important to remember that these lateral deviations are associated with similar deviations of the nasal septum.

After this, a more quantitative measurement of the deformity, is made from a set of photographs, which are an absolute necessity in this type of surgery because:

(1) They form the most easily and quickly comprehensible record which is much more satisfactory than any written description of the nose.

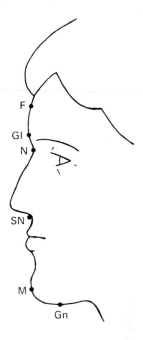

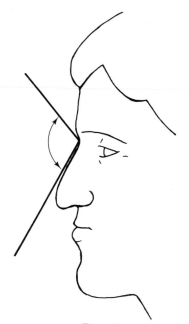

Figure 6.33 Integumental points. F Frontale, Gl Glabella, N Nasion, SN Subnasion, M Mental point, Gn Gnathion

Figure 6.34 Naso–frontal angle

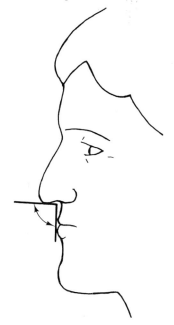

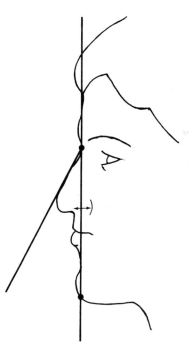

Figure 6.35 Naso–labial angle

Figure 6.36 Angle of nasal projection

(2) They form an excellent means of comparison between the pre- and post-operative condition. They can be used to remind the patient of his original appearance which is quite often forgotten.

(3) They may well be indispensable should any medico–legal problems ensue.

Standardized views are vital, and all the photographs should be taken under identical conditions of lighting. Black-and-white photographs suffice, and there should be a full frontal view, lateral views taken from both sides with the face in repose, a lateral view taken with the patient laughing, and a basal nostril view. The forehead should always be fully exposed, and not covered by a forward-directed hair style. Some latent deformities only become apparent when the individual is laughing as this produces changes in the relation of the tip of the nose to the dorsum. This particularly applies to convexities or humps in the supra-tip region.

Pre-operative planning

The next step is to make a detailed analysis of the deformity from the photographs, and then plan the changes which should be effected to correct them.

I think that this can best be illustrated by a specific example. One starts by drawing horizontal lines across the frontal photograph at the level of the hairline, eyebrow, naso–labial junction, and at the lower border of the chin. The three parts of the face are roughly of equal width, and are therefore within the limits of a normal proportion (*Figure 6.37*). Vertical lines are dropped from the inner canthus on each side and through the saggital plane. As can be seen, the nose is grossly deviated in the form of a classic 'S'-shaped deformity. On the lateral views, the various angles are measured. The naso–frontal angle is within normal limits, but the naso–labial angle is only 80 degrees instead of the normal 90 degrees, and this will therefore need correction. The angle of the nasal projection is 38 degrees, which is within normal limits. A rather unsightly nasal hump is also seen with a drooping tip, and this must be corrected (*Figures 6.38, 6.39,* and *6.40*). In the basal photograph, one draws a line through the points where the alae join the cheek. A line is also drawn through the sagittal plane, and two further lines drawn at a tangent to the main axis of the alar cartilage. Using this technique, it can be seen that there is a gross deviation of the nose to the right (*Figure 6.41*).

The objectives of this operation are therefore to:

(1) straighten the nasal septum,
(2) straighten the external nasal pyramid,
(3) lower the nasal hump,
(4) elevate the nasal tip.

Physical and psychological contraindications

Any chronic infective condition, such as sinusitis, should of course be cured before embarking on a septo–rhinoplasty. This operation is an elective procedure, and the operative risk should be minimal. This type of surgery should not be performed on any patient whose general condition significantly increases the operative risk. It is important to establish if there is any hypersensitivity to drugs, and in particular to

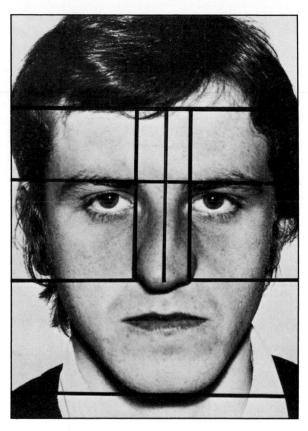

Figure 6.37 Anterior view showing 'S' deviation of nose

strapping, as this is vitally important in the post-operative splinting of the nose. A careful examination of the skin covering the nose is extremely important. After performing a reduction rhinoplasty, one relies on the skin to drape over the newer smaller nasal skeleton in order to produce a satisfactory result. The natural elasticity is normally adequate for this purpose, but there is a loss of cutaneous elasticity with advancing years, and one should be very cautious about operating on a patient over 50, especially when any radical change of nasal shape is contemplated. Similarly, there are hazards in operating on younger patients who are badly afflicted with acne. Here, the skin is often thick and greasy and it reacts very badly to the undermining required in this form of surgery. One can almost get a subcutaneous keloid formation, which could completely ruin the end result, even when the skeletal rhinoplasty technique has been perfect.

Psychological factors are of importance in any form of surgery which has a cosmetic element. Usually this is minimal in the functional type of septo–rhinoplasty which tends to be referred to the ear, nose and throat surgeon. These problems are more frequently found in the purely cosmetic type of case. There is no contraindication to operating on neurotics, whose psychological state often improves after a successful septo–rhinoplasty. It is, however, most important not to operate on psychotics, particularly if they are of the paranoid variety. If there is any doubt on this point, the patient should be referred to a psychiatrist before being accepted for operative treatment.

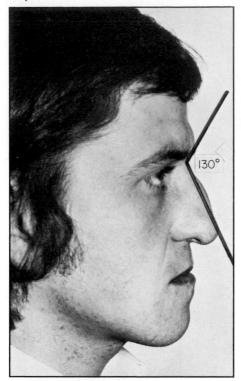

Figure 6.38 Lateral view showing nasal hump and normal fronto–nasal angle

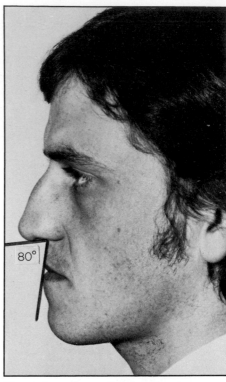

Figure 6.39 Lateral view showing acute naso–labial angle and retracted columella

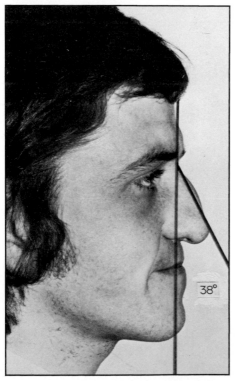

Figure 6.40 Lateral view showing normal angle of nasal projection

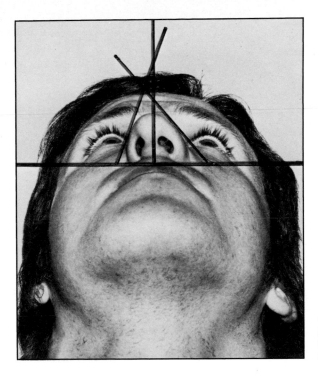

Figure 6.41 Basal view showing gross septal deviation to the left and deviation of the nasal tip to the right

Anaesthesia for septo–rhinoplasty

This type of surgery can be performed under either general or local anaesthesia. Bleeding is usually more profuse under general anaesthesia but this can be reduced to acceptable levels by the pre-operative packing of the nose with cocaine and adrenaline and/or the use of a hypotensive technique.

In the USA, most of these operations are performed using a local nerve block type of anaesthesia (*see Figure 6.42*). This must of course be supplemented by local anaesthesia to the nasal cavities, a subject which has previously been discussed in the section on septal surgery.

Operative technique

We have diagnosed the nasal deformity and have decided what basic changes are required. We are now in a position to decide on the best operative techniques which will enable us to achieve these objectives. The actual operation should be carefully planned long before the first incision is made. For this purpose the nose can be conveniently divided into three parts:

(1) the septum and turbinates;
(2) the nasal tip;
(3) the bony pyramid and upper cartilaginous vault.

It is my practice to perform the septal surgery first as the septum plays such a key role in the support of the nasal pyramid, and is also of primary importance when the nose has to be straightened. The operative details of septal surgery have already been fully considered.

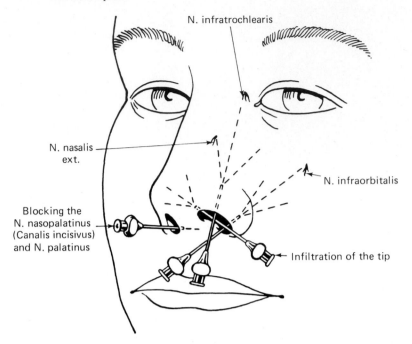

N. infratrochlearis

N. nasalis ext.

N. infraorbitalis

Blocking the N. nasopalatinus (Canalis incisivus) and N. palatinus

Infiltration of the tip

Figure 6.42   Regional nerve block anaesthesia for rhinoplasty. (From Denecke and Meyer, 1967. Reproduced by kind permission of Springer-Verlag (New York) Inc.)

Any work on the nasal tip which may be required should then be performed for the reasons given below, and finally the bony pyramid and upper cartilaginous vault are corrected.

The nasal tip

It may then be necessary to:

(1) change the shape of the nasal tip; and/or
(2) alter the position of the nasal tip.

Correction of the shape of the tip

The main structural frame of the lower cartilaginous vault is formed by the alar cartilage, and the basis of all tip surgery is to correct the defect by modifying the shape, size and position of these cartilages as may be required. The ideal tip in the Caucasian nose should be delicately sculptured and well defined. It should be separated from the main dorsum of the nose by a faint suggestion of a supra-tip depression, and below should sweep gracefully in a convex fashion into the columella. The nasal tip when viewed from below should form an equilateral triangle. Many noses are marred by a rounded, bulbous, poorly defined tip. This deformity is usually associated with an abnormally wide angle at the dome between the lateral and medial crura of the alar cartilage. The objective is to narrow this angle, either by incising the cartilage at the dome, or by removal of cartilage at this point.

The simplest and most conservative method of achieving this is to make a vertical incision through the cartilage of the dome area (*Figures 6.43,* and *6.44*). The effect is increased by removing an inverted triangular piece of cartilage from the dome area (*Figure 6.45*). With either of these techniques there is no alteration in the amount of tip

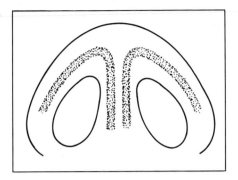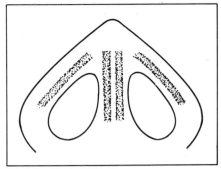

Figure 6.43   A more pointed nasal tip can be produced by incising the alar cartilages in the dome area

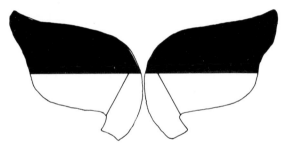

Figure 6.44   The alar cartilages seen from the front. Narrowing of the tip produced by removal of the upper half of the lateral crura (black area) and incision through the dome area to correct bulbosity of the tip, which is made more pointed

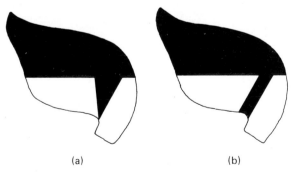

(a)   (b)

Figure 6.45   (a) Greater narrowing of the tip without loss of projection can be obtained by the removal of an inverted triangle of cartilage from the dome area. (b) Greater narrowing of the tip with loss of projection can be obtained by the removal of a complete strip of cartilage from the dome area

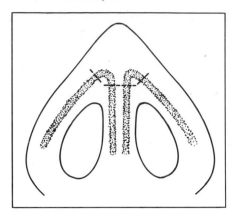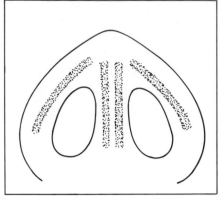

Figure 6.46   A reduction of tip projection can be effected by excision of cartilage from the dome area

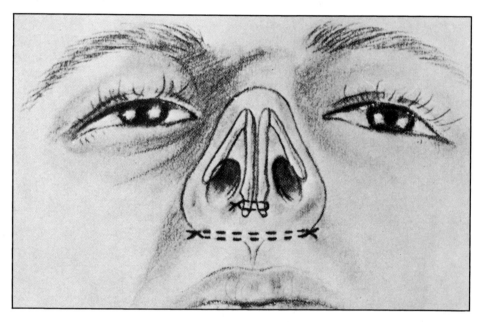

Figure 6.47   Narrowing the base of the nasal tip by basal and columellar bunching sutures. (From Hinderer, 1971. Reproduced by kind permission of Aesculapius Publishing Co.)

projection. Removal of an entire segment of the dome cartilage will produce a more pointed tip (*Figures 6.45* and *6.46*), but this technique should only be used when it is necessary to combine this effect with some loss of tip projection. The bulbosity and widening of the tip may extend posteriorly to its base and need correction. The lateral crura of the alar cartilage have often an outer convexity which contributes to the width of this part of the nose. Removal of the upper portion of the lateral crus will usually help narrow this part of the nose (*see Figures 6.44* and *6.45*). Narrowing the base of the tip can be achieved with a nasal bunching suture (*see Figure 6.47*). These are inserted through small incisions in the alar facial groove, through which some undermining of the subcutaneous tissue is performed. A straight Keith needle can then be passed through the tissues at the base of the nose; 2/0 chromic catgut is usually used. It is often necessary to narrow the posterior part of the columella. This is achieved by the use of a columellar bunching suture (*see Figure 6.47*).

Correction of the tip position

(*1*) *Reduction of tip projection* The tip projection can be reduced by excising a whole segment of cartilage in the region of the alar dome and then suturing the cut ends together with 3/0 chromic catgut (*see Figure 6.46*).

(*2*) *Increasing tip projection* This is rather difficult to achieve and it is rarely possible to increase tip projection by more than about 2–4 mm. The best known method is probably the Goldman (1953) method. The basis of this method is to produce increased tip projection by elongation of the medial crura. This is obtained at the expense of the lateral crura which are completely divided a few millimetres lateral to the dome area. The cartilage medial to the incision is then mobilized, straightened and placed in the sagittal plane, and stitched to its companion on the other side. Frequently, however, the cartilage is too flimsy and must be strengthened by the support of a cartilage baton which is usually obtained from the nasal septum (*see Figure 6.48*).

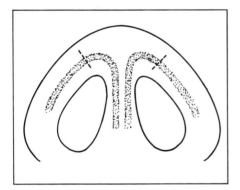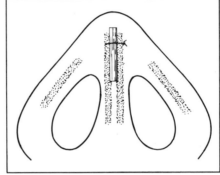

Figure 6.48 The Goldman tip. This technique enables the tip projection to be increased

(*3*) *Elevation of the tip* The nasal tip is raised by rotating the alar cartilage upwards around a posterior pivot (*see Figure 6.49*). The cartilage above and behind this pivot in the lateral crus will prevent this rotation, and it is, therefore, necessary to divide the rim just anterior to the pivot, and to remove the horizontal segment of cartilage above this line in order to permit the easy rotation of the tip upwards. This rotation of the alar cartilage is combined with shortening of the nose. This involves, of course, both shortening the medial wall which is the septum, and the lateral wall. This is achieved by removal of a caudal strip from the septal cartilage (*see Figure 6.50*), and by the removal also of an equal width of tissue from the lower border of the upper lateral cartilages (*see Figure 6.51*).

This is the general anatomical basis of tip surgery. There is also a general surgical principle which we must consider before going on to the actual details of the surgical technique. Vestibular skin must not be sacrificed, particularly if there has been much

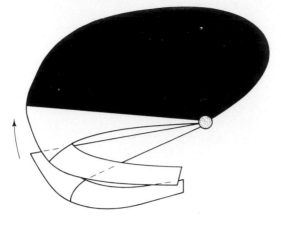

Figure 6.49   Elevation of the nasal tip by upward rotation of the alar cartilage

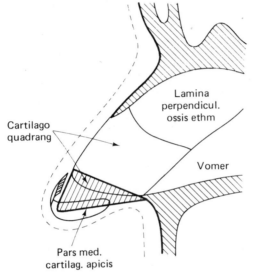

Lamina
perpendicul.
ossis ethm

Cartilago
quadrang

Vomer

Pars med.
cartilag. apicis

Figure 6.50   Shortening the nasal septum by resection of its lower border. (From J. Joseph, 1933. Reproduced by kind permission of Verlag Curt Kabitzsch)

removal of cartilage, otherwise post-operative fibrosis will lead to the development of a so-called 'pinched tip'. In this type of surgery, it is best to start with the septum first, and then to go on with the problems of the external nasal pyramid. Here it is advisable to start the work on the nasal tip because this is often one of the more delicate and demanding steps in the operation. It is, therefore, easier for this to be done before the more haemorrhagic stage of the operation which occurs when the osteotomies are performed. It is also necessary to establish the final position of the tip before any dorsal hump is lowered for reasons which are given later.

Exposure of the alar cartilages
The first step of tip surgery is to expose the alar cartilages, and this is best done by what is called the 'luxation method'. One starts with an 'inter-cartilaginous' incision between the lower border of the upper lateral cartilage and the upper border of the lateral crus of the alar cartilage; that is at the internal nares (*see Figure 6.23*). The 'transfixation' incision is made at the lower border of the septal cartilage and is extended forwards and laterally to join the anterior part of the inter-cartilaginous

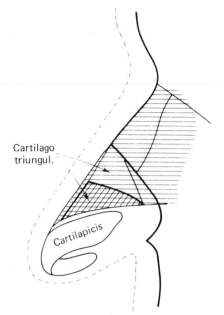

Cartilago
triungul.

Cartilapicis

Figure 6.51 Shortening the lateral nasal
wall by resection of the lower borders of
the upper lateral cartilages. (From J.
Joseph, 1933. Reproduced by kind permission of Verlag Curt Kabitzsch)

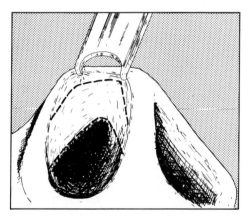

Figure 6.52 The rim and intercartilaginous
incisions used to expose the alar cartilages

incision. Exposure is improved by the use of a thimble retractor, and the left mid-
finger should be used to support the tissue being incised. This enables one to assess the
depth of the incision more accurately, thus avoiding any buttonholing in the skin. The
septal parts of the incision on both sides are united, so that the membranous and
cartilaginous septum are completely separated in this area. The inter-cartilaginous
incision is not only needed to assist in the exposure of the alar cartilage, but it is also
used to provide access to the skeletal framework of both the bony pyramid and the
upper cartilaginous vault.

A vestibular rim incision is then made. This should follow the lower border of the
alar cartilage, and is usually started about half-way along the alar margin on its
medial surface about 3 mm above the lower border of the nostril (*see Figure 6.52*). It is
important that the skin of the vestibule is incised exactly perpendicularly with a knife,
and that the incision should follow the lower border of the lateral crus particularly in
the region of the soft triangle (*see Figure 6.53*). If the incision is made into the soft

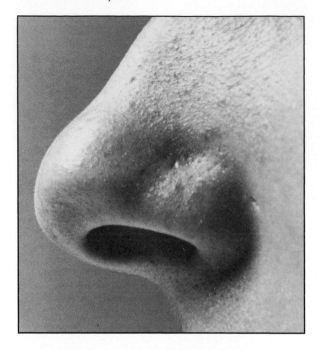

Figure 6.53 The Soft Triangle. There is a triangular facet on the antero–inferior surface of the nasal tip which is formed by a skin fold without any cartilaginous support

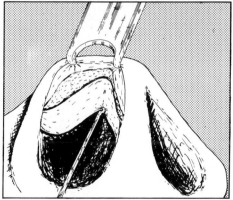

Figure 6.54 Exposure of the alar cartilage by the luxation technique

triangle, healing is often associated with an unpleasant notching effect, and one loses that pleasant facet on the lower surface of the nasal tip. The incision is then continued medially and posteriorly beyond the soft triangle region down to the medial crus. The lateral end of the incision may be extended to the posterior half of the ala where the lower border of the cartilage diverges from the rim, and the incision must also turn away from the nostril rim to correspond with this divergence. The lower border of the cartilage is visible through the marginal incision, and then the skin of the ala and the nasal tip, together with its subcutaneous connective and fatty tissue is elevated off the underlying cartilage by blunt scissors dissection. The slightly curved Knapp scissors are probably best for this purpose. The dissection is accomplished by an opening–closing movement of the scissors. The dissection is continued upwards in this plane until the inter-cartilaginous incision is reached. The skin and subcutaneous tissue in this area are now separated from a bridge flap formed by the alar cartilage and its lining vestibular skin. When this has been done the bridge flap is grasped with a pair of dissecting forceps and luxated out of the nostrils. This movement is similar to that of a bucket handle *(see Figure 6.54)*. The bridge flap can then be supported on a flat elevator which has been placed between it and the rim of the alar skin. All fat and connective tissue is then carefully removed from the exposed cartilage, which can then be incised, resected and remodelled as desired *(see Figure 6.55)*. Afterwards the bridge

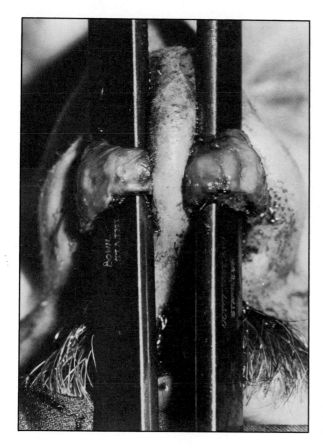

Figure 6.55   Exposure of the alar cartilages prior to incision and remodelling

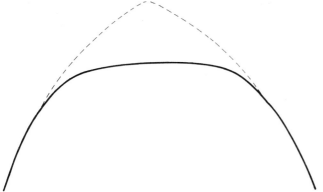

Figure 6.56   Truncated cone left after lowering of a nasal hump

flap is pushed back into the nostril and will be stitched back in place at the end of the operation.

The great merit of the luxation technique is that the whole of the alar cartilage, with the exception of the posterior part of the medial crus, lies exposed for the surgeon to inspect and re-model as required. Symmetrical excisions can easily be made, and what is more important still, the surgeon can see exactly what amount of cartilage he is leaving.

Surgery of the bony and cartilaginous dorsum

The bony and cartilaginous dorsum are best considered as a single unit because:

(1) The nasal bones overlap the upper lateral cartilages and are firmly united to them. This means that any displacement of the nasal bone almost invariably carries with it the attached upper lateral cartilage.
(2) Dorsal humps almost always include bony and cartilaginous elements.

Surgical indications

The most common indications for performing rhinoplastic procedures in this region include:

(1) The lowering of nasal humps. This procedure is usually termed reduction rhinoplasty.
(2) Alteration in the shape of the bony and cartilaginous dorsum. It is frequently necessary to straighten a deviated dorsum and to alter the width of this part of the nose. Following the removal of a nasal hump, one is left with a wide, flat dorsum which on cross-section has the shape of a truncated cone (*see Figure 6.56*). It is therefore usually necessary to include the narrowing of the nose as the second step in a conventional reduction rhinoplasty.
(3) Augmentation of the dorsum. Augmentation of the dorsum may be necessary to correct depressions or 'saddling' deformities in this region.

Methods of hump reduction

(1) Hump removal. The removal of a nasal hump through an endo–nasal incision was first performed by Roe of Rochester, New York in 1889, and this is still by far the commonest technique used today.
(2) Backward displacement of the hump. Later Cottle (1954) described the 'push-down' technique which involves the backward displacement of the hump following the removal of a strip from the nasal septum and infracturing of the nasal bones. Cottle maintains that removal of the nasal hump is often followed by an 'open-roof syndrome', in which vasomotor changes occur in the nose, usually following changes in temperature. He claims that this can be prevented by the use of his 'push-down' technique. I find it much more difficult to obtain good cosmetic results by using Cottle's technique and there appears to be very little risk of the 'open-roof syndrome' following hump removal.
(3) Hump removal and then replacement. More recently Skoog (1966) has advocated that the hump should be first radically removed, and then stripped of its mucosal lining, reduced in bulk, and finally replaced with a free autograft. He claims that this produces a smoother dorsum.

General principles of hump removal

(1) The nasal hump is a male characteristic and a small hump is therefore often acceptable in a man but not in a woman. A man can look somewhat emasculated with a scooped out dorsum but this type of nose will often suit a pretty girl. It is therefore necessary to be less radical in lowering the male nasal dorsum.

(3) It is best to delay the hump removal until after the tip work has been completed. This is because one has two important landmarks to consider in estimating the extent of hump removal, namely the nasion above and the tip below, and the final degree of tip projection will only be known with certainty after the completion of this stage of the rhinoplasty. Lipsett (1959) has shown that it is extremely difficult to plan the extent of the hump removal until the final position of the tip has been established, and that there is a grave risk of excessive hump removal if these two stages of the operation are reversed (*see Figure 6.57*).

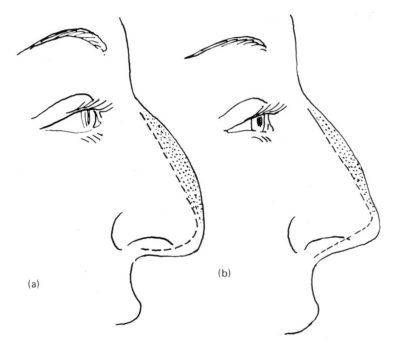

(a)

(b)

Figure 6.57 (a) Excessive hump lowering occurs if this stage of the operation is performed before elevation of the nasal tip. (b) Correct amount of hump lowering which can only be accurately determined after the final position of the tip has been established. (From Lipsett. Reproduced by kind permission of *Archives of Otolaryngology*)

(3) Due allowance must be made for the variation and thickness of the skin and subcutaneous tissue covering the nasal dorsum (*see Figure 6.58*). Wright (1967) has emphasized that the nasal skin is quite thick over the nasion, thin over the rhinion and thicker again over the supra-tip region. In order to obtain the straight nasal profile, it is necessary to retain a slight hump at the level of the rhinion. The commonest mistake made by the novice is to remove too much of the bony hump

and too little of the cartilaginous hump. This results in a supra-tip convexity which is called the 'polly' or the 'parrot beak' deformity, and which often makes a nose look worse than before the operation (*see Figure 6.59*). To compensate for the thicker skin of the supra-tip area, it is necessary to lower the cartilaginous dorsum radically at this level.

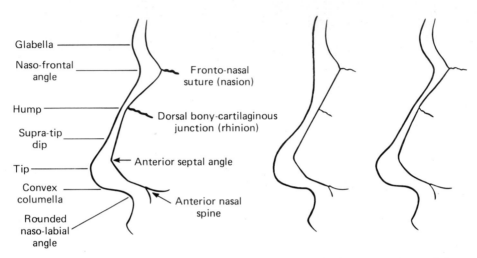

Figure 6.58   Allowance must be made for the varying skin thickness over the nasal dorsum when a hump is lowered. (From Bernstein, 1973. Reproduced by kind permission of W. B. Saunders Co.)

Technique of hump removal

It is first necessary to uncover the skeletal framework of the nasal dorsum. A pair of Knapp scissors is inserted through the inter-cartilaginous incision (*see Figure 6.24*), and the skin is undermined by a combination of spreading and cutting movements. Usually, the plane of dissection should be as close as possible to the cartilaginous and bony framework, because most of the blood vessels lie more superficially, and can thus be avoided. The skin is undermined over the upper lateral cartilages until the lower border of the nasal bones has been reached. It is then necessary to incise the periosteum covering the nasal bones with a sharp Joseph elevator (*see Figure 6.60*) and the elevation is then continued upwards at a sub-periosteal level (*see Figure 6.61*). It is most important not to let the elevator slip under the nasal bones, as it may then detach the upper lateral cartilage from its main anchorage, and thus cause a subsequent depression in this area. In the midline, the periosteum enters the median suture, and here a knife or a pair of very sharp scissors will have to be used. After the early stage of the dissection has been completed, the use of an Aufricht speculum enables one to have reasonable visual control over this stage of the operation. The elevation is continued upwards over the nasal bones and the adjacent frontal process of the maxilla to just beyond the level of the nasion, but not widely over the frontal process of the maxilla, because the splinting support of the soft tissues on the bony lateral walls of the nose will be required later after the medial, transverse and lateral osteotomies have been performed It is most important that all strands of connective tissue between the skeletal framework and the subcutaneous tissues are divided, otherwise of course the ultimate removal of the bony hump will be more difficult and traumatic.

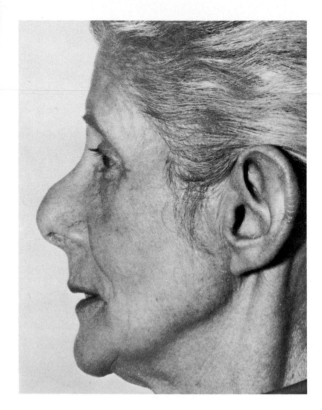

Figure 6.59 A 'polly beak' nose. This followed a reduction rhinoplasty which had been performed over 20 years previously

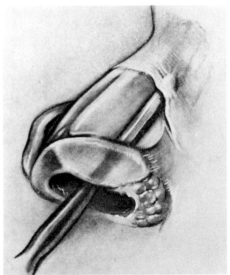

Figure 6.60 Incising periosteum with Joseph periosteal elevator. (From Seltzer and reproduced by kind permission of J. B. Lippincott & Co.)

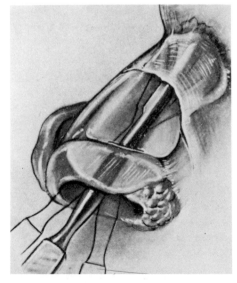

Figure 6.61 Completing the elevation of the periosteum over the nasal bones. (From Seltzer and reproduced by kind permission of J. B. Lippincott & Co.)

The bony hump can be removed by chisels, saws, bone forceps or drills, and very small humps can be removed with a rasp. Good results can be obtained by any technique once it has been mastered. It is much safer to perform a staged or graduated removal of the hump. 'One piece' concept is dangerous and it can easily lead to too much removal of bony hump and the development of 'polly beak' deformity. For this reason, the safest instrument to use is a rasp because it cuts slowly and it is possible to detect errors at an early stage and to compensate for them. A rasp can also be used to lower the lateral convexities on the nasal dorsum. When using a saw or chisel, it is necessary to allow for the thickness of the instrument, otherwise too much bone will be removed. For the larger hump, I personally favour the use of a guarded chisel and the progress of the instrument can be regularly checked by palpating its lateral guards through the subcutaneous tissues. After the chisel has reached the level of the nasion, it is possible to remove the hump, and final adjustments can then be made by using a rasp. The rasp, chisel and saw can only be effectively used on rigid bone, and it is for this reason that the hump removal must precede the mobilization of the lateral bony walls of the nose which occurs after osteotomies have been performed. The cartilaginous dorsum must be lowered with either a knife or sharp angulated scissors. Initially, the bony and cartilaginous elements of the dorsum are lined up and then afterwards a little extra is taken off the cartilage. Minor adjustments may be necessary after the osteotomies have been performed. A final inspection of the skeletal dorsum is then made and it may be necessary to remove any irregularities. This can be best done at the level of the bony dorsum by using Kaplin's scissors, and at the level of the cartilaginous dorsum with Fomon's angulated scissors.

Osteotomies

Mobilization of the lateral nasal walls is necessary before one can either straighten the nose or alter its width. This is achieved by performing lateral, medial and transverse osteotomies (*see Figure 6.62*). Complete osteotomies are particularly important following old fractures because the membranous bone which forms the bony pyramid does not produce much callus and often heals by fibrous union. Minimal mobilization and reduction often stretches the fibrous tissue and initially completely corrects the deformity, but recurrence occurs with the subsequent contraction of the fibrous tissue. Radical mobilization with slight over-correction and splinting, is therefore necessary to deal effectively with this type of problem. If the nose has both a hump and a lateral deviation, the hump should be removed obliquely to restore the equalization of the lateral walls of the nose.

Sometimes when the hump is very large, and extends up to the region of the nasion, the actual hump removal effectively produces a satisfactory medial osteotomy. This is, however, unusual and one more commonly has to separate the bony septum from the lateral wall, by a few blows on a chisel, which is directed parallel to the midline of the nose. The osteotomy, for reasons which will be given later, should be confined to the thin nasal bone and should not extend into the thick upper central mass of bone at the root of the nose. As soon as the chisel begins to enter the thicker bone, the sound of the mallet striking the chisel becomes dull, and this indicates that a sufficient depth of bone has been penetrated. The lateral osteotomy is usually performed through a small stab incision in the nasal vestibule, just in front of the anterior end of the inferior turbinate (*see Figure 6.63*). Some surgeons prefer to perform the lateral osteotomy through an extended inter-cartilaginous incision, through a sublabial incision or

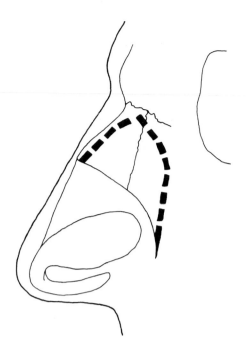

Figure 6.62   Lateral, medial and transverse osteotomies

sometimes through a small external incision in the alar facial crease. The incision is extended on to the periosteum covering the piriform aperture, which is then divided and a Joseph elevator is used to make a subperiosteal tunnel along the base of the lateral wall of the nose to a point immediately in front of the attachment of the medial canthus. It is also advisable to elevate the muco–periosteum off the inner aspect so that it is less likely to be torn during the actual osteotomy. The osteotomy can be made with a guarded chisel or by using Joseph saws. The upper part of the osteotomy is best made with a curved chisel which is directed towards the midline so that part at any rate of the transverse osteotomy can be performed at this stage. The actual location of the chisel during the osteotomy can be easily determined by palpating the elevated lateral guard. It is usually then possible to complete easily the transverse osteotomy by fracturing the intact bone which extends towards the nasion. Simple digital pressure with the thumb is usually sufficient but in more resistant cases, Walsham's forceps can be used, first to outfracture, and then to infracture the lateral nasal wall.

One has now completely mobilized the lateral nasal wall and the segments are then repositioned as required to correct the deformity. The best way to narrow the nose is to displace the lateral walls medially and posteriorly so that they become locked between the outer borders of the lateral osteotomies (*see Figure 6.64*). If the nose is deviated, the lateral wall on the deviated side is narrower and some equalization of disparity will be necessary. The wider side can be narrowed by multiple osteotomies or by trimming the bone along its medial border with a pair of Kaplin's scissors. In a deviated nose, this asymmetry involves the upper lateral cartilages and it is therefore also necessary to trim the excess width of the lateral cartilages on the side opposite to the deviation with a pair of Fomon scissors.

The osteotomy should be performed through thin bone, avoiding the extremely dense, solid bone, which is situated at the root of the nose above. Attempts to perform

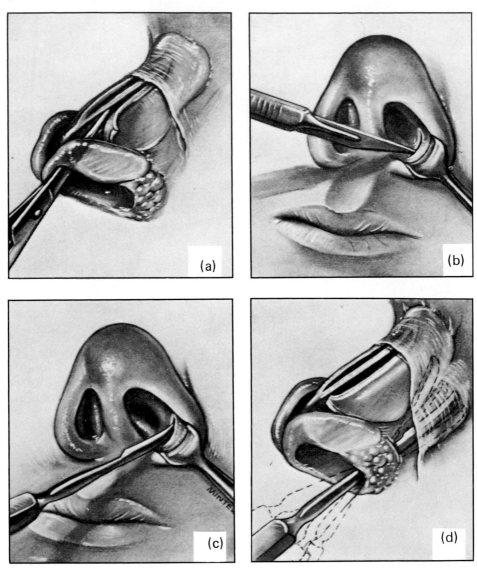

Figure 6.63   (a) Medial osteotomies; (b) incision just anterior to inferior turbinate for the lateral osteotomy; (c) and (d) elevation of the periosteum along the line of the lateral oesteotomy. (From Seltzer and reproduced by kind permission of J. B. Lippincott & Co.)

the osteotomies through this dense bone, usually result in the so-called 'rocker' (*see Figure 6.65*). Here, the transverse osteotomy is oblique, and when an attempt is made to displace the mobilized lateral wall medially, the inward movement of the upper fragment is resisted by the sloping edge of bone which extends to the upper margin of the transverse osteotomy. A fulcrum is established at the lower border of this bone, and when the lower part of the nasal bone is displaced medially, the upper part moves outwards, and this actually causes a widening at the level of the nasion.

Sometimes the solid dense central bony triangle at the root of the nose does need correction after the performance of the osteotomy, and this can usually be done with

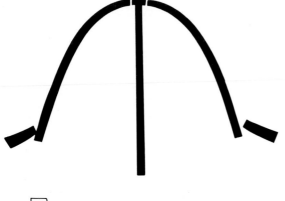

Figure 6.64 Bony pyramid narrowed by locking the lateral nasal
bone between the outer margins of
the lateral osteotomies

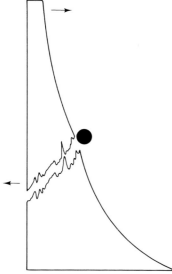

Figure 6.65 'Rocker' formation which occurs when the
transverse osteotomies are performed too high

either a rasp, a chisel, or a dental drill. Once the osteotomies have been performed, it
is necessary to re-check the hump removal, and make any final adjustments that are
required with a sharp angulated bone or cartilage scissors. Sometimes, however, there
are still minor irregularities and depressions which are best corrected by the insertion
of crushed cartilage grafts over them. Septal cartilage, preferably autogenous, can be
placed in a Cottle crusher and then inserted through the intercartilaginous incision
over the affected part of the dorsum.

Augmentation rhinoplasty

(1) Supra-tip saddling   Supra-tip saddling occurs when the septal support to the
dorsum has been lost either by trauma or disease. The bony pyramid is unaffected
although the supra-tip depression may give the erroneous impression of a 'pseudo'
bony hump. Treatment involves the augmentation of the depression with autogenous
cartilage grafts taken from the septum (*see Figure 6.66*). These can be inserted through
the inter-cartilaginous incision. If there is an actual bony hump present, this can be
removed and then replaced in the supra-tip area as a free graft.

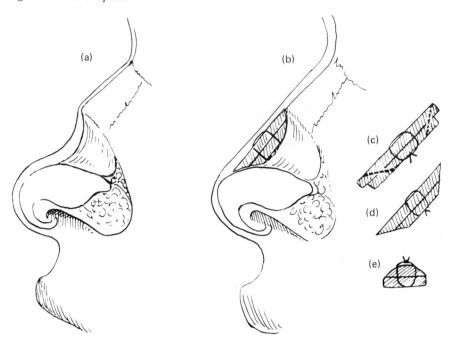

Figure 6.66   The augmentation of a supra-tip depression with autogenous cartilage grafts. (From Converse and reproduced by kind permission of W. B. Saunders & Co.)

(2) Extensive saddling   When the saddling is extensive and involves the bony pyramid, there is not enough local tissue available to effect a repair and it is necessary to use some extra-nasal material in the form of either cancellous bone or rib cartilage. The use of alloplastic implants for this purpose has not infrequently been followed by extrusion and scarring of the skin over the nasal dorsum (*Figure 6.67*). Extensive saddling is usually associated with widening of the dorsum and bulbosity of the tip. It is therefore often necessary to correct the tip and narrow the nasal pyramid and this is usually best done as a primary procedure at least three months before the augmentation rhinoplasty is performed. The graft needs to be completely surrounded by the tissues of the nose after it has been inserted into the dorsum, and the multiple intranasal incisions associated with the correction of these multiple defects, may well result in some exposure of the graft and imperil its vitality. It is therefore much safer to stage these two procedures.

Post-operative splinting and care

Outer splints
Outer splints are very important as the various segments of the nasal framework have been separated and mobilized, and their deformities corrected. They can then be positioned to produce a well-shaped nose, and this process has been likened by Trent Smith to 'the potter modelling clay'. The nose must be immobilized in the corrected position by splints during the healing phase. The pressure of the splints also minimizes

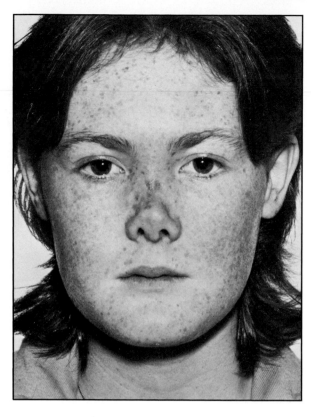

Figure 6.67   Scarring of the nasal dorsum following a fistula which developed after a Silastic implant had been inserted to augment the nasal dorsum

the risk of subcutaneous haematoma formation. It is best to start putting horizontal bands of Blenderm over the nose. These should overlap, as herniation of the skin and subcutaneous tissues can occur through any gaps left between these strips, and this can progress to skin necrosis and ugly scarring. A vertical loop is used to narrow the tip, and also to prevent drooping. After the application of the skin splints, the nose should be protected by an outer splint made either of plaster of paris, metal or dental stent. Finally, a gauze bolster is placed under the nose.

Post-operative care
After the operation, the nose is disturbed as little as possible; if there is a lot of bruising around the eyes, cold compresses are applied locally. The first main dressing takes place on the seventh day, when both the outer and skin splints are carefully removed. The outer splint should then be re-applied for another 10–14 days. They can then be removed, and after this period of time, the bone has reunited firmly enough to withstand moderate trauma.

Ulceration and perforation of the septum

These are usually different stages in the same pathological process, and apart from the traumatic cases, septal perforations are usually preceded by ulceration. The energetic and successful treatment of a septal ulcer will therefore prevent the development of a perforation, and this is particularly important in the case of children, as the development of a perforated septum in the growing nose will often retard growth both of the nose and of the mid third of the face.

Causes of septal perforations

(1) Trauma
    (a) Surgical
    (b) Repeated cautery
    (c) Digital trauma ('nose picking')
(2) Malignant disease
    (a) Malignant tumours
    (b) Malignant granuloma (Wegener's)
(3) Chronic infections
    (a) Syphilis
    (b) Tuberculosis
(4) Poisons
    (a) Industrial
    (b) Cocaine addicts
(5) Idiopathic

Apart from syphilis which normally attacks the bony septum, most perforations are usually found anteriorly in the septal cartilage. Unfortunately most are iatrogenic in origin and usually occur as a complication of septal surgery, particularly when the Killian SMR technique is used. Although the septoplasty operation does not give complete immunity against this complication, perforations are a rarity following this operation. Perforations result from mucoperichondrial tears, particularly when they are bilateral and overlapping. Gross post-traumatic fibrosis increases this risk, and the site of the perforation is usually along the line of the chondro–vomerine suture where the anatomy of the perichondrial and periosteal layers also increases the difficulties of flap elevation. When mishaps of this kind occur during an SMR, every effort should be made to prevent this complication by inserting a bony or cartilaginous autograft between the torn flaps and also by closing the tears with catgut sutures (*see Figure 6.27*). Repeated cautery of the septum can lead to perforations. The risk is much greater when both sides of the septum are cauterized at one sitting, and it is therefore wise to have an interval of 3–4 weeks between the two treatments. In my experience, patients who suffer from Osler's disease are lucky to escape this complication.

Septal perforations are sometimes occupational in origin and the commonest such cause is penetration of the nasal mucosa by one of the hexavalent forms of chromium. In addition to its role in plating processes, this metal is used in certain tanning, dyeing and photographic processes. Workers engaged in the manufacture of bichromates are particularly at risk. Other causes include exposure to anhydrous sodium carbonate (soda ash), arsenic and its compounds, organic compounds of mercury, particularly mercury fulminate, alkaline dusts such as soap powders, hydrofluoric acid and fluorides, capsaicin, the pungent active principle of capsicum (chillies), vanadium, dimethyl sulphate, cocaine and other drugs taken as snuff, copper salts (rarely), and lime (rarely).

The incidence of chrome perforation among platers has been greatly reduced by the use of exhaust ventilation and seromists. The highest incidence of chrome perforation is found in chemical workers engaged in the production of chromates. In one such factory in the UK, 236 out of 480 workers had chrome perforations. There was no obvious relationship between the incidence of the perforation and the length of exposure. There are suspicions that some at least of these perforations were self-induced, because the monetary award for this occupational disease is often considered to far outweigh the resulting minimal disability.

Symptoms and signs

Apart from the traumatic causes, septal perforations are usually preceded by ulceration. There are often four well-marked stages, starting with redness and congestion of the mucosa producing irritation and rhinorrhoea. Shortly afterwards the mucosa becomes blanched and anaemic then later undergoes necrosis as shown by the development of tough adherent crusts over the affected area. Finally the crusting extends into the substance of the cartilage and a perforation results. Septal perforations are quite often asymptomatic, but the development of large crusts may cause obstruction and the separation of these crusts may lead to bleeding. Patients not infrequently complain of abnormal dryness in the nose, and sometimes of a dull discomfort over the bony dorsum. The passage of respiratory air often produces a whistling noise. Crusting problems are usually much worse when there is any interference with the normal respiratory air currents, as may occur with such obstructive lesions as septal deviations behind the perforations.

Diagnosis

The history is of importance in the diagnosis of traumatic and occupational cases. When the edge of the lesion looks raised or hypertrophic, a biopsy should be performed to exclude malignancy. A biopsy is also useful in suspected cases of Wegener's granuloma. Serological tests for syphilis should always be performed if the lesion is involving the bony septum, and an ESR is invariably raised in cases of Wegener's granuloma; this can be a useful confirmatory diagnostic test for this condition, together with the biopsy.

Treatment

The first objective in the management of septal ulcers and perforations is to cure the causative disease process. Conditions such as malignant tumours, malignant granuloma, and chronic infections are dealt with in other chapters of the book. In the occupational cases, it will be necessary to obtain the cooperation of the industrial medical officer to prevent further exposure to the toxic agent. Most recent cases have occurred when the exhaust ventilation system in the chrome plant has become defective.

The second objective is to encourage natural healing of the lesion, and if this does

not occur, to consider performing a surgical repair. The patient must be told to treat
his nose with great care, and to avoid such traumatizing actions as vigorous blowing
and nose picking. The patient should also apply twice daily some Cicatrin cream on
the tip of the little finger to the lesion. This treatment will heal most ulcers, although
the original area will often permanently remain white, dry and scarred.

Perforations never heal spontaneously, but fortunately most of them do not cause
symptoms, and therefore do not require any treatment. Crusting and bleeding are the
main problems associated with the more troublesome minority of septal perforations.
Less severe cases can be satisfactorily controlled by the use of a Coll. Alk. nasal douche,
but should this prove to be inadequate, the closure of the perforation, either by filling
it with an obturator, or by means of a surgical operation, will have to be considered.

Obturators (*see Figure 6.68*) are a simple, safe, and reliable method of closing almost
any septal perforation. This method can be used to close really large perforations, and
the author has dealt with defects up to 4 cm in diameter by this technique. Cooperation
of a dental prosthetics department is essential, and the author has been fortunate in
obtaining the help of Dr Davenport, who has evolved a technique in which a Silastic
obturator is made from an impression taken in silicone rubber. Over 20 septal
perforations have now been closed by this technique, and apart from one early case in
which minor modifications were necessary, an excellent fit was always obtained.
Crusting was not completely eliminated with the larger perforations, but the crusts
were always much more easily controlled by the use of a nasal douche.

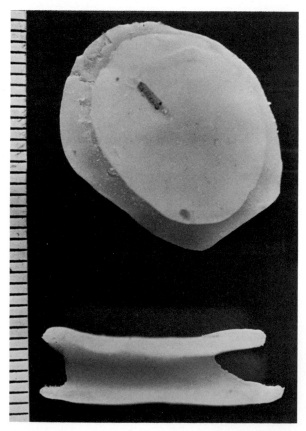

Figure 6.68   A Silastic obturator
for the closure of a septal perforation. There is a millimetre scale
on the left side

The operative closure of septal perforations is a rather unsatisfactory chapter in the subject of nasal surgery. This form of treatment can be considered for the more anterior and smaller lesions. It is difficult to assess the results of surgery from a study of the literature, because late results are rarely given. It would appear, however, that at least one-third of the operations are primary failures, and that up to another third

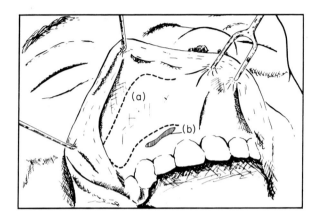

Figure 6.69   Closure of a septal perforation by a labial flap. (a) Design of labial flap; (b) small incision in floor of nose. (From Tipton. Reproduced by kind permission of *Plastic and Reconstructive Surgery*)

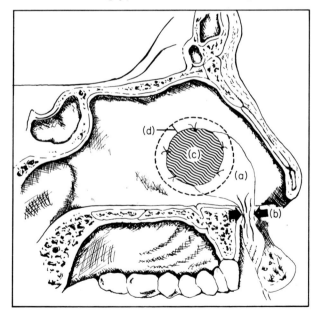

Figure 6.70   Labial flap in place closing off the septal perforation (c) with its distal edges tucked in under the edges of the septal mucosa around the defect (d). (From Tipton. Reproduced by kind permission of *Plastic and Reconstructive Surgery*)

will re-perforate during the next 18 months. It would therefore appear that closure of the perforation with an obturator is the initial treatment of choice, and that operative techniques are only indicated in those rare cases where the obturator proved to be unsatisfactory. Many different methods have been described for the closure of septal perforations. Most techniques require the elevation of mucoperichondrial flaps, and this is often very difficult because the Killian type of SMR operation has usually previously been performed. Seiffert (1967) and Ismail (1964) have both advocated the use of turbinate tissue. Probably the most reliable and generally applicable method involves the closure of the perforation with a pedicle flap of buccal mucosa from the inner margin of the upper lip. This technique has been advocated by both Tipton (1970) and Tardy (1973). The flap is elevated and is then brought up through a small stab incision in the floor of the nasal vestibule up to the septal perforation where it is sutured in place (*see Figures 6.69* and *70*). Four to six weeks later the bridge of the flap can be divided quite simply under a local anaesthetic.

References

Beekhuis, G. Jan. (1973) 'Nasal Septoplasty', *Otolaryngologic Clinics of North America*, **6**, 693

Bernstein, L. (1973a) 'Early Submucous Resection of Nasal Septal Cartilage', *Archives of Otolaryngology* **97**, 273

Bernstein, L. (1973b) 'Submucous operations on the Nasal Septum', *Otolaryngologic Clinics of North America* **6**, 675

Briant, D. (1977) Personal communication

Chassaignac, C. (1851) *Gazette des Hopitaux*, Paris 419

Cottle, M. H. (1954) 'Nasal Roof Repair and Hump Removal', *Archives of Otolaryngology* **60**, 408

Cottle, M. H. (1968) 'Rhino–sphygmo-manometry and aid in physical diagnosis', *International Rhinology* **6**, 7

Cottle, M. H., Fischer, G. G., Gaynon, I. E. and Loring, R. M. (1958) 'The "Maxilla–Pre-maxilla" Approach to Extensive Nasal Septum Surgery', *Archives of Otolaryngology* **68**, 301

Curtiss, E. S. (1952) 'Postural Nerve Block for Intranasal operations, *Lancet* **1**, 989

Diefenbach, J. (1845) *Die operative chirurgie.* Liepzig 366

Douek, E. (1974) *The Sense of Smell and its Abnormalities* London; Churchill Livingstone

Fomon, S. (1970) *Rhinoplasty—New Concepts*, pp. 1–40. Springfield, Illinois, Charles C. Thomas

Fomon, S., Gilbert, J. G., Silver, A. G. and Syracuse, V. R. (1948) 'Plastic repair of the obstructing Nasal Septum', *Archives of Otolaryngology* **47**, 7

Freer, O. (1902) 'The correction of deflections of the Nasal Septum with a minimum of Traumation', *Journal of the American Medical Association* **38**, 636

Fry, J. H. (1969) 'The Pathology and treatment of Haematoma of the Nasal Septum', *British Journal of Plastic Surgery* **22**, 331

Fuchs, P. (1969) 'Experimental production of growth disturbance by using a caudally based vomerine flap in rabbits' *Transactions of the 4th International Congress of Plastic Reconstructive Surgery*, pp. 484–488. Amsterdam

Galloway, T. (1946) Referred to by Bolotow, Fomon, Pullen and Syracuse. 'Plastic repair of the deflected Nasal Septum', *Archives of Laryngology* **44**, 141

Goldman, I. B. (1953) 'New technique of corrective surgery of the nasal tip', *Archives of Otolaryngology* **53**, 183

Gray, L. P. (1972) In *Modern Trends in Diseases of the Ear, Nose and Throat* Ed. by Ellis, M. pp. 219–236 London; Butterworths

Hartenstrom, D. F. (1970) *Facial Growth Effects of Nasal Septal Cartilage Resection in Beagle Pups.* (Thesis) University of Iowa, Iowa City

Hayton, C. H. (1948) Quoted by St. Clair Thomson and V. E. Negus *Diseases of the Nose and Throat* p. 193 London; Cassell

Hirsch, O. (1952) 'Symptoms and Treatment of Pituitary Tumours' *Archives of Otolaryngology* **55**, 268

Ismail, H. K. (1964) 'Closure of septal perforations. A new technique', *Journal of Laryngology and Otology* **78**, 620

Jeppesen, F. and Windfeld, I. (1972) 'Dislocation of the Nasal Septal Cartilage in the Newborn', *Acta Obstetrica Gynecologica, Scandinavica* **51**, 5

Killian, G. (1904) 'Die submucöse Fensterresektion der Nasen-scheidewand', *Archiv für Laryngologie und Rhinologie* **16**, 362

Langenbeck, B. (1843) *Handbuch der Anatomie.* Gottingen

Lipsett, E. M. (1959) 'A new approach to surgery of the lower cartilaginous vault', *Archives of Otolaryngology* **70**, 42

Metzenbaum, M. (1929) 'Replacement of the lower end of the dislocated cartilage versus submucous resection of the dislocated end of the septal cartilage' *Archives of Otolaryngology* **9**, 282

Metzenbaum, M (1936) 'Dislocation of the lower end of the septal cartilage', *Archives of Otolaryngology*, **24**, 78

Minnis, N. L. and Morrison, A. W. (1971) 'Trans-Septal Approach for Vidian Neurectomy', *Journal of Laryngology and Otology* **85**, 255

Moffett, A. J. (1941) 'Postural Instillation–A Method of Inducing Local Anaesthesia in the nose', *Journal of Laryngology and Otology* **56**, 429

Peer, L. (1937) 'An operation to repair lateral displacement of the lower border of the Septal Cartilage', *Archives of Otolaryngology* **25**, 475

Roe, J. O. (1899) 'Correction of Nasal Deformities by subcutaneous operation', *American Medical Quarterly* **1**, 56

Rubrecht, W. (1868) *Weiner medis Wochenschrift* **18**, 1157

Sarnat, B. G. and Wexler, M. R. (1966) 'Growth of the face and jaws after resection of the septal cartilage in the rabbit', *American Journal of Anatomy* **118**, 755

Seiffert, A. (1967) Quoted in *Plastic Surgery of Head and Neck* Denecke, H. J., and Meyer, R. p. 139 New York; Springer-Verlag

Selzer, A. P. *Plastic Surgery of the Nose*. Philadelphia; J. B. Lippincott & Co.

Shalom, A. S. (1963) 'The Anterior Ethmoid Nerve Syndrome' *Journal of Laryngology and Otology* **77**, 315

Skoog, T. (1966) 'A Method of Hump Reduction in Rhinoplasty', *Archives of Otolaryngology* **83**, 283

Sluder, G. (1927) *Nasal Neurology, Headaches and Eye Disorders* London; Kimpton

Tardy, M. E. (1973) 'Septal Perforations', *Otolaryngology Clinic of North America* **6**, 711

Tipton, J. B. (1970) 'Closure of large septal perforation with a labial-buccal flap', *Plastic and Reconstructive Surgery* **46**, 514

Wright, W. K. (1967) 'Study on hump removal in Rhinoplasty', *Laryngoscope* **77**, 508

7 Foreign bodies in the nose: rhinoliths

Joselen Ransome

Foreign bodies in the nose do not feature largely in otolaryngological literature: yet on occasions they may constitute a considerable challenge to both the diagnostic and surgical skills of the otolaryngologist.

Aetiology

Mode of entry

Foreign bodies may enter the nose through:

(1) *the anterior naris* (the most common way);
(2) *the posterior naris*, during vomiting, coughing and regurgitation, or in patients with palatal incompetence—when the foreign body will consist of stomach, oesophageal or mouth contents, and occasionally a roundworm (ascaris);
(3) *penetrating wounds* and nasal surgery;
(4) *a palatal perforation* as in cleft palate or following a gumma of the hard palate or surgery of the palate for malignant disease;
(5) *sequestration of bone in situ* after trauma (which may be operative), and syphilis;
(6) *calcification in situ* of inspissated mucopus or of exogenous foreign material, leading to the formation of a rhinolith.

Types of patients

Children constitute a large majority of patients with foreign bodies in the nose. The foreign body will be whatever small object the child encounters in the world he explores, and it will usually be introduced through the anterior naris. Children with cleft palate will also have food from the mouth entering the nose, and occasionally exogenous material which the child is exploring with the mouth. Children of low socio–economic groups living in tropical climates may also be the victims of myiasis (diseases due to maggots, larvae and flies).

Adults with foreign bodies in the nose are usually *mentally disturbed* if they have been inserted through the anterior naris, but may also be the victims of *penetrating injuries*, for instance caused by bullets and shrapnel, or of *operations on the nose*, in which swabs, or particles of tissue or instruments may be left behind.

Debilitating diseases such as diabetes and syphilis, and also patients with ozaena, and *low socio–economic status* may predispose to myiasis in tropical climates.

Site of foreign body

If it has been inserted by the patient it is more commonly in the right nasal cavity, since right-handedness predominates in the general population. The foreign body may be in any part of the nasal fossa.

Types of foreign body

Foreign bodies in the nose may be

(1) animate,
(2) inanimate: (i)   vegetable,
                (ii)   mineral,
                (iii) arising from surgery,
                (iv)   sequestra,
                (v)   rhinoliths.

(1) Animate
Maggots, screw worms and their larvae, and black carpet beetles may all infest the nose in tropical climates (myiasis), and occasionally a roundworm (ascaris) may be coughed or regurgitated through the posterior naris.

(2) Inanimate
(i) *Vegetable* foreign bodies are commonly peas, beans, dried pulses and nuts. (ii) *Mineral* matter may be pieces of pencils, paper, sponge, pieces from metal and plastic toys, washers, nuts, nails, screws, buttons, studs, plasticine, pebbles, beads and cotton wool, to name but a few. (iii) *Arising from surgery*: pieces of polyps, bone, cartilage, swabs, instruments or packs may be left behind. (iv) *Sequestra* occur in syphilis and neoplasm, and after trauma. (v) *Rhinoliths* occur *in situ*—see above and below.

Pathology

Some foreign bodies are inert and may remain in the nose for years without mucosal changes. Many however lead to inflammation and infection of the mucous membrane, which in turn leads to *foetid mucopurulent discharge* and epistaxis, these symptoms being *unilateral*, except with animate infestations. Ultimately granulation tissue is formed, and there may be ulceration of the mucosa, and occasionally necrosis of bone or cartilage.

These changes tend to bring about impaction of the foreign body, which may not be visible on either anterior or posterior rhinoscopy because of surrounding oedema, granulations and discharge. This is particularly so with vegetable foreign bodies which not only absorb water from the tissues and swell, but also evoke a very brisk inflammatory reaction. Occasionally the inflammatory reaction is sufficient to produce toxaemia.

Maggots and screw worms attack both nasal cavities and may give rise to a severe inflammatory reaction. During maturation, larvae burrow into the tissues. The mature larva of the screw worm has rings round the body, giving the appearance of a screw. If untreated they may attack nasal bone and cartilage and also involve the sinuses, orbits, adjoining skin, meninges, and brain (Gupta and Nema, 1970). Ascaris produces less inflammation but gives the patient a feeling of irritation and movement in the nose.

Sharp foreign bodies may occasionally penetrate the sinuses and give rise to sinusitis.

If a foreign body is buried in granulations or firmly impacted, it may act as a nucleus for concretion to occur, i.e. it receives a coating of calcium and magnesium phosphate and carbonate and becomes a *rhinolith*. Occasionally this process may occur round an area of inspissated mucopus, or even a blood clot. Rhinoliths usually form near the floor of the nose and are radio-opaque.

Symptoms and signs

1. Mineral and vegetable foreign bodies

These generally give rise to a *unilateral foetid discharge*, usually mucopurulent and sometimes blood-stained. There is frequently unilateral nasal obstruction, and there may be pain, epistaxis, and sneezing. A few foreign bodies are inert and give either no symptoms, or unilateral nasal obstruction if large enough.

Examination of the nose shows reddened congested mucosa, mucopus and sometimes granulations, ulceration and necrosis. The foreign body may or may not be visible, depending on its size and nature, and on the degree of surrounding oedema.

2. Animate foreign bodies

The symptoms are often bilateral, and nasal obstruction, headaches and sero-sanguineous foetid discharge may occur within a few days of infestation. In the larval stage pyrexia may occur. The patient has a constant feeling of formication in the nose. In poor communities the patients adapt surprisingly well to the condition, and instead of being driven to despair, have to be prodded into seeking treatment, on the grounds that complications may occur.

Examination shows marked swelling of the mucosa, which is fragile and bleeds easily. In heavy infestations there is an appearance of constant motion, which on closer inspection is seen to be due to masses of worms, which are firmly attached and difficult to remove. In long-standing infestation there may be destruction of bone and cartilage.

Due to secondary infection and bone destruction complications are not rare, and patients may present with orbital infection or meningitis. In the rare cases of ascaris in the nose, the worm is large (6–10 in) and easy to remove. There is minimal mucosal reaction.

3. Rhinoliths

As they increase in size slowly and are relatively inert, rhinoliths are initially symptomless, and later cause nasal obstruction if they become large enough. They may be discovered when a cause is sought for an unresolved sinus infection.

Examination of the nasal cavity shows a brown or greyish irregular mass, usually near the floor of the nose, which feels stony hard and gritty on probing. *X-rays* will reveal the extent of the rhinolith, which may attain a very large size, and may occasionally extend into the antrum.

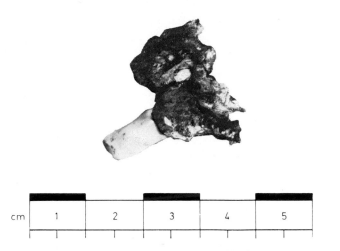

cm   1   2   3   4   5

Figure 7.1   Rhinolith from a case described by Mr. R. McNab Jones

Diagnosis

(1) With *animate* foreign bodies, the diagnosis is usually all too apparent on inspection.
(2) With *inanimate* foreign bodies, the suspicion usually arises because of a unilateral purulent nasal discharge, and in children this must be regarded as due to a foreign body until proved otherwise. Frequently the foreign body will be seen on anterior rhinoscopy (and sometimes on posterior rhinoscopy), but on occasions the mucosal oedema or granulations will hide the foreign body. In cooperative adults and older children the nose should be sprayed with a vasoconstrictor to shrink the mucosa, and then the fossa examined again, and if necessary gently probed. If a foreign body is still not found, the nose should be x-rayed as many foreign bodies are radio-opaque. In younger children or very apprehensive adults it may be necessary for the search to be carried out under a general anaesthetic, and this procedure is described below.
Other conditions to be excluded are neoplasm (by biopsy of granulations), unilateral

sinusitis (by x-ray), syphilitic necrosis (by serology), diphtheria (by nasal swab) and unilateral choanal atresia (by passing a catheter through the nasal fossa, or by x-ray after instilling a contrast medium).

Management

1. Animate foreign bodies

Infestations with maggots and screw worms are treated by instilling a 25 per cent chloroform solution into the nasal cavities. This is repeated two or three times a week for about six weeks until all larvae are killed. After each treatment the patient blows his nose to clear it of dead worms and larvae. Sometimes treatment is given under general anaesthesia (with a cuffed endotracheal tube and throat pack), when repeated irrigation followed by suction can be carried out.

Ascaris is managed by removal of the worm with forceps, then treatment of the general condition with piperazine, and with magnesium sulphate purges to clear dead worms from the bowel.

2. Inanimate foreign bodies

The following applies to *all inanimate foreign bodies except rhinoliths.*

If the foreign body is easily seen and the patient is a cooperative older child or adult, it is usually possible to remove the foreign body through the anterior naris, either with no anaesthetic or after spraying with 5 or 10 per cent cocaine solution.

The patient is placed in the usual upright position for routine ENT examination, and the nasal fossa illuminated with a head mirror or fibre-light headlight. It is important that the light source should be very bright. The following instruments should be available: nasal speculum, curved hook, Jobson Horne probe, selection of angled crocodile forceps, and angled nasal dressing forceps of various sizes, nasal sucker and source of suction. Also a jar to receive specimens to send to the pathology department should be prepared.

The nasal speculum is inserted with the left hand, and with the right hand the curved hook is passed beyond the object and the tip rotated to rest just posterior to the object. The object is then gently drawn forwards and removed completely, or brought almost to the nasal vestibule and then removed with forceps. The above technique should be used whenever there is a risk of displacing the object backwards into the nasopharynx, as with spherical objects such as beads. Rough semi-impacted objects such as bits of paper and sponge, and objects placed very near the vestibule, can be removed directly with forceps.

A *general anaesthetic* will be required in the following circumstances: (i) if the patient is uncooperative or very apprehensive; (ii) if there is likely to be troublesome bleeding, for instance if the foreign body is firmly embedded in granulation tissue; (iii) if the foreign body is posteriorly placed with a risk of pushing it back into the nasopharynx; (iv) if a foreign body is strongly suspected but cannot be found, and more extensive examination of the nose is required, with the opportunity to deal with whatever is found. It must be emphasized that there is *no need for haste* on these occasions. The foreign body may have been in the nose for a considerable period and it is important to wait for ideal facilities, especially an experienced anaesthetist. Unskilled manipulation in adverse conditions can lead to inhalation of the foreign body or of blood.

The patient is anaesthetized and a cuffed oral endotracheal tube inserted and a pharyngeal pack. With the patient in the usual position for nasal surgery, the nose is examined using a nasal speculum, headlight, and suction to remove secretions. The affected nasal fossa is then sprayed with 1 ml of a mixture of 5 per cent cocaine and 1/1000 adrenaline (50 per cent of each), to minimize bleeding. After waiting for this to take effect, the nose is then examined again, and the foreign body is gently withdrawn.

If it is wedged posteriorly and cannot be brought out through the anterior naris, it is occasionally necessary to push the foreign body backwards into the nasopharynx. Before doing so the patient is placed in the tonsil position, a Boyle Davis gag is inserted, and the palate gently retracted with a soft catheter passed through the unaffected side of the nose and out through the mouth. An assistant holds the catheter while the surgeon pushes back the foreign body, at the same time watching the nasopharynx with a small laryngeal mirror. The foreign body cannot fall into the larynx because of the patient's position and the cuffed tube, and can readily be picked out of the nasopharynx with curved forceps.

Rhinoliths

These present a different problem as they are impacted and often large. It may be necessary to break up the rhinolith within the nasal fossa with forceps, and then remove it piecemeal. This procedure should be carried out under a general anaesthetic. Rarely a rhinolith is so large that it can only be removed through a lateral rhinotomy approach. Occasionally one may even extend into the antrum, in which case a Caldwell–Luc approach is required.

References

Gupta, S. K. and Nema, H. V. (1970). *Journal of Laryngology*, **84**, 454

McNab Jones, R. (1971). *Scott-Brown's Diseases of the Ear, Nose and Throat*, 3rd edn. Volume 3, p. 41. London; Butterworths

8 Epistaxis
O H Shaheen

History

Epistaxis is mentioned in medical literature dating back to very early times. Hippocrates (fifth century B.C.) was probably the first to appreciate that pressure on the alae nasi was an effective method of controlling nose bleeds, although in some cases he resorted to nasal packing and the application of cold fomentations to the shaved head. He regarded the complaint as being primarily of young persons, and was the first to describe vicarious menstruation.

Ali Ibn Rabban Al-Tabiri (A.D. 850) devoted a chapter of his massive work *The Paradise of Wisdome* to epistaxis. In it he wrote 'The complaint of nose bleeding is due to swelling of a vein and its rupture, or perhaps a reduction in the force which confines the blood within'. He implied that some of the medications inserted into the nose owed their efficacy as much to their temperature as to their pharmacological properties.

Morgagni (1769) recognized 'the extremely turgid blood vessels about that part where the alae nasi are formed with the bone, about the finger's breadth more or less from the bottom of the nostril'. He was reported to have stopped nose bleeds by introducing his finger and 'pressing that part whereupon the blood ceased to flow, so that it was not even discharged by the posterior nostril into the fauces'. Morgagni drew his inspiration from his former teacher Valsalva and for this reason Little's area is referred to as 'Locus Valsalvae' in Italian circles. Morgagni's records also contain the suggestion previously entertained by Valsalva that nasal haemorrhage might be arterial in origin for it was his practice to 'syringe the nose with cold water and to apply the spirit of wine, especially to contract the mouths of swollen arteries'.

Mahomed (1880–81) who pioneered the development of the sphygmomanometer stated that 'the frequency with which severe epistaxis occurs in old people with high arterial pressure is striking and for them very fortunate for if their noses did not bleed their brains would'. In 1879 Little published his case reports in the *Hospital Gazette* (Rainey, 1952) in which he identified the site of bleeding as being at the caudal end of the septum, and a year later Kiesselbach made similar observations. However, even after the introduction of modern histological methods, investigations into the mechanism of epistaxis were few and relatively uninformative, so that until recently very little was known about the pathology of nasal blood vessels.

The first attempts at arterial ligation were in 1868 (Bartlett and McKittrick, 1917) when Pilz of Bresslau tied the common carotid artery, and it was much later that external carotid ligations were performed for the control of nose bleeds. Seiffert (1928) introduced ligation of the internal maxillary artery via a transantral approach and Goodyear (1937) was the first to tie the anterior ethmoidal artery.

Vascular anatomy of the nose

Textbook descriptions of the vascular anatomy of the human nose are based on Zuckerkandl's original and comprehensive studies of the subject (1892). Basically, the nose is vascularized by the internal and external carotid arteries via their respective branches, there being a confluence of the two systems at a certain level within the nose, and more especially at the caudal end of the septum where a number of arteries anastamose with each other (Little's area).

With the exception of Little's area the middle turbinate has been regarded by clinicians for a long time as the dividing line between the internal and external carotid distributions, with a corresponding imaginary line of demarcation at the same level on the nasal septum (Weddell *et al.*, 1946). This landmark has served as a guide in deciding which of the two areas is responsible for the epistaxis, and has allegedly helped the surgeon to decide which artery to ligate in severe cases of epistaxis.

The dividing line between the two carotid distributions may not however coincide exactly with the level of the middle turbinate. The work of Zuckerkandl (1892) and Burnham (1935) indicates that the blood supply to the turbinate is derived exclusively from the external carotid artery and that anastomosis between the two carotid distributions occurs above and anterior to its attachment to the lateral nasal wall, and not within it. They also described an artery to the superior turbinate and meatus, with a corresponding vessel on the septum, both of which originate from the nasopalatine branch of the sphenopalatine artery (external carotid).

Shaheen (1967) confirmed the presence of a branch from the nasopalatine artery supplying the superior meatus, turbinate and corresponding septum by x-raying the excised nasal fossae of cadavers which had been previously injected with barium–gelatin mixtures (*Figure 8.1*). It would seem therefore that the area designated as receiving blood from the internal carotid artery is smaller than previously supposed. Certainly the gross disproportion between the diameters of the anterior ethmoidal artery and the sphenopalatine at their points of entry into the nose would corroborate this view. The surgeon who lacerates the anterior ethmoidal artery in an external ethmoidectomy rarely has difficulties with haemorrhage; and similarly those who deliberately ligate this vessel for epistaxis are always impressed by its small size, whereas by contrast the terminal segment of the internal maxillary artery is a much larger vessel (*Figures 8.2a* and *8.2b*). The calibre of the posterior ethmoidal artery is also small so that its contribution to the nasal blood supply is unlikely to be significant even if it varies reciprocally in size with the anterior ethmoidal vessel as suggested by Batson (1935).

It is noteworthy that the anterior ethmoidal artery was found to be absent unilaterally in 14 per cent of cadaver dissections, and bilaterally in 2.5 per cent of cases, the canal being either imperforate or filled with fibrous tissues or nerves (Shaheen, 1967).

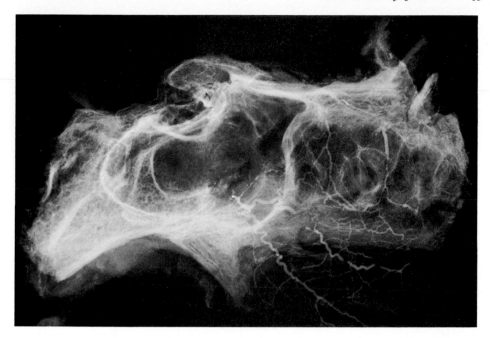

Figure 8.1   The branch from the nasopalatine artery which supplies the superior turbinate and equivalent area of the nasal septum, anastamosing with the arcades formed by the ethmoidal vessels

This supports the contention that these vessels contribute very little to the blood supply of the nose, even if a somewhat larger posterior ethmoidal artery is found doubling for the missing anterior vessel and running a similar course to it, as sometimes happens. In this connection, the surgeon who sets out to ligate the ethmoidal vessels should be aware that when the anterior vessel is missing the posterior ethmoidal artery may arise directly from the circle of Willis and so may not be encountered in the orbit at all. This arrangement conforms much more to the state of affairs in early embryonic life when the posterior ethmoidal artery is the dominant vessel of the nose, dwarfing not only the anterior ethmoidal artery but the nasopalatine vessel as well (Shaheen, 1967) (*Figure 8.3*).

Burnham (1935) in his description of the anatomy of the lateral nasal wall claimed that the arteries to the inferior and middle turbinates and their respective branches lay partly embedded in the bone of these structures. In the case of the inferior turbinate, he found that the bony canals containing the branches of the inferior turbinate artery extended along the central three-fifths of the bone. The middle turbinate artery and its branches were protected by a bony covering in the posterior half of the concha. Thus a considerable segment of both of these arteries and their branches are unlikely to give rise to epistaxis even if rupture occurs. By the time they have emerged from their bony channels to lie beneath the mucous membrane, they will have diminished considerably in size.

Ogura and Senturia (1949) found in a series of patients with epistaxis that the bleeding point arose on the lateral nasal wall in 28 out of 88 cases, and other authors have similarly implicated the lateral wall as a common site for bleeding. Shaheen

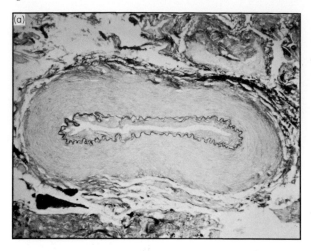

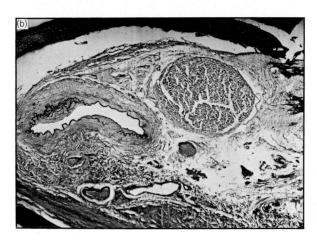

Figure 8.2 (a, b)   The maxillary artery and anterior ethmoidal neurovascular bundle at their points of entry in the nose (magnification ×80 reduced by half in printing)

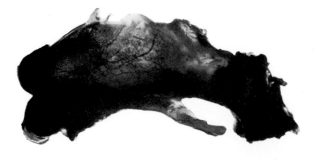

Figure 8.3   The nasal septum of a three months old fetus which had been injected with a silicose elastomer, showing the dominance of the ethmoidal vessels and in particular the posterior ethmoidal artery

(1967) on the other hand was unable to find any cases of bleeding from the lateral wall of the nose in 117 cases, and his anatomical dissections and serial sections of the nose confirmed the findings of Burnham (1935) (*Figure 8.4*).

The vast majority of patients who suffer from arterial epistaxis bleed from the nasal septum, and chiefly from the area where anastomosis of the nasopalatine, greater palatine, anterior ethmoidal, and coronary arteries takes place (*Figure 8.5*). This plexus was originally described by James Little and it is important to note that bleeding from it is arterial in origin and not venous as some reports suggest. The venous bleeding which is common in young persons arises from the vein which lies immediately behind the columella at the anterior edge of Little's area. It runs vertically downwards and crosses the floor of the nose obliquely before joining the venous plexus on the lateral wall of the nose (*Figure 8.6*).

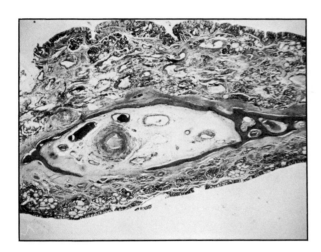

Figure 8.4 The middle turbinate artery in transverse section, encased in its shell of bone (magnification × 25 reduced by a fourth in printing)

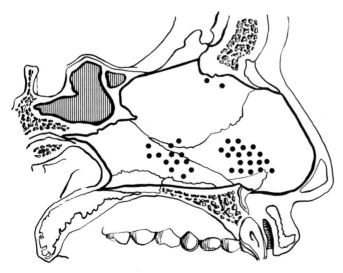

Figure 8.5 Scattergram of bleeding points showing the large number of arterial ruptures which occur in Little's area

The dynamics of the nasal circulation depend to a large extent on the presence of arterio–arterial anastomoses between the various arteries which contribute to the vascular supply of the nose. The branches of the anterior and posterior ethmoidal arteries join in a series of arcades in the upper one third of the nose (*Figure 8.1*) and the branches of the sphenopalatine artery anastomose with those of the ethmoidal arteries above the level of the middle turbinate. Opposing heads of pressure meet in the anastomoses with a sharp interface between the two, which can be displaced by dropping the pressure in one or other of the opposing systems. Shaheen (1967) demonstrated by means of dye injections into the carotid vessels of live humans, that the dispersion of dye in the nasal mucous membrane could be affected by dropping the pressure in the system not being injected. For instance, dye injected into the internal carotid artery failed to appear in the nose, confirming the poor contribution of the ethmoidal vessels, but when the external carotid was occluded at the time of injection the entire upper half of the nose was suffused with dye from above downwards (*Figure 8.7*). The rapidity with which such dye displacement takes place, confirms the importance of the arterio–arterial anastomoses in the nose.

The importance of possible anastomoses across the midline must also not be overlooked, either at the nasopharyngeal end or between the two anterior ethmoidal arteries at the crista galli.

These observations could well explain the many documented reports of failed ligation in which surgeons surmized, probably incorrectly, that they had tied the wrong vessel simply because bleeding had not stopped after ligation.

The arterio–venous anastomoses which are present at the anterior end of the inferior turbinate and septum at a microscopical level are probably of little importance in the aetiology and persistence of epistaxis, but their precise role is as yet far from clear.

Clinical manifestations

The prevalence of epistaxis in random samples of the population was found in one study to be between 10 and 12 per cent (Shaheen, 1967). The age distribution shows an increase in frequency between the ages of 15 and 25 years, and later from 45 to 65 years (*Figure 8.8*) but with little difference between the sexes.

In only a small number of cases can epistaxis be attributed to a well-defined primary cause such as a blood dyscrasia, a blood vessel abnormality, or local nasal pathology. In the majority of cases bleeding arises from an artery or a vein without any obvious abnormality to account for it. Hence the terms spontaneous or idiopathic epistaxis which have been coined to cover this, the commonest category of epistaxis.

Certain contributory factors may be implicated in the onset of bleeding in cases of so-called spontaneous epistaxis such as nose blowing, sneezing, coughing, straining, pregnancy, coryza and sinusitis. They all share one thing in common, namely a sudden rise in vascular pressure.

Venous epistaxis from the retro–columellar vein tends to occur in subjects under the age of 35, whereas arterial epistaxis occurs in the older age groups. The duration of

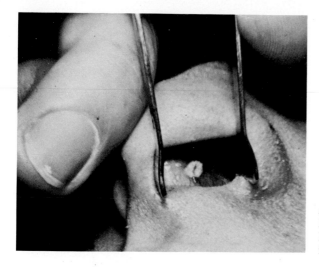

Figure 8.6 The retro–columellar vein at the anterior end of
Little's area which causes bleeding in young persons

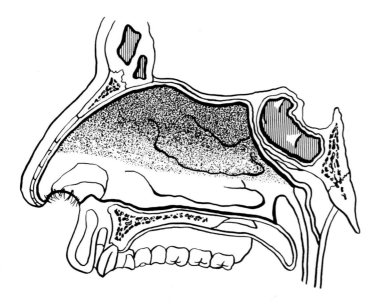

Figure 8.7 Diffusion of dye from above downwards when the internal
carotid artery is injected with dye while the external carotid artery is
occluded

bleeding as might be expected is short-lived in venous epistaxis, and quite prolonged
in bleeding of arterial origin (*Figure 8.9*). Furthermore, there is an inverse relationship
between the frequency and duration of epistaxis, the more severe arterial haemorrhages
recurring rarely more than once or twice (*Figure 8.10*). No correlation can be
established between the prevalence of epistaxis in random samples of the population,
and their blood pressure status (*Figures 8.11a* and *8.11b*), although there is some
correlation between the severity of epistaxis and the degree of vessel wall disease as
judged by retinoscopy (Shaheen, 1967). The finding of a high proportion of subjects

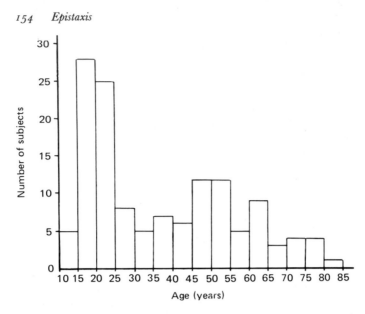

Figure 8.8   Age distribution of subjects of both sexes with a history of epistaxis taken from a population survey

Duration of nose-bleeding in subjects
over and under the age of 35 years

	10 min or under	*Over 10 min and under 2 h*	*Over 2 h*
Subjects over 35 years	10	18	44
Subjects under 35 years	28	13	4

Figure 8.9   The striking difference in duration between venous and arterial epistaxis

with high blood pressures in hospital practice (*Figure 8.12*) signifies not that hypertension causes epistaxis, but rather that patients with higher blood pressures have more severe or persistent bleeding and are therefore eligible for hospitalization.

The pathology of nasal arteries

Examination of the medium and smaller nasal arteries of persons dying in middle and old age has shown that these are subject to a progressive replacement of the muscle tissue in the tunica media by collagen (Shaheen, 1967). This change varies from interstitial fibrosis (*Figure 8.13*) to almost complete replacement of the muscle by scar tissue (*Figure 8.14*). It seems that persons giving a history of epistaxis exhibited the more severe changes, but this is not to say that these changes are necessarily responsible

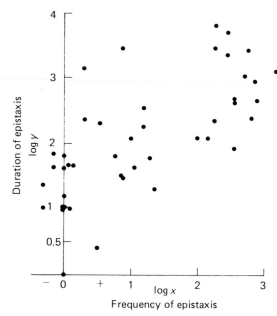

Figure 8.10   The inverse relationship between duration of haemorrhage as expressed by average
duration of episodes and the frequency of haemorrhage as expressed by length of history divided by
number of episodes

for vessel rupture. They could however account for the lengthy duration of arterial
haemorrhages, presumably because of a failure of the vessel to contract down in the
absence of sufficient muscle in the tunica media.

It is also apparent that larger vessels of the calibre of the maxillary artery are prone
to calcification (Mönkeberg's sclerosis). The resulting lack of elasticity could well
contribute to the pathogenesis of small vessel rupture by the creation of a local systolic
hypertension.

The precise mechanism of bleeding is thought to be a dissecting aneurysm of the
nasopalatine artery or one of its branches, but it is not clear what initiates the process
of dissection (*Figure 8.15*).

It is also a mystery as to why bleeding occurs from the retro–columellar vein in
young subjects. Careful inspection of the site shortly after a bleed sometimes reveals a
tiny area of local ballooning overlying the vein, and this could possibly signify an area
of vessel wall weakening, perhaps as a result of localized ischaemic processes.

Clinical management of spontaneous epistaxis

The young person with recurrent bleeding

After taking a careful history to establish that bleeding is not secondary to systemic
disease, the nose is examined for signs of recent bleeding and for local abnormalities.
In the absence of any obvious local disease, attention is turned to the septum which

will often reveal an engorged vein at the anterior end of Little's area just behind the columella. If bleeding has been quite recent, there may be a microaneurysm to be seen in the mucosa overlying the vein. Topical anaesthesia with 5 per cent cocaine followed by cauterization with a silver nitrate stick will suffice to control most cases of epistaxis.

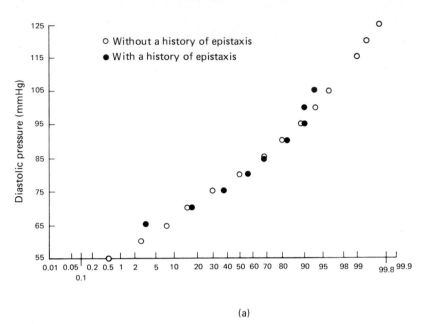

(a)

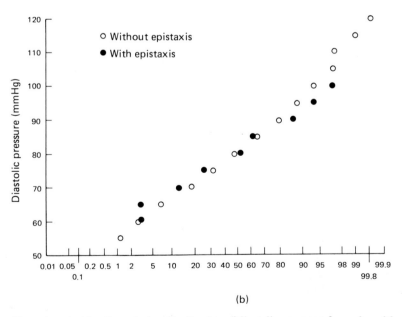

(b)

Figure 8.11 (a, b)   Cumulative distribution of diastolic pressures for males with or without a history of epistaxis taken from two population surveys

Age – sex adjusted diastolic pressures for subjects
of both sexes attending hospital with epistaxis

Diastolic pressures (mmHg)	Number of subjects
65	2
70	0
75	3
80	7
85	7
90	5
95	8
100	10
105	7
110	5
115	6
120	6
125	3
130	1
135	0
140	2

Figure 8.12   The blood pressure distribution of subjects attending hospital with epistaxis. Pressures adjusted to a standard reference age for both sexes

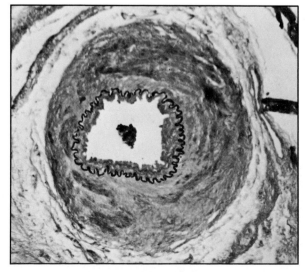

Figure 8.13   Interstitial fibrosis of the tunica media of a nasal artery seen in transverse section (magnification × 110, reduced by one third in printing)

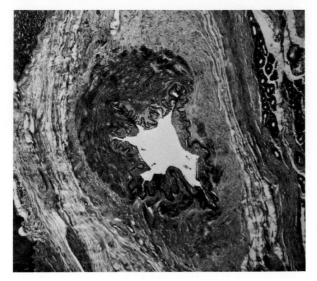

Figure 8.14 Severe segmental loss of muscular tissue with replacement by collagen in the tunica media of a nasal artery seen in transverse section (magnification × 90, reduced by one third in printing)

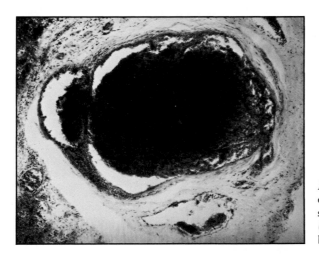

Figure 8.15 Transverse section of the nasopalatine artery to show a dissecting aneurysm (magnification × 120, reduced by one third in printing)

However, some are particularly obstinate and require more than one application of a caustic, in which case it may be more useful to use trichloracetic acid in preference. Great care must be taken to ensure that none of the acid comes into contact with the nasal vestibule as this will leave a particularly painful burn. There are some patients who bleed in spite of seemingly adequate attempts at cauterization, and the best policy is to coagulate the offending vessel with the diathermy under general anaesthesia. Galvanocautery under local anaesthesia is not to be recommended in children, and even adults find the experience unpleasant. The sight of the heated filament, the sensation of heat within the nose, and the smell of charred flesh are off-putting to all but the hardiest individual.

Treatment of a nose bleed in young persons

Pinching the nostrils is the time honoured method of stopping venous bleeding from the caudal end of the septum. Once bleeding has ceased, the nose can be cocainized and cauterized, although the vessel may bleed during the process of applying the caustic. Perseverance is required until bleeding finally stops.

Treatment of recurrent bleeding in older subjects

Epistaxis in older persons does not recur with the same frequency as it does in younger people. Some patients only have the one major bleed, and when examined afterwards there may be very little to see. In such cases there is nothing to be gained by cauterizing Little's area, unless it is certain that bleeding previously originated from this part of the septum.

Assessment of the cardiovascular system is important, however, and the patient should be referred to a physician if any abnormality such as hypertension is discovered. This is not so much to prevent further epistaxis, as to protect the individual from the harmful effects of the raised blood pressure.

Management of a nose bleed in elderly persons

Observations of the patient's pulse, blood pressure, and general condition are made in order to gauge the extent of blood loss. Estimation of the packed-cell volume in conjunction with the haemoglobin will also guide the clinician as to the need for replacing lost blood. At the same time the bleeding and clotting times and platelet count should be investigated to rule out blood dyscrasias.

The nose is examined, preferably with the patient sitting upright in a chair. A plastic cover is draped around his neck and a bowl placed in his hands. Inspection of the nose may show a spurting blood vessel on the nasal septum but usually the site of bleeding is smothered in blood. Cocainizing the nose with a 5 per cent spray serves two purposes, namely to allow the introduction of a catheter so that the blood can be sucked away, and to stop bleeding by vasoconstriction. This gives the examiner the opportunity of locating the site of bleeding, but if this has stopped, suspect areas can be rubbed with orange sticks coated with cotton wool to try and make the vessel bleed again.

The bleeding point is cauterized if accessible, but quite frequently it is situated far back on the septum or behind a spur so that cauterization is technically impossible.

If the bleeding persists, the nose should be packed, preferably with ribbon gauze medicated with a suitable antiseptic such as bismuth–iodine–paraffin. This can be left undisturbed for several days without fear of the patient developing complications. The old fashioned method of controlling epistaxis by sitting the patient up with a cork between his teeth (Trotter's method) and allowing him to bleed until be became hypotensive is to be deprecated. Death from coronary thrombosis secondary to hypotension is a well-recognized complication of epistaxis and regularly appears in the Registrar-General's mortality statistics. It must be emphasized that old patients with poor hearts and circulations do not tolerate severe and prolonged blood loss.

Some clinicians prefer to insert an inflatable balloon in preference to ribbon gauze which is abrasive to the nasal mucosa. However, inflatable balloons will not adapt themselves readily to the irregular contours of the nose, and are therefore less reliable in the control of epistaxis.

After two to three days the packing can be removed, and in most instances bleeding will have stopped completely. In cases of recurrent bleeding, however, the pack will have to be re-inserted. Patients in this category, together with those suffering from prolonged bleeding and unfit persons, should always be hospitalized. They should be nursed sitting up and sedated to allay their anxiety and lower their blood pressure. The choice of sedative is a matter of individual preference, but opiates such as Omnopon are popular, although they may sometimes make the patient vomit, and diazepam by injection is also effective. If bleeding persists in spite of adequate packing, serious consideration must be given to the need for arterial ligation. There is some evidence to suggest that submucous resection of the septum may be helpful when bleeding originates from behind a prominent septal spur.

Arterial ligation

The patient who continues to bleed every time the pack is removed or who keeps on bleeding with the pack *in situ* will generally have to be transfused. If over a period of four to five days bleeding has not stopped, arterial ligation should be performed. In the absence of definite knowledge about the whereabouts of the bleeding point, it is reasonable to interrupt the external carotid system since this supplies as much as 90 per cent of the nasal mucosa. Bleeding from the ethmoidal region is in fact very uncommon and is rarely of a severity to merit arterial ligation, in spite of the occasional report describing severe ethmoidal bleeding.

Although interruption of the internal maxillary artery has become fashionable, it is by no means certain that this is necessarily more effective than ligation of the external carotid artery. Being nearer to the source of bleeding, the drop in blood pressure in that part of the nose supplied by the maxillary artery is greater than after tying the external carotid. In that sense dividing the maxillary artery should in theory be more effective, but as was mentioned previously, the drop in pressure almost certainly encourages the displacement of blood from other areas of the nose through arterial anastomoses, with the possibility of bleeding persisting. By contrast ligation of the external carotid artery does not produce quite the same blood pressure reduction distally and is therefore less effective in controlling bleeding, although blood flow from the ethmoidal to the nasopalatine areas may in fact be less. If bleeding persists after ligation of the maxillary artery it is logical to proceed to interruption of the anterior ethmoidal artery with the prospect of arresting the bleeding permanently. The addition of ethmoidal artery ligation to external carotid ligation for persistent haemorrhage is less likely to be as effective, since the cause of the persistent bleeding in this case is probably inadequate drop of pressure in the distal external carotid rather than displacement of blood from one area of the nose to another. In cases of hypertension, it would be reasonable to ligate the maxillary and anterior ethmoidal arteries empirically at the same sitting.

Ligation of the internal maxillary artery

This operation is usually performed under general anaesthesia. A sublabial incision is made and as large an opening as possible is made in the anterior antral wall without compromising the infra-orbital nerve. The thin posterior bony wall of the antrum is shattered gently with a gouge and removed piecemeal with punch forceps to reveal the underlying periosteum on the posterior wall of the maxilla. This is incised horizontally from side to side and the fat of the pterygo–palatine fossa teased out with long straight artery forceps until the tortuous maxillary artery is seen. The artery is divided between clips as close to the sphenopalatine foramen as possible and clips are placed on any large adjacent branches. The creation of an antrostomy is optional.

Ligation of the anterior ethmoidal artery

This is performed through an external ethmoidectomy type of incision. After ligating branches of the angular vein, the incision is deepened down to the periosteum which is then incised in the line of the incision. The periosteum is elevated posteriorly, first off the lacrimal fossa, then the lamina papyracea of the ethmoid. The medial orbital periosteum is retracted laterally together with the lacrimal sac and held out of the way by a self retaining retractor (Talbot). The artery is identified as a funnelling of orbital periosteum into the ethmoid labyrinth at the junction of the medial and superior walls of the orbit about half-way back from the orbital margin. It is coagulated and divided, and the incision closed without drainage.

Unusual causes of epistaxis

Osler's disease (*see Plate 3a, facing p. 16*)

This is a familial hereditary complaint in which sufferers develop prominent telangiectatic formations recognized as red spots on the lips and the mucous membrane of the mouth, especially the tongue, as well as telangiectases on the face and in the nose. The defects in the nose are liable to cause severe nose bleeds, and bleeding is rarely from one site alone. The condition may be complicated by the presence of lesions in the gut which may bleed, or arteriovenous malformations in the lungs.

Harrison (1957) has shown that high doses of oestrogen will lessen the frequency and severity of nose bleeding, probably by inducing a squamous metaplasia of the nasal mucous membrane. However this form of treatment is inappropriate in male patients, and could well be dangerous if prescribed over a long period of time.

Saunders (1963) advocated excising the mucous membrane of the anterior part of the septum and lateral nasal wall and its replacement by a split skin graft which is laid on the perichondrium and sewn into position. This treatment is effective temporarily but bleeding usually recurs months or years later. Radiotherapy is also successful for a time in controlling the nose bleeds. The bleeding from this condition is frequently severe and often requires multiple transfusions of blood. The disease is sometimes complicated at a later stage by the development of hypertension with its sequelae.

Bleeding diatheses

Epistaxis may be a manifestation of a clotting defect, increased fragility of capillaries, or a deficiency in platelets. A history of prolonged bleeding after trauma or dental extraction is suggestive, or alternatively bruising or bleeding into joints. When suspected the patient should be stripped and a search made for signs of purpura, bruising and swollen joints. A Hess's test and platelet count are carried out, and the bleeding and clotting times are measured. If required, specific tests for deficiences of the factors responsible for coagulation can be performed to rule out such diseases as Christmas disease and haemophilia. In elderly subjects Waldenström's macroglobulin-aemia should be excluded.

The treatment depends to a large extent on the individual cause of the blood dyscrasia but in the short term blood transfusion may be necessary.

Nasopharyngeal angiofibroma

This arises in male adolescents and is thought by some to be a vascular malformation. It is characterized not infrequently by severe haemorrhages resulting in anaemia, local sepsis, and debility. The diagnosis is confirmed by arteriography and the correct treatment is surgical removal.

References

Bartlett, W. and McKittrick, O. F. (1917). *Annals of Surgery*, **65**, 715

Batson, O. V. (1935). *Annals of Otology, Rhinology and Laryngology*, **44**, 939

Burnham, H. H. (1935). *Journal of Laryngology*, **50**, 569

Goodyear, H. M. (1937). *Laryngoscope*, **47**, 97

Harrison, D. F. N. (1957). *Journal of Laryngology*, **71**, 577

Hippocrates. Translation by Jones, W. H. S. (1923–31). *Aphorisms* V33, **4**, 167. Airs, Waters, and Places IV, **1**, 79. (Wellcome Historical Museum)

Ibn Rabban Al-Tabiri, A. (A.D. 850). *Paradise of Wisdome*. Book 4, Maquala 3, Chapter 9

Mahomed, F. A. (1880–81). *Guy's Hospital Reports*, **25**, 295

Morgagni, J. B. (1769). *The seats and causes of diseases investigated by anatomy* (1761). Translated by Alexander, B. Letter XIV. Articles 24, 23, 25 (Book 1, p. 336–340). (Wellcome Historical Museum)

Ogura, J. H. and Senturia, B. H. (1949). *Laryngoscope*, **59**, 743

Rainey, J. J. (1952). *Archives of Otolaryngology*, **55**, 451

Saunders, W. H. (1963). *Journal of Laryngology*, **77**, 69

Seiffert, A. (1928). *Zeitschrift für Hals—Nasen—, und Ohrenheilkunde*, **22**, 323

Shaheen, O. H. (1967). Thesis for the Master of Surgery in the University of London.

Weddell, G., Macbeth, R. G., Sharp, H. S. and Calvert, C. A. (1946). *British Journal of Surgery*, **33**, 387

Zuckerkandl, E. (1892). *Normale and Pathologische Anatomie der Nasenhöhle*. (W. Braumuller)

9 Acute and chronic inflammations of the nasal cavities
Neil Weir

ACUTE INFECTIVE RHINITIS

The term acute infective rhinitis is taken to mean an acute viral or bacterial infection of the nasal mucous membrane. It is exceedingly common and is a manifestation of the common cold, influenzal infections of the upper respiratory tract, the exanthems and certain specific infections. It can also occur as a secondary response to local irritants and trauma.

The common cold (coryza)

Incidence

The common cold is probably the commonest viral infection in man. The incidence is variable but it is estimated that the average young adult has two to three colds a year (Smiley, 1924) although some give a figure as high as seven (Hope Simpson, 1958). Colds occur most frequently in children and least in patients over 55 years of age (US Public Health Service, 1927). Children of early school age are the most susceptible to colds while immunity to droplet infection is gradually being acquired. In the adult severe colds can lead to much absenteeism and consequent economic loss.

Predisposing factors

Climate The frequency of colds is surprisingly constant in all parts of the globe, with the exception of the extreme north and south (Paul and Freese, 1933). In the USA a statistical study by questionnaire showed that epidemics of colds were synchronous in all localities, and that the frequency rose to three peaks, the first late in October, the second early in January and the third in March.

Environment, temperature, chills and humidity That the ideal environment for maximum resistance may be found in life under perfect conditions of humidity, temperature and ventilation is suggested by Kerr and Lagen (1933–34), who exposed, under these conditions, groups of susceptible men in the same room with subjects in the early stages of a cold, and in some they even inoculated cold filtrates into the conjunctival sac without obtaining a single transfer.

There is widespread belief that chilling may precipitate a cold in an individual; however, attempts to demonstrate such an effect experimentally have given negative results (Andrewes, 1950).

Chill may act in two ways: (1) by lowering general resistance to infection; and (2) by causing reflex vasoconstriction of the nasal mucous membrane.

The normal temperature of the mucous membrane of the nose has been shown to vary between 33 and 34°C. Chilling of the body surface may reduce the temperature of the nasal mucosa by as much as 6 °C (Mudd, Goldman and Grant, 1921).

The optimal relative humidity of the atmosphere is 45 per cent. A lowering of relative humidity to 15 per cent, as may easily occur when the relatively dry cold outside air in winter is heated indoors by radiators, withdraws more water than the nasal mucosa can supply, and causes drying of the mucous blanket.

Excessive humidity is also harmful, as it reduces the evaporation of sweat from the skin and, owing to the high conductivity of water vapour, a slight lowering of temperature produces severe chilling, with the effects described above.

Hope Simpson (1958) demonstrated a striking correlation between increase in the frequency of colds in a group of families and falls in the temperature of the soil. Humidity also affects the survival of viruses (Tyrrell and Bynde, 1961). Common cold viruses prefer high humidity. Influenza viruses survive better in dry air.

Fatigue, fitness and exercise   Locke (1937) assessed the fitness of subjects by their oxygen consumption under standard exercise, and found that 64 per cent of those with fitness above 0.6 had only one cold a year, while 80 per cent of those below 0.5 had four colds a year. However, colds very often hit the man who is feeling very fit on his return from holiday (Andrewes and Tyrell, 1965).

Nutrition   The lowering of resistance by hunger and under-nutrition has been shown by Cruickshank (1942), who found that the death rate in measles, pertussis, influenza and bronchopneumonia amongst poor children was five times greater than amongst the better-off.

Dietetic   Certain hypersensitive individuals suffer from nasal turgescence, stuffiness and excessive secretion, with lowered resistance to colds when they take wheat, citrus fruits and sucrose in their diet (Jarvis, 1938).

Vitamin deficiency   Deficiencies of vitamins A and C from their importance in tissue oxygenation, and vitamin D from its effect on calcium metabolism and the permeability of the vascular endothelium, all play a part in maintaining local resistance to infection (Ruskin, 1938; Macbeth, 1943). Deficiencies of these vitamins increase susceptibility to infection. Claims that vitamins, particularly vitamin C, are effective in preventing colds are not supported by controlled trials (Andrewes and Tyrell, 1965).

Nasal obstruction   Deviation of the nasal septum, hypertrophy of the turbinates, enlarged adenoids, polypi, scars and adhesions all interfere with ventilation and the free passage of air through the nasal chambers, and with the secretion and movement of the mucous blanket, and thus predispose to infection.

Foci of chronic infection   Foci of infection in the sinuses, nasopharynx or pharynx, by decreasing tissue resistance, favour infection. In children chronic adenoiditis, tonsillitis and sinusitis; in adults chronic sinusitis and tonsillitis are the most important.

The pH of nasal secretion   A drift to the acid side is associated with few bacteria, while an alkaline drift is associated with many bacteria in the nasal secretion.

     Rhinoviruses (common cold) are destroyed by an acid pH (Ketler, Hamparian and Hilleman, 1962).

General diseases   Any general disease, but particularly renal, hepatic and blood disorders, diabetes mellitus and tuberculosis may lower general resistance to colds.

Endocrine factors   In hypothyroid cases there is pallor, with boggy swelling of the turbinates, associated with undue susceptibility to colds (Harkness, 1937). Hyper-thyroidism causes vasomotor instability, and chills after sweating, which predispose to colds. It also induces hypertrophy of the lymphoid tissue in the nasopharynx, which provides a nidus for the lodgment of organisms.

Causative agents

Viruses

In general it may be said that in communities the causative agent of the common cold is ubiquitous, but that infection occurs only when an individual's resistance is lowered, or when he is subjected to an overwhelming concentration and virulence of the causative agent. It is generally accepted that the common cold is due to infection with filtrable viruses, followed by secondary infection with bacteria.

     In spite of the rapid advances in virology and the isolation, identification and even culture of many viruses, it is still uncertain what proportion of respiratory illnesses is caused by them.

     Andrewes (1947) reported successful transmission of colds by filtered nasal washings in 50 per cent of experiments on humans, and an active virus has been stored for a year at $-76\,°C$.

     There are five groups of pathogenic respiratory viruses (Stuart-Harris, 1963):

(1) The influenza viruses discussed below.
(2) The picorna viruses subdivided into four groups: (a) Coxsackie virus; (b) Reo virus; (c) ECHO virus; (d) rhinovirus (common cold).
(3) Respiratory syncytial viruses (RS)—these produce typical colds but in small children can cause more severe illness of the lower respiratory tract.
(4) Para-influenzal viruses—also are mainly pathogenic in children.
(5) Adenoviruses. These can be isolated from tonsils and adenoids removed surgically in 50–90 per cent (Zaiman, Balducci and Tyrrell, 1955; Israel, 1962), and in which they cause chronic infection. They also cause acute respiratory infection, chiefly involving the pharynx.

The para-influenzal, RS and rhinoviruses are present in the community at all times. Probably subclinical infections are common.

In the nose the rhinoviruses are by far the most common and most important invaders and are rarely found in the absence of infection. They are unusual in that they prefer to multiply at 33 °C, and will not attack or damage cells at 37 °C. Some will grow only on human kidney cells and are identified as 'H' strains; others will grow on monkey kidney and are identified as 'M' strains (Andrewes *et al.*, 1961). It is thought that seven or more serotypes of 'M' strains and 50 or more serotypes of 'H' strains exist.

Mode of transmission

Droplet and dust   In talking, sneezing and coughing innumerable infected droplets are sprayed out which fall to the ground at distances of 0.9–1.8 m. Bedmaking, house dust and the manipulation of handkerchiefs also contribute large numbers of airborne particles (Dumbell, Lovelock and Lowbury, 1948).

Droplet nuclei   Droplet nuclei are small droplets which evaporate as they fall, and shrink to less than 0.1 mm in diameter. In this form they remain suspended in the air as mist, and drift on the air currents for as long as two days, and thus have a much wider range than that of droplets (Wells and Wells, 1936). These will transport viruses, but are too small to carry the larger bacteria.

Contact   The causative organism may be transmitted by kissing, food, fingers and fomites.

Incubation period

This varies from 1–3 days. In inoculation experiments it has been 24 h or less (Dochez, Mills and Kneeland, 1936; Dochez, Shibley and Mills, 1930).

Duration of infectivity

Colds have been transmitted the day before symptoms developed (Long, Bliss and Carpenter, 1932) but the maximum infectivity occurs during the first few days and diminishes rapidly after the symptoms abate.

Local defences and mode of infection

Nose
The local defences of the nose consist of:

(1) The vibrissae in the nasal vestibule.
(2) The mucous blanket, with its lysozyme content.
(3) The resistance of the epithelial cells.

(4) Interferon.
(5) pH of the secretions.

Nasopharynx
The mucosa of the nasopharynx differs from that of the nose in the presence of lymphoid tissue, which is of the first importance in protecting the body against organisms. It is here that organisms are held while immunity is built up, and in this the lymphoid cells play an important part.

The vibrissae entangle and filter out the majority of particles from the ingoing air. The remaining particles, droplets and droplet nuclei become entangled by the mucous blanket, and are rapidly swept away through the nose and nasopharynx to the pharynx to be swallowed. Particles the size of bacteria are not soluble in mucus and the rate of flow of the blanket is such that they are carried away before they have time to penetrate to the underlying epithelial cells. Bodies as small as viruses, however, are soluble in the mucus, and can penetrate the blanket with great facility. Any factor which retards or breaks the continuity of the blanket will allow the infective agent to penetrate to the epithelium.

Cilia are extremely susceptible to drying. Subjection to dry conditions for a few minutes destroys them, and they cannot subsequently be revived. Paralysis of the cilia arrests the streaming of the mucous blanket, and through the supernatant dried mucus at this spot organisms can penetrate and infect the underlying epithelium.

If chilling accompanies or follows the drying, the resistance of the nasal epithelium itself is depressed by the reflex vasoconstriction and fall of temperature.

The mucous blanket also contains lysozyme of such activity that, when diluted one part in a thousand, it will still dissolve 75 per cent of bacteria within an hour (Fleming, 1929). During the early stages of a cold the lysozyme content is reduced. The initial invasion occurs most commonly in the nasopharyngeal mucous membrane, but may take place on one side of the nose, or in the pharynx or larynx.

Immunity

Specific neutralizing antibodies are found in the blood and are of major importance in resistance. They are usually specific and do not confer immunity to other strains. They can be increased by vaccination. Their site of formation is probably in lymphoid tissue.

Interferon (protein) is the natural defence of the cell to foreign nucleic acid (Issacs, Cox and Rotem, 1963). It has probably wide virus-inhibiting properties but it is inactivated by oxygen. Tests in man have not shown protection from respiratory virus infection.

In humans a high immunity usually lasts for a month after attack, and thereafter falls rapidly. Antibodies to the 'M' strains of rhinoviruses seem to persist in the serum for longer periods.

Pathology

In the earliest stage of invasion there is transient vasoconstriction. This is followed by vasodilatation, oedema and increased activity of the seromucinous glands and goblet cells (*Figure 9.1*).

Leucocytic infiltration of the tissues follows, with swelling and desquamation of the epithelial cells. The secretion is at first clear, watery and sterile, with a few epithelial and pus cells, but later it becomes coloured and viscid, stiffens on a handkerchief and contains many pus cells and bacteria. The toxins produced in the mucous membrane

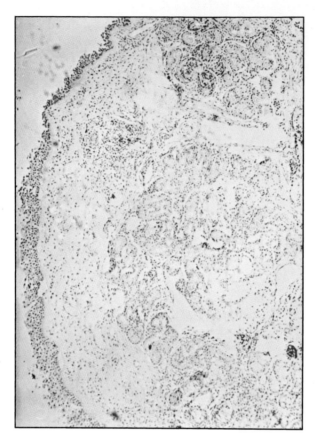

Figure 9.1 The nasal mucous membrane in acute rhinitis showing general oedema and hyperaemia with swelling of the seromucinous glands, desquamation of the epithelium, and cellular infiltration (× 100)

are swiftly taken up by the lymphatics, and passing through the cervical lymph glands and ducts reach the blood stream.

Resolution takes place by a reversal of these processes, and by proliferation of the remaining tissue cells to replace those that have been destroyed.

The lysozyme content is reduced in the early stages (Hilding, 1934). The average pH of the nasal mucus lies between 5.5 and 6.5 (Fabricant, 1941). During an acute rhinitis the reaction becomes alkaline, and during resolution it returns to neutral (Tweedie, 1934).

Bacteriology

Cultures from the normal mucous membrane of the posterior areas of the nose are usually sterile, provided that they are not contaminated from the vestibule and anterior areas. Cultures from the anterior nares show staphylococci in 43 per cent of normal individuals.

In the first three days of a common cold the cultures from the posterior areas may be sterile, but after the third day pure or mixed cultures of streptococci, pneumococci, *Haemophilus influenzae*, or staphylococci are often shown (Tweedie, 1934).

Clinical picture

The course of a cold may be described in four stages.

Prodromal or ischaemic stage   This lasts for a few hours, and represents the stage of local invasion and general nasal ischaemia. The familiar hot, dry or tickling spot is felt at the site of the invasion, while the general nasal airway seems unusually patent.

Early reaction and irritation   The infection which is at first localized spreads to the adjacent mucous membranes through the lymphatics, and also over the surface. This process may take a few hours or days. The site of invasion is often the first to recover, while the disease is still active in those areas which have been affected later. The throat is dry and sore on swallowing, and there is sneezing, watery nasal discharge and obstruction. The mucous membrane is red and swollen. General symptoms of mild toxaemia and fever now appear.

Stage of venous stasis and secondary infection   After the second day the colour of the mucosa becomes dusky, with a bluish tinge, the discharge thickens, diminishes and becomes mucopurulent. The obstruction and toxaemia are at their maximum.

Resolution   The symptoms and signs gradually diminish, and after 5–10 days recovery takes place.

Complications

Nasopharyngitis and pharyngitis   The nasopharynx and pharynx are invariably infected to some extent in every cold.

Sinusitis   Sinusitis is one of the most common complications, but the sinuses are not invaded during the course of an uncomplicated cold.

Pharyngotympanic salpingitis, otitis media and mastoiditis   The infection ascends from the nasopharynx, invading the pharyngotympanic tube, middle ear and mastoid cells in sequence. It may be arrested at any point of the ascent.

Lymphadenitis   This is usually transient, and affects the retropharyngeal and deep cervical group.

Tonsillitis   A mild inflammation usually accompanies a cold, but parenchymatous or follicular tonsillitis is considered as a complication.

Lower respiratory complications   Laryngotracheitis, bronchitis, pneumonia and asthma constitute the group of lower respiratory complications.

Gastroenteritis   Swallowed secretion may cause acute gastroenteritis, with anorexia, vomiting and diarrhoea (McGibbon and Hall, 1947) but this complication is rare except in infants.

Other complications   Nephritis and rheumatism are allergic and toxaemic manifestations.

Diagnosis

Allergic, vasomotor or hypersensitive rhinitis should be excluded.

In vasomotor or allergic rhinitis there may be a history of sensitivity to chilling, bright light, or changes of temperature, or an individual or family history of allergy. The allergen may be identifiable from the history, or by specific tests. The attack is of sudden explosive onset, and often lasts for only a few minutes or hours, with frequent relapses. The paroxysms of sneezing and nasal discharge are excessive; the discharge is clear, with relatively little mucin, and does not stiffen on a handkerchief. The general symptoms of infection are absent.

Microscopical examination of the discharge shows that the cells are scanty, and eosinophils may be seen among them. It is important to remember that the two conditions may be combined, and that there may be allergy to the infecting organisms (bacterial allergy). More commonly the infection is secondary to the allergic obstruction.

The causative agent of the acute rhinitis must be identified from the history and bacteriological examination. The local and general signs and symptoms do not differ greatly with different organisms except in the specific forms.

Prevention

Simple measures   Dusty rooms, crowded rooms and public vehicles should be avoided. Patients with colds should use paper handkershiefs, and burn them at once to prevent the massive distribution of infected particles (Dumbell, Lovelock and Lowbury, 1948). Gargling with antiseptic solutions after exposure to infection is of doubtful value and the use of local nasal applications is harmful owing to interference with ciliary activity.

Strict measures   Included in the strict measures are the following: (1) isolation; (2) masking in room and kitchen, with special cleanliness of clothes and hands; (3) exclusion of any attendant suffering from a cold; and (4) sterilization of fomites.

Prophylaxis

A multitude of different measures have been used, but statistically only continued courses of ultraviolet light (Sherman, 1938) have given a significant reduction in the incidence.

The methods may be classified into the following three groups.

Maintaining a high level of resistance

A full balanced diet is necessary, with adequate vitamin and mineral supplements. The severity of colds is slightly reduced after administration of vitamins A and D throughout the winter (Sherman, 1938).

Vitamin C is only of proven value in cases of severe deficiency, with lowered general resistance (Harkness, 1937; Macbeth, 1943). It may be administered also as calcium ascorbate (Ruskin, 1938).

Avoidance of fatigue, of sudden changes of temperature, and of contaminated, dusty or too dry or humid atmospheres, and the maintenance of physical fitness are also factors in the maintenance of resistance.

Treatment of local predisposing conditions

The normal airway should be restored and local infective lesions treated. In a controlled trial of immediate adenotonsillectomy versus a two-year postponement of the operation, Mawson and his colleagues (1967) found a noticeable reduction in the frequency of colds in the operated group, especially during the first post-operative year. However, children transferred from the control group to the operated group, because of severity of symptoms, were found to be more susceptible to head colds and cough in the post-operative period than other children (Mawson, Adlington and Evans, 1968).

Artificial production of immunity

Vaccines   These may be administered by the following routes: (1) parenteral; (2) oral (Thomson, Thomson and Morrison, 1948); (3) nasal (Walsh and Cannon, 1938).

The majority of controlled investigations of vaccines have failed to show any reduction of the incidence of colds, but a number report some reduction in the severity, duration and complications (Council on Pharmacy and Chemistry, and Council on Industrial Health, 1944).

Ritchie (1958), working with autogenous vaccines, found that colds passed from the prodromal to the fully-developed stage in 62 per cent of controls compared with 13 per cent in the vaccinated group. The difficulty in producing vaccines lies in the multiplicity of serologic types of rhinoviruses. By reducing the severity of secondary bacterial invasion they are, nevertheless, particularly useful in the allergic subject who is specially susceptible to colds.

Treatment

There is no known specific treatment for the common cold, but general and local supportive and palliative treatment can mitigate the severity and complications. There are so many different varieties of colds, so many different individual reactions to them, and so many different individual responses to treatment, that no hard and fast therapeutic rules can be laid down.

General treatment is directed to providing the best conditions for rest, both general and local, and at the same time supplying heat and the maximum blood flow to the infected tissues. Unfortunately the majority of patients are not willing to submit to full-scale treatment for a cold of moderate severity, and modifications must be made, according to the circumstances.

Complete rest, both general and for the upper respiratory tract, necessitates confinement to bed in an even temperature of 65–70 °C, with a humidity of 45 per cent.

Heat, both local and general, is provided at first by a hot bath. Inhalations of Menthol or Tincture of Benzoin (BP), (one teaspoonful in a pint of steaming water), may be soothing and will apply heat directly to the mucous membrane of the nose.

Analgesics and antipyretics, such as acetylsalicylic acid, may be valuable for the general malaise, aching and feverishness of the cold. Codeine compounds are more effective as sedatives. Both should be combined with a copious fluid intake.

Antihistamines have not been shown to fully reduce or abolish the symptoms of colds but they can be particularly effective in the allergic patient who is often unduly susceptible to colds. Antihistamines can be usefully combined with an analgesic.

Alcohol is a sedative which is the chief justification for the faith placed in whisky as a treatment in the early stages of a cold. It is also a vasodilator and counteracts the discomfort of the peripheral vasoconstriction at that stage.

Local vasoconstrictors should be used sparingly as the excessive use of any vasoconstrictor agent should be avoided on the grounds of interference with ciliary activity, mucosal blood flow and local tissue resistance. Temporary relief from Benzedrine or 0.25–0.5 per cent ephedrine in isotonic saline may be used occasionally, particularly if it enables a child to sleep or a baby to suckle.

Antibiotics do not appear to influence the course of a cold and therefore should only be used, and then in full doses, if complications develop such as middle-ear infection, sinusitis, tonsillitis, bronchitis or pneumonia.

Influenzal rhinitis

Influenzal rhinitis occurs in association with an infection by one of the influenza viruses. There are three main groups of virus unrelated antigenically (A, B and C).

Influenza A virus which has undergone several mutations since its discovery in 1933 has been responsible for pandemics of the disease. The original A virus has since been replaced by different strains, A^1 (1946) and later A^2 (1957). It is indeed unfortunate that the virus is subject to antigenic change for there is little or no cross-immunity and an entire population may find itself susceptible to the 'new' virus. Influenza B and C viruses are less liable to antigenic variation. The virology of these infections and its particular interest to the otolaryngologist have been described in some detail by Dudgeon (1969) and also by Anderson (1969).

The characteristic lesion is a varying degree of necrosis of the ciliated epithelium of the upper respiratory tract (nose and in some cases, trachea). For a time there may even be replacement by transitional epithelium, and secondary bacterial invasion is inevitable.

In some cases of influenza the rhinitic manifestations are not marked or are overshadowed by tracheal, gastrointestinal, pulmonary or general symptoms. But in others severe coryza is simulated and in some of the pandemics many cases have been complicated by epistaxis.

Preventive treatment by the injection of immunizing vaccines is generally applied to those persons leading institutional lives, where the risk of infection is greater, or to the elderly or infirm, particularly those with chronic pulmonary or heart disease, renal disorders or diabetes, where any complication is likely to be more serious. A recent estimate of the mortality among the elderly in England and Wales, based on calculations of excess mortality suggests that in each winter between 1967 and 1973 an average of about 11 000 elderly people died directly or indirectly from the effects of influenza (Clifford *et al.*, 1977). Nevertheless, the vaccines are not a panacea, for not only do they have a tendency to toxicity but the immunity which they confer is transient.

Two types of vaccine are currently being produced. The conventional 'killed' vaccine is prepared to cover the anticipated mutations. [In 1977/78 these were A/Victoria/3/75 and B/HongKong/8/73 (Influvac).] Surface antigen vaccines are an alternative and are less inclined to produce side effects such as fever and sore arms. They are prepared by extracting the essential immunizing components of killed vaccines, purifying them and rendering them sufficiently antigenic by incorporating an adjuvant such as aluminium hydroxide (Fluvirin). This process reduces the viral protein content to one-tenth of that of the conventional vaccines.

Recently specific chemotherapeutic agents have been developed for the prophylaxis and treatment of influenza. Amantidine (Symmetrel) is thought to impair the uncoating of a virus once it has entered the host and may also impair viral penetration of the host cell wall. It is notably effective against influenza A.

Treatment of the established case is along general lines and consists of rest, analgesics and in severe cases prophylactic antibiotics. Local nasal treatment is not advocated.

Rhinitis of the exanthems

In measles, scarlet fever, pertussis and the enteric group, typhus, smallpox and chicken-pox, an acute rhinitis occurs in the prodromal and early stages. The local condition does not differ from that described in the common cold.

Differential diagnosis depends on the associated specific signs and symptoms. Secondary bacterial rhinitis is common, and often very severe and of suppurative type, and complications are more frequent than after the common cold.

Specific rhinitis

Acute nasal diphtheria

Definition
An acute infective rhinitis due to the *Corynebacterium diphtheriae*.

Clinical picture

Nasal diphtheria may be primary or secondary to the faucial form. In the latter case it indicates a severe attack. There is often a transient simple rhinitis in the early stage of faucial diphtheria, but no membrane forms and it passes off in a few days.

The acute form differs from the chronic form described under fibrinous rhinitis on p. 190 in the short duration, pyrexia and general toxaemia, adenitis and subsequent paralysis. In this country immunization has practically eliminated diphtheria but the occasional case might arise from immigrants who have not been immunized.

Treatment

C. diphtheriae is sensitive to penicillin, and a course of four or five days' intramuscular and local penicillin should be given in addition to the full doses of the antitoxin intravenously. Antitoxin neutralizes the toxins, while penicillin shortens the disease but does not neutralize the toxins.

There is a tendency for the *C. diphtheriae* to persist in the nose for weeks after such an attack. Isolation should be continued until the cultures from three successive daily swabs have been negative.

Acute syphilis

The condition of acute syphilis is dealt with under the heading of 'Nasal Syphilis', p. 181.

Erysipelas

In erysipelas of the external nose the nasal mucous membrane may become secondarily infected by the streptococcus from the skin. The infection responds rapidly to penicillin.

Glanders

Acute glanders differs from the chronic form described on p. 198 only in the rapidity of onset and the severity of both local and general manifestations. There is marked fever and prostration, and a pustular rash develops resembling smallpox. The nasal mucosa is greatly swollen, and later ulcers form and may destroy the septum and turbinates. The lymph glands are swollen and inflamed, and may suppurate. Death usually follows within a few weeks.

Diagnosis

Glanders is most likely to be confused with smallpox, typhus fever, erysipelas, impetigo or syphilis.

Anthrax

Primary anthrax of the nose with malignant pustule formation has been described.

Candidiasis (Moniliasis)

This subject is dealt with on p. 203.

Gonorrhoea

Rhinitis due to infection with *Neisseria gonorrhoeae* is certainly rare. Unlike the conjunctivae the nasal mucous membrane has a high resistance to this infection. One or two doubtful cases of purulent rhinitis in infants have been said to be due to gonorrhoea, but their authenticity has been doubted. The infection responds to penicillin or to co-trimoxazole (Septrin).

Common pathogens

A primary rhinitis due to the common pathogenic bacteria is indistinguishable clinically from that of a common cold, with secondary infection by these organisms.

Local irritants and trauma

In this group there is a simple catarrhal reaction in the nasal mucous membrane with particularly severe irritation amounting in some cases to actual neuralgic pain in the nose and face. Sneezing and copious watery discharge are important features. The reaction follows immediately on the exposure and persists while that lasts. In most cases it passes off rapidly afterwards, unless the causative agent has produced some destruction of the epithelium, in which case regeneration and healing may take some days before it is complete. The period of recovery depends on the severity and degree of subsequent secondary infection.

Foreign bodies

This subject is dealt with in Chapter 7.

CHRONIC INFECTIVE RHINITIS

There are many forms of chronic rhinitis and not a little confusion has arisen from the fact that the term has been taken by different authorities to include different conditions. In the present section the accent has been laid on 'infection', and the conditions referred to are either the result of, or associated with the latter.

Hypertrophic rhinitis

Hypertrophic rhinitis occasionally arises as a result of chronic infection in the nose or paranasal sinuses. Several decades ago infection was considered to be the most likely aetiological factor in chronic hypertrophic rhinitis, but, nowadays, though the condition is still common, infection is a relatively infrequent cause.

For this reason hypertrophic rhinitis is dealt with in detail in Chapter 10. However, if the turbinates are grossly enlarged by redundant masses of fibrous mucous membrane, and chronic sinus infection is present as well, both conditions—the mucosal hypertrophy and the sinus infection—require treatment.

Atrophic rhinitis

Atrophic rhinitis is a chronic nasal disease characterized by progressive atrophy of the mucosa and underlying bone of the turbinates and the presence of a viscid secretion which rapidly dries and forms crusts which emit a characteristic foul odour sometimes called ozaena (a stench). There is an abnormal patency of the nasal passages.

Aetiology

The aetiology of atrophic rhinitis is still unknown. In the past numerous organisms have been cited as the cause, among which are (1) *Coccobacillus* (Loewenberg, 1894); (2) *Bacillus mucosus* (Abel, 1895); (3) *Coccobacillus foetidus ozaena*;(4) diphtheroid bacilli, and (5) *Klebsiella ozaenae* (Henriksen and Gundersen, 1959). It is true that these organisms may be found in cultures but there is little evidence that they cause the disease.

Other factors which have been regarded as possible causes are chronic sinusitis, excessive surgical destruction of the nasal mucous membrane and syphilis.

Atrophic rhinitis usually commences at puberty and is much more common in females than males; thus it is generally accepted that endocrine imbalance may play a part. Heredity is an important factor and there appears to be a racial influence in that the yellow races, Latin races and American Negroes are relatively susceptible whereas the incidence is low in natives of equatorial Africa. Poor nutrition is undoubtedly a factor in the development of the condition and Bernát (1965) considers that atrophic rhinitis is an iron-deficiency disease.

Atrophic rhinitis is now relatively rare and the incidence of chronic nasal infection has also decreased. It therefore seems probable that in the past atrophic rhinitis was due to an inflammatory process which produced an endarteritis and periarteritis of terminal arterioles (Ruskin, 1942; Taylor and Young, 1961). Harrison (1957) in a study of patients suffering from familial haemorrhagic telangectasia showed that prolonged oestrogen therapy in man produces metaplasia of the columnar ciliated nasal epithelium to stratified squamous epithelium. However, if raised oestrogen levels are an aetiological factor, why do pregnant women with vasomotor imbalance due to increased circulating oestrogens not develop atrophic rhinitis? Atrophic rhinitis is likely to result from a number of separate factors working simultaneously.

Pathology

Most authors agree that there are patches of metaplasia from columnar ciliated to squamous epithelium (*Figure 9.2*), that there is a decrease in the number and size of the compound alveolar glands, and that there are dilated capillaries; but some (Taylor and Young, 1961) were unable to demonstrate endarteritis and periarteritis of the terminal arterioles. It is possible, therefore, that there are two types of atrophic rhinitis:

(1) Type 1, characterized by endarteritis and periarteritis of the terminal arterioles, which is the result of chronic infection and which might benefit from the vasodilator effect of oestrogen therapy.
(2) Type 2, in which there is vasodilatation of the capillaries, which might be made worse with oestrogen therapy.

It seems likely that in the past the majority of cases were of Type 1.

Taylor and Young (1961) also found that the endothelial cells lining the dilated capillaries had more cytoplasm than normal capillaries and showed a positive reaction for alkaline phosphatase which suggested to them the presence of active absorption of bone which is a feature of atrophic rhinitis.

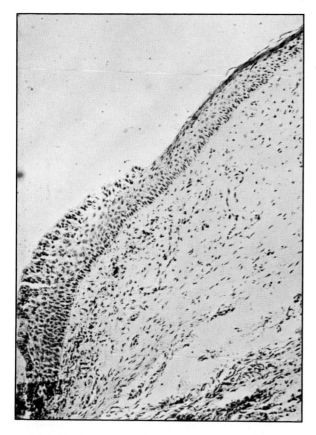

Figure 9.2 The nasal mucous membrane in atrophic rhinitis, showing metaplasia of the epithelium from columnar-ciliated to squamous type, and fibrosis of the tunica propria

Clinical picture

The presenting symptoms are most commonly nasal obstruction, headache and epistaxis. Anosmia may be present and the patient is often only made aware of the loathsome effluvium surrounding her by the reluctance of others to come within her vicinity. Sometimes the symptoms are mainly pharyngeal and are caused by the pharyngitis sicca which often accompanies the condition or by choking when detached crusts slip from the nasopharynx into the oropharynx.

Clinical examination of the morose and dejected patient confirms the presence of foetor in all but the earliest cases and the nasal cavities are found to be lined with green, yellow and black crusts. Even before the removal of the latter the enormous capacity of the nasal passages is apparent and their detachment reveals a bleeding and ulcerated mucosa and shrivelled turbinates.

Investigations

Before embarking on treatment it is advisable to exclude the presence of sepsis in the paranasal sinuses by radiology, and if necessary by proof puncture. Swabs from the nasal secretions may be cultured but whilst of interest, the results are unlikely to be of great value in the management of the case. Serological tests to exclude syphilis are essential as syphilis is certainly the most likely condition to be confused with atrophic rhinitis. The blood picture, serum proteins and iron should also be checked.

Treatment

Conservative treatment
In the first place the patient should be instructed to douche the nose twice daily with an alkaline solution prepared by dissolving in 280 ml ($\frac{1}{2}$ pint) warm water a teaspoonful of the following powder:

Sodium bicarbonate	28.4 g
Sodium biborate	28.4 g
Sodium chloride	56.7 g

It may be necessary for the nasal cavities to be syringed with this solution in some cases and in the most resistant cases plugging of the nostrils with cotton wool tampons for periods of up to 1 h prior to douching or syringing may be necessary to loosen the crusts. Certainly regular nasal cleansing is the basis of the conservative treatment in atrophic rhinitis and it may be of some consolation that if the patient is prepared to carry out this simple treatment with unfailing regularity freedom from offensive effluvia may almost always be achieved. Unhappily however many of the patients are inadequate and unprepared to cooperate fully.

Following the removal of crusts it is customary to apply, for example, 25 per cent glucose in glycerine, which inhibits the proteolytic organisms, or oestradiol in arachis oil 10 000 units/ml. The place of oestrogen therapy has been discussed above. The use of potassium iodide by mouth with the object of increasing nasal secretion has been suggested. Autogenous vaccines may be given. Sinha, Sardana and Rjvanshi (1977) have reported promising results using tissue therapy with systemic human placental extracts, which gave an 80 per cent improvement in two years, and submucosal intranasal injection of human placental extracts which produced 93.3 per cent relief over the same period of time.

Surgical treatment

Numerous attempts to relieve the condition surgically have been made in the past. These include submucous injections of paraffin, and operations aimed at displacing the lateral nasal walls medially (Lautenslager's operation). More recently Teflon strips, polythene and cartilage have been inserted after flaps of mucoperichondrium were raised from the septum or mucoperiosteum from the floor or lateral walls. Wilson (1964) has reported good results from the submucosal injection of a suspension of powered Teflon in 50 per cent glycerine paste.

Repeated stellate ganglion blocks have been employed with some success by Sharma and Sardana (1966) who advocate cervical sympathectomy or blockade as a possible first line of treatment. Previously, however, autonomic surgery for atrophic rhinitis had proved disappointing.

Encouraging results have been obtained following the closure of one or both nostrils by plastic surgery (Young, 1967). Young's method is to raise folds of skin inside the nostril and suture the folds together with the object of complete interruption of the air flow. After periods varying from months to several years the nostrils have been reopened revealing absence of crusting and normal mucosa. Sinha, Sardana and Rjvanshi (1977) found that bilateral closure was not tolerated by some patients who disliked mouth-breathing and a nasal voice. However, partial nostril closure leaving a 3 mm hole was well tolerated and gave similar results with no recurrence of disease over a two-year period. Any further increase in size of the hole rapidly decreased their success rate.

Rhinitis sicca

Rhinitis sicca is the term often reserved for a dry, mildly atrophic anterior rhinitis which does not progress to the full clinical picture of atrophic rhinitis given in the previous section. The causes are not well defined but it is generally recognized that the condition occurs in alcoholism, anaemia, nutritional and constitutional diseases and in those engaged in dry, hot and dusty occupations.

The pathology resembles that of early atrophic rhinitis; indeed some authorities would not distinguish the two as separate entities. There is deficiency and inactivity of the seromucinous glands, metaplasia of the columnar ciliated epithelium to cuboidal or squamous epithelium and deficiency of the mucous blanket. A penetrating ulcer of the anterior part of the cartilaginous septum may be present.

The patient complains of discomfort, irritation and sometimes epistaxis and crusting but the crusts are thin and dry and do not as a rule extend to the posterior part of the nasal cavities as do the crusts of atrophic rhinitis; neither do they emit a characteristic foetor.

Clinical examination reveals a dry, whitish or glazed mucous membrane sometimes accompanied by crusting or complicated by a septal perforation.

As in atrophic rhinitis the patient should be investigated with a view to excluding nutritional deficiencies or local infection.

In treating the disorder all possible causes should be removed and if necessary iron and vitamins administered. Locally, douching with the solution advocated for the treatment of atrophic rhinitis is undoubtedly of value, but the time-honoured treatment with oily drops and sprays is to be deprecated owing to the danger of inhalation lipoid pneumonia and paraffin granuloma. These sinister conditions have been recognized for a number of years and their pathology is clearly described by Spencer (1968).

Rhinitis caseosa

Rhinitis caseosa (nasal cholesteatoma) is a chronic inflammation of the nose associated with the formation of granulation tissue and an accumulation of offensive cheesy material resembling cholesteatoma.

The condition is rare and, according to Meyersburg, Bernstein and Mezz (1936), unilateral. These authors surveyed the condition fully and found that it is slightly more common in males and could occur at any age between nine and 80. They considered it to be a consequence of chronic sinusitis, but numerous theories have been advanced regarding its causation. It has been considered to be due to fungal infection, the presence of a foreign body or the distintegration of nasal polypi.

Microscopical examination of the caseous debris shows keratinous material, numerous organisms and sometimes cholesterin crystals. The lining mucous membrane shows chronic inflammatory changes.

Clinical examination in the early stages merely reveals that one side of the nose is filled with whitish debris but later the bone is invaded, the soft tissues of the face are inflamed and abscesses may form and burst through the skin.

Careful investigation by means of radiology and histological examination is necessary to exclude the presence of coexistent conditions such as sinus infection or malignant disease, and treatment consists of thorough removal of the debris by douching or surgery. Surprisingly perhaps, the prognosis is extremely good provided care is taken to follow up the patient and deal with any signs of stagnating discharge.

Gangosa

Gangosa (rhinopharyngitis mutilans; gangreangosa; kaninloma) is a slowly progressive ulceration and necrosis of the palate, nose and pharynx. As a disease it appears to be a separate entity but it may be clinically indistinguishable from tertiary yaws (see 'Yaws', p. 196); thus there may arise a certain amount of confusion.

The geographical incidence of the specific form is limited to the Pacific Islands, Ceylon and equatorial Africa. Gangosa affects males and females of all ages and is associated with dirty and insanitary conditions. It is extremely rare in the white races but has been reported. The cause and mode of spread are unknown; no specific organisms have been found in the tissues or in the discharge.

The disease commences as a small painless nodule in the middle of the palate. This perforates into the nose and spreads intermittently destroying all structures including the nose, palate, orbit and its contents and even the entire face. Pain is absent.

The disease may be steadily progressive, or may be arrested at any stage, the resulting scars resembling those of burns. Most cases survive (Arrowsmith, 1921; Myerson, 1933). Serological tests for syphilis are negative and there is no response to anti-syphilitic treatment.

NASAL SYPHILIS

Primary syphilis

Chancres of the nose are very rare. They constitute 1 per cent of all extragenital chancres (Bulkley, 1894). Extragenital chancres constitute 5 per cent of the total. The vestibule is the site of infection.

The histological appearances of the syphilitic lesion are characterized by oedema, and infiltration of the stroma with lymphocytes, plasma cells and endothelial cells. The perivascular cuffing by these cells and the endarteritis reduce the lumen of the blood vessels, and result in necrosis and ulceration.

The symptoms appear 3–4 weeks after contact, and at first there is swelling, irritation and pain. Ulceration and fungation may follow. The pre-auricular or submandibular lymph nodes enlarge, with firm induration around them. Malaise with raised temperature may occur. The lesion usually disappears spontaneously in 6–10 weeks.

The following will be useful in establishment of diagnosis.

(1) Cultures from the surface of the lesion will be negative.
(2) Smears examined by dark-ground illumination or after staining should show the spirochaete, *Treponema pallidum.*
(3) Serological tests for syphilis may be positive, except in the earliest cases, or in those cases already having antibiotics. Serological tests in current use include: (a) Venereal Disease Reference Laboratory (VDRL) titres; (b) *Treponema pallidum* haemagglutination test (TPHA); (c) Fluorescent treponemal antibody test (FTA);
(d) *Treponema pallidum* immobilization test (TPI); (e) Wassermann and Kahn complement fixation tests.
(4) A biopsy may be performed in doubtful cases. The microscopical appearances are characteristic.

Owing to its rarity and the fact that the chancre does not present a typical appearance, the diagnosis is often overlooked and may not be suggested until secondary manifestations are seen. The hardness and relative painlessness of the nodule, with early and great enlargement of the lymphatic glands, should suggest the diagnosis.

It has to be differentiated from malignant neoplasms and furunculosis. Malignant neoplasms are progressive, and occur in the later age groups. Furunculosis is painful and suppuration follows. The syphilitic lesion usually disappears spontaneously in 6–10 weeks.

General anti-syphilitic treatment, with intramuscular penicillin, should be given at once, and the chancre may be cleansed with 1 : 2000 solution of perchloride of mercury and the surface smeared with 2 per cent yellow mercuric oxide ointment.

Secondary syphilis

Secondary symptoms appear 6–10 weeks after inoculation. The most common manifestation is a simple catarrhal rhinitis. Clinically this does not show any special characteristic, except in its persistence. There may be crusting and fissuring of the nasal vestibule.

Secondary syphilis is rarely recognized in the nose, as mucous patches hardly ever occur on such a thin attentuated mucous membrane.

The diagnosis is usually suggested by the appearance of other secondary lesions, particularly the development of mucous patches in the pharynx, roseolar or papular rashes, pyrexia and the shotty enlargement of many lymph nodes. The scar of the primary lesion may be visible. Serological tests for syphilis are positive. The response to anti-syphilitic treatment is so rapid as to be of diagnostic value.

The condition responds to general anti-syphilitic treatment.

Tertiary syphilis

This is the stage most commonly encountered in the nose. The pathological lesion is the gumma, invading mucous membrane, periosteum or bone.

The bony portion of the septum is the site most commonly attacked. More rarely the lateral nasal wall, frontal sinus, nasal bones or floor of the nose are invaded. Pain and headache (which is always worse at night), swelling and obstruction are the early symptoms. The swelling may be diffuse or localized, and offensive discharge, bleeding and crusting follow, but the pain is then relieved. The olfactory acuity diminishes. In neglected cases, perforation of the affected nasal wall, and collapse of the bony support of the nose may occur. Ultimately there may be severe scarring, and secondary atrophic rhinitis.

The earliest stage of simple swelling is not often seen. Later there is a diffuse or localized submucosal swelling, and infiltration. The surface is red, and may be nodular. The lesion is usually unilateral but if the septum is involved the swelling is seen on both sides. Tenderness of the nasal bridge is a characteristic sign. As a rule, when first seen, ulceration has already taken place, and a putrid-smelling discharge is escaping from the crusted surface. The crusts should be removed, and bare bone may be felt with a probe. The margins of the ulcers are irregular, overhanging and indurated.

The following are special aids to diagnosis.

(1) There is no shrinkage with vasoconstrictors.
(2) Radiographs show rarefaction of bone, with blurring of the cortical outline.
(3) Serological tests for syphilis are positive in 90 per cent of cases.
(4) Biopsy shows the typical syphilitic histological appearances.

This stage has the following complications and sequelae.

(1) Secondary infection with pyogenic organisms.
(2) Sequestration.
(3) Perforation of the septum, palate or nasal walls.
(4) Collapse of the nasal bridge, and deformity of the face.
(5) Scarring and stenosis of the nasal passages.
(6) Atrophic rhinitis.
(7) Intracranial complications from involvement of the meninges.

Differential diagnosis

A gumma should be suspected when there is a firm reddened nodular swelling of the bony portion of the septum or nasal wall, with obstruction, nocturnal pain and tenderness of the nasal bridge. Ulceration, foetor and necrosis of bone practically confirm the diagnosis. Serological tests for syphilis are positive. Other blood changes are absent, and the response to treatment is rapid.

In all cases of doubt a biopsy should be performed, as the histological appearances in syphilis and in all the conditions given below are characteristic.

Yaws differs from syphilis only in its origin in tropical countries, the onset in childhood by extragenital infection, and the gross skin lesions. Serological tests for syphilis are usually positive and the lesions respond to anti-syphilitic treatment.

Lupus vulgaris affects mainly the anterior cartilaginous portion of the septum and anterior ends of the turbinates. There may be associated nodules in the skin. Apple-jelly nodules may be seen, and there is no special odour.

In *tuberculosis* the course is rapid, and the skin is not affected. Typical signs of tuberculosis may be present in the lungs.

Sarcoid resembles tuberculosis, but does not caseate; nodules appear in the skin and other organs. There is anergy to tuberculin, and the Kveim-Siltzbach skin test is usually positive.

In *atrophic rhinitis* the foetor is characteristically offensive and nauseating. The mucosa does not ulcerate deeply, and there is no bone necrosis.

Leprosy occurs only in certain countries, is painless and develops very slowly. Nodules may be present in the skin, and deformity is severe in the late stages.

Areas of anaesthesia may be present. The *Mycobacillus leprae* may be seen in the discharge.

Scleroma occurs in patients of Central European, Asian, American and African origin. It is slow, painless and does not ulcerate. Stenosis and adhesions are characteristic. Associated lesions are found in the nasopharynx and larynx.

Chronic glanders closely resembles tertiary syphilis, but there is an intermittent pyrexia, and *Loefflerella mallei* may be cultured from the discharge.

Leishmaniasis occurs chiefly in South American countries. It commences as a nodule on the septum, which spreads slowly, destroying cartilage, but not bone. It is followed by fibrosis, and scarring. The histology is characteristic, and the Leishman–Donovan bodies can be identified. Response to tartar emetic is rapid.

Benign neoplasms grow slowly, and are painless. Ulceration and bleeding are rare, except in angioma.

A *malignant neoplasm* is at first unilateral. It grows steadily and ulcerates superficially, and the surface is hard and friable, and bleeds readily on probing. Radiographs show invasion and destruction of bone.

A sequestrum must be distinguished from a foreign body or a rhinolith by probing. The first is always attached deeply at some point, the second and third can always be moved, if only to a slight extent. When bone necrosis is present, only the silent form of osteomyelitis requires to be excluded. In this the swelling is more diffuse; it is associated with sinusitis, there are general signs of infection and a leucocytosis. Radiographs show the typical worm-eaten appearance of the bone.

A septal perforation due to gumma is situated posteriorly on the vomer or ethmoid. When due to rhinitis sicca, trauma, lupus vulgaris, leprosy or chrome ulceration it affects the anterior cartilaginous portion.

Treatment

General treatment
General anti-syphilitic treatment is given.

Local treatment
The nasal passages must be cleared of crusts and discharge by copious alkaline douches every morning, and repeated if necessary two or three times a day. Dilute mercuric nitrate ointment should be applied freely to the nasal vestibules.

Sequestra should be removed with great care. The free portion may be removed piecemeal, but any firmly attached portion should be allowed to separate naturally, as avulsion may cause severe haemorrhage or damage adjacent tissues (for treatment of atrophic rhinitis, see p. 176).

Perforations of the palate and deformities of the face may be repaired by plastic operations.

Gummas respond rapidly to general anti-syphilitic treatment, but atrophic rhinitis and deformity may persist after the disease is cured.

Hereditary or congenital syphilis

In congenital syphilis any of the lesions described under the secondary and tertiary forms of syphilis of the nose may occur.

In the infant, 'snuffles' is the most common lesion. This begins about the third week of life, but may appear as late as three months after birth. At first it appears as a simple catarrhal rhinitis. In a short time it becomes purulent, with secondary fissuring and excoriation of the nasal vestibules and upper lip. The obstruction may be so severe as to interfere seriously with suckling and nutrition.

Gummatous and destructive lesions occur most commonly at puberty in the 'latent' form of the disease. Mucous membrane, periosteum and bone may all be affected. The resulting ulceration and destruction lead ultimately to atrophy of the mucous membrane, secondary atrophic rhinitis, and sinking of the nasal bridge, producing the saddle-nose deformity.

Serological tests for syphilis of the patient and parent are positive; biopsy shows the characteristic syphilitic histological picture.

There may be a pre-natal and family history of syphilis, miscarriages or stillbirths. Snuffles should be suspected when a severe rhinitis with excoriation of the nares develops about the third week of life, and interferes with suckling. A common cold infection at this age may often produce a severe rhinitis but there is usually a definite history of exposure to infection; serological tests for syphilis are negative, and cultures may show virulent pyogenic organisms. When obstruction dominates the picture congenital atresia of the choanae or adenoid hypertrophy must be excluded by sounding the nasal passages with a rubber catheter.

In the tertiary form the diagnosis rests on the presence of other stigmas, particularly Hutchinson's teeth and Moon's teeth, interstitial keratitis, corneal opacities, sensorineural deafness and the serological reactions.

Treatment

In snuffles the airway must be restored for suckling. The discharge is removed by gentle suction and irrigation, and drops of o.1 per cent Privine, or o.5 per cent ephedrine in normal saline solution, should be inserted into the nose, with the head hyperextended, before feeding.

In the tertiary forms simple nasal toilet by syringing with isotonic alkaline douche solution will remove the crusts and discharge, and yellow mercuric oxide ointment may be applied frequently to the nasal vestibules.

In both forms anti-syphilitic treatment is essential and rapidly arrests the disease, but the destruction and deformity remain.

Tuberculosis

Tuberculosis of the nose is very rare. It may be nodular or ulcerative. It affects the cartilaginous portion of the nasal septum, and has been reported on the lateral nasal wall. It may be primary (Havens, 1931) but is usually secondary to tuberculosis of the lungs.

The symptoms are discharge, slight pain and partial obstruction. On examination a bright red nodular thickening, with or without ulceration, is seen on the septum. Tuberculosis follows a relatively rapid course, and ulceration leads to perforation of the septum.

Bacteriological examination of the discharge shows tubercle bacilli, and biopsy will confirm the typical appearance of tuberculosis.

Nasal douches may be used to remove the discharge and crusts. Treatment is with antituberculous drugs (rifampicin, ethambutol, INAH, streptomycin, PAS, in planned schedule for long-term therapy).

Lupus vulgaris

Lupus vulgaris is an indolent and chronic form of tuberculous infection which affects the skin and mucous membrane.

It is twice as common in females as in males, and is developed most often in early adult life. It is a disease mainly of northern climates, and is rare in the tropics. The mucocutaneous junction of the nasal septum is the most common site of inoculation as this is frequently exposed to trauma in patients who have the habit of picking the nose. The nasal lesion is frequently associated with, or a precursor of, nodules on the face.

Sections of tissue show the characteristic appearance of a tuberculous granuloma. In the centre at first there is a collection of reticulo-endothelial cells which soon necrose and coalesce. Around this necrotic centre there is a ring of living reticulo–endothelial cells, and around this ring are lymphocytes, plasma cells and fibroblasts; scattered throughout the tubercle are found giant cells, with a peripheral arrangement of nuclei (*Figure 9.3*).

The early symptoms are those of nasal discharge and obstruction followed by crusting and occasional epistaxis. When the ulceration is established there may be slight foetor and soreness. Ulceration may be followed by fibrosis and contraction, with distortion of the alae nasi. When the turbinates are extensively involved the ciliated epithelium is not renewed and atrophic rhinitis may develop.

The course is very slow, and may last for a lifetime with periods of regression and healing, alternating with periods of active extension, depending to a great extent on the general health of the patient.

The typical early lesion is a reddish firm nodule at the mucocutaneous junction of the nasal septum. In more advanced cases, there may be extensive involvement of the floor of the nose and the turbinates, spreading backwards from the primary site. The surface shows superficial ulcers and crusts. The septum may perforate, but only in the cartilaginous portion, and there is no sinking of the nasal bridge.

If the disease spreads forwards there may be external scarring and distortion of the nasal vestibules, tip and alae nasi, and nodules may be seen in the skin of the face.

Blanching, bacterial examination and biopsy are of use in diagnosis.

(1) To show apple-jelly nodules, the blood is expressed from adjoining tissues by pressure with a glass slide on the skin, or shrinkage with cocaine and adrenaline on the mucous membrane, thus making the pinkish lupus nodules more evident by contrast.
(2) Bacteriological examination of the discharge may show tubercle bacilli.
(3) Biopsy will confirm the typical histological picture. For differential diagnosis, see 'Tertiary Syphilis' (p. 182).

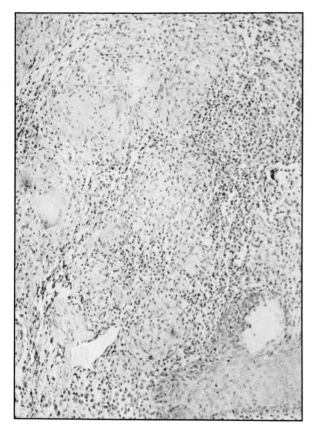

Figure 9.3 Lupus vulgaris, showing giant cells, and zones of reticulo-endothelial cells, lymphocytes, plasma cells and fibroblasts (× 200)

Complications

(1) Pulmonary tuberculosis develops in a small proportion of cases.
(2) Dacryocystitis, corneal ulceration, nasopharyngeal lupus, and lupus of the face may occur.
(3) Atrophic rhinitis may be a sequel.
(4) Epithelioma may develop in the infected tissue.

Sudden increase in size and hardness of one area, and, in the elderly patient, an increased tendency to bleed should arouse the suspicion that a malignant change had supervened. A biopsy should be taken, and the tissue examined histologically.

Treatment consists of specific anti-tubercular therapy and calciferol (vitamin D_2), 150 000 units daily for 3–6 months. Plastic repair of deformities of the nose may be required when the disease has been arrested.

Sarcoidosis (Boeck's sarcoid) *(see Plate 3b, facing p. 16)*

Sarcoidosis is a chronic systemic disease of unknown cause which is clinically characterized by involvement of virtually every organ with a non-caseating granulomatous inflammation which closely resembles tuberculosis without caseation. The tubercle consists of a collection of pale-staining epithelioid cells, sometimes surrounded by a thin layer of lymphocytes. Giant cells are present and, in older lesions, contain asteroid intracytoplasmic inclusion bodies which stain with haematoxylin (Shaumann bodies). This histological picture is not, however, specific for sarcoidosis as it may be seen in other granulomas, for example tuberculosis, leprosy or berylliosis. Before confirming the diagnosis it is therefore important to exclude these other causes.

Nasal sarcoidosis was first described by Boeck (1905), and confirmed by biopsy by Kistner and Robertson (1938).

Aetiology

Two hypotheses have been advanced (Gordon *et al.*, 1976):

(1) That sarcoid is a special form of tuberculosis which is the result of an altered bacillus with an atypical host response. Tuberculosis is known to precede, occur with or follow clinical sarcoidosis. However, tubercle bacilli have been reported in only a few cases.
(2) That an unidentified organism or agent is responsible, for example pine pollen, wood dust, beryllium and silica or tubercle bacilli, *M. leprae*, a protozoon, virus or fungus.

Incidence

Sarcoidosis occurs all over the world but is more prevalent in rural south-eastern USA and Scandinavian countries. Coloured races are more affected than white, and females more than males. Nasal sarcoidosis occurs in 3–20 per cent of systemic cases. The median age of onset is 25 years, and 50 per cent of cases occur below the age of 30 years.

Clinical picture

Presenting symptoms include nasal discharge, which ranges from serosanguineous to mucopurulent, nasal obstruction and epistaxes. There may be a secondary sinusitis due either to superadded infection or to involvement by the disease. Nasal skin and bone lesions are asymptomatic. There may be a general swelling of the bridge of the nose with discoloration of the overlying skin (Black, 1966).

Examination of the nasal mucosa may reveal tiny 1 mm yellow nodules surrounded by hyperaemic boggy mucosa. Alternatively the mucosa may be dry, ulcerated and covered with crusts. The anterior septum and inferior turbinates are the most commonly involved areas. Adhesions may develop between them resulting in stenosis of the anterior nares. Septal perforations may arise spontaneously or may occur following septal surgery in the unrecognized case. Nasal skin lesions appear as elevated, yellowish, dry, scaling, discrete nodules or plaques. These may coalesce to form large bluish red granulomas, separated by normal skin, over the tip, alae, columella or dorsum. Violaceous, diffuse bulbous affliction of the nasal tip area in conjunction with other skin and pulmonary lesions was separately described by Besmer in 1889 as *Lupus pernio* (Gordon *et al.*, 1976) and as a manifestation of chronic multi-system sarcoidosis (James, 1959). Weiss (1960) believes that skin and mucosal lesions are complete, separate independent lesions.

Nasal lesions may be associated with other lesions in the head and neck which may include tonsil, tongue, salivary glands, lacrimal glands, bronchial mucosa, paranasal sinuses, nasopharynx, or larynx. Heerfordt's syndrome describes a transient bilateral facial palsy associated with fever, parotid enlargement and uveal tract disease.

Diagnosis

The histological picture is described above. Culture and stains for acid-fast bacilli and fungi should be negative. There is usually an anergy to the tuberculin skin test but pulmonary tuberculosis develops during the course of the disease in 10 per cent of cases and tuberculin hypersensitivity then develops. The Kveim–Siltzbach skin test (in which a subcutaneous injection of a suspension from a lesion in another case is followed by the development of a sarcoid nodule) is usually positive in all mucosal cases, and is an invaluable aid in the differential diagnosis of granulomas in the nose.

The radiographic changes in cases of involvement of the nasal bones are characteristic and consist of cystic, punched-out lesions with thinning of the cortex of the bone and a reticular pattern in the medulla (Curtis, 1964). Hilar node involvement is shown in radiographs of the chest, and bone cysts are seen in radiographs of the hands and feet.

Serum and urinary calcium levels should be measured to exclude hypercalcaemia.

Differential diagnosis

(1) Lupus vulgaris.
(2) Syphilitic gumma.
(3) Leprosy.
(4) Berylliosis.
(5) Histoplasmosis.
(6) Blastomycosis.

Treatment

There is no specific therapy. Chloroquine has been used for skin involvement but its long-term use is precluded by irreversible retinal changes. Depot steroids (McKelvie, Gresson and Pokhrel, 1968) produce a marked decrease in the size of mucosal lesions but there is little improvement in the reduction in size of lesions in patients with systemic disease. Steroid nasal sprays are beneficial. Atrophic rhinitis may develop as a result of the disease or secondary to depot steroids.

It is important to determine which features of the disease are indicative of the likely development of chronic sarcoidosis with life-threatening pulmonary and renal involvement.

Progressive eye or pulmonary involvement, hypercalcaemia or CNS signs are indicators of chronic sarcoidosis. In these cases treatment with systemic steroids, commencing in high doses and gradually reducing to a low maintenance dose, is indicated.

Chronic diphtheritic rhinitis

Chronic diphtheritic rhinitis (fibrinous rhinitis) is an inflammation of the nasal mucous membrane, due to the *Corynebacterium diphtheriae*. Diphtheria is now extremely rare in this country. More commonly a fibrinous rhinitis may be caused by the pneumococcus, staphylococcus or streptococcus and is seen very occasionally in debilitated children.

All the changes of a severe chronic inflammation are seen and on the surface there is extensive necrosis and defoliation of the epithelium. The area is covered with a membrane of fibrin and entangled cells. The fibres of fibrin extend deeply into the submucosa and this accounts for the tenacity of its adhesion, and for the bleeding when the membrane is removed. The corynebacteria and pneumococci cause the formation of an adherent membrane, but staphylococci and streptococci produce only a superficial membrane which can be stripped off easily.

The local symptoms are obstruction, and discharge which is watery at first and later becomes bloodstained and mucopurulent. The course of the disease is slow, and may go on for three months, and ends in spontaneous recovery. Paralysis, toxaemia and other general symptoms are absent.

The anterior nares may be excoriated by the acrid discharge. The nasal mucosa is generally congested and swollen, and the inferior turbinates, floor of the nose and sometimes the septum are covered with a greyish adherent membrane. After removing this a raw bleeding surface remains.

Bacteriological examination of the nasal discharge should never be omitted, and if *C. diphtheriae* is present the organism should be tested for virulence.

Treatment consists of systemic antibiotics and nasal toilet. Systemic antitoxin is unnecessary but in the past local application of antitoxin has been found beneficial. The patient should in all cases be isolated.

Rhinoscleroma

Rhinoscleroma, or scleroma, is a progressive granulomatous disease commencing in the nose and eventually extending into the nasopharynx and oropharynx, the larynx and sometimes the trachea and bronchi (Friedmann, 1966).

Scleroma may occur at any age and in either sex. It is seen mainly in central and south-eastern Europe, North Africa, Pakistan and Indonesia, Central and South America. It may be seen anywhere in the world and people of any race may be affected. There is in most patients one common factor—a poor standard of domestic hygiene.

Pathology

Although there is still controversy over the precise pathogenesis of scleroma it is now generally agreed that the causative organism is the Gram-negative Frisch bacillus (*Klebsiella rhinoscleromatis*). That this organism was a secondary invader following an initial filterable virus infection is disputed by the work of Fisher and Dimling (1964), who failed to reveal virus-like particles or inclusion bodies on electron microscopy. Steffen and Smith (1961) successfully recovered the organism from the lungs of mice previously inoculated with *K. rhinoscleromatis*, and Sinha, Pandhi and Prakash (1969) isolated it in 60 per cent of their cases.

Histologically (*Figure 9.4*) granulomatous tissue infiltrates the submucosa and is characterized by the presence of an accumulation of plasma cells, lymphocytes and eosinophils amongst which are scattered large foam cells (*Mikulicz cells*), which have a central nucleus and a vacuolated cytoplasm containing Frisch bacilli (*Figure 9.5*) and *Russell bodies*, the latter resembling plasma cells and having an eccentric nucleus and deep eosin-staining cytoplasm.

Mikulicz cell

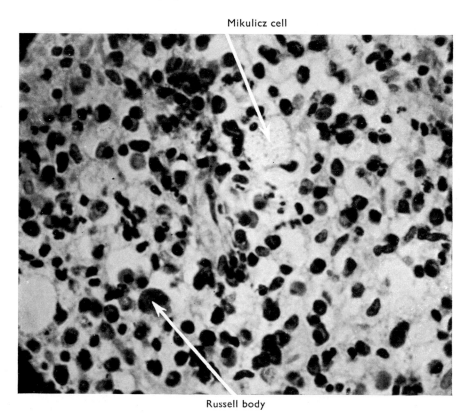

Russell body

Figure 9.4   Scleroma, showing infiltration with plasma cells, lymphocytes, eosinophils, Russell bodies and Mikulicz cells (× 800)

Friedmann, as a result of an electron microscope study, suggests the transformation of plasma cells into Russell bodies. The name Mott cell has been suggested for this type of plasma cell, Russell bodies being formed in the Mott cell through the coalescence of secretory droplets (Friedmann, 1963). The histochemical studies of Gonzalez-Angulo *et al.* (1965) indicates a high content of mucopolysaccharides around the walls

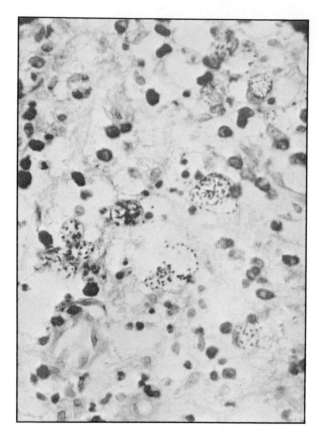

Figure 9.5 Scleroma, showing Frisch bacilli in the vacuoles of the Mikulicz cells (× 800)

of the *Klebsiella* and infer that this may be responsible for the protection of the organism against both antibiotic therapy and the patient's own antibodies.

Clinical picture

There are three recognized stages of this chronic and progressive disease.

(1) *The atrophic stage.* Changes occur in the mucous membrane of the floor of the nose, septum or turbinates which resemble atrophic rhinitis, with crust formation and foul-smelling discharge (*Figure 9.6*).

(2) *Granulation or nodular stage.* Non-ulcerative nodules develop which at first are bluish red and rubbery and later become paler and harder.

(3) *Cicatrizing stage.* Adhesions and stenosis distort the normal anatomy. The disease may extend to the maxillary sinus (Mossallam and Attia, 1956; Yassin and Safwat, 1966), the lacrimal sac (Badraway, 1962), the nasopharynx, hard palate, trachea and main bronchi. Spread to lymph nodes has been reported but is extremely uncommon and is thought to be prevented by early fibrous tissue deposition blocking the lymphatics (Badraway and El-Shennawy, 1974). Bone may be extensively involved (Badraway, 1966). Malignant change is uncommon but can occur (Yassin and Safwat, 1966).

Treatment

Once the diagnosis has been confirmed by biopsy, treatment must be intense and prolonged in order to eradicate the disease completely. Bactericidal antibiotics in large doses given for a minimum of 4–6 weeks are continued until two consecutive cultures from biopsy material are proved to be negative (Ssali, 1975). In practice the best results have been obtained from ampicillin or co-trimoxazole (Septrin), vibramycin and streptomycin. These drugs may if necessary be combined.

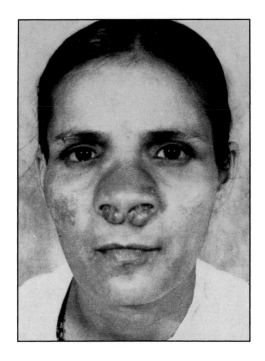

Figure 9.6 A case of rhinoscleroma. (Reproduced by courtesy of Dr. Rege, Bombay)

Chemotherapy may be combined with surgery to re-establish the airway without causing further atrophic changes. This is most effectively achieved by discrete removal of granulations and dilatation of the airways combined with the insertion of polythene tubes for 6–8 weeks (Ssali, 1975).

In late cases where the disease has been eradicated plastic reconstructive surgery may be required.

Leprosy

Leprosy is a chronic granulomatous disease caused by *Mycobacterium leprae*, an acid-fast bacillus morphologically similar to *M. tuberculosis*. Although *M. leprae* cannot yet be cultured on an artificial medium it can, nevertheless, be inoculated into experimental animals, particularly immunologically deficient mice (Rees, 1966), to produce a disease similar to that in man.

Worldwide, 12–15 million people suffer from some form of this disease which is particularly prevalent in India, Central Africa, and Central and South America.

Three main types of leprosy are recognized (Barton *et al.*, 1976).

(1) *Tuberculoid leprosy* in which solitary lesions cause anaesthetic cutaneous 'patches' with involvement of one or more related sensory or motor nerves with possible paralysis of muscles. Cutaneous patches may extend as far as the nasal vestibule but nasal mucosa is not involved bacteriologically or histologically. Isolated cranial nerve palsies (for example, fifth and seventh) may occur.

(2) *Lepromatous leprosy*, in which there is diffuse infiltration of skin, nerves and mucosal surfaces. *M. leprae* tends to favour an environment where the temperature is lower than central (core) temperature. Thus cutaneous infiltration on the face is most apparent on the edges of the pinna, chin, nose and brow. Nasal mucosal involvement occurs early in the disease process and is present in 97 per cent of patients with lepromatous leprosy (Barton *et al.*, 1973). The nasal discharge in these patients, who frequently have minimal systemic signs, contains millions of potentially infectious bacilli and therefore suggests that this is the principle route of spread of infection. Most commonly there is crust formation, nasal obstruction and blood-stained discharge. Hyposmia may be demonstrated in over 40 per cent of patients with lepromatous leprosy (Barton *et al.*, 1974).

(3) *Borderline leprosy*. The first two types are probably immunologically stable. Patients with borderline leprosy with poor resistance may develop the lepromatous type or less commonly, as the disease is modified by treatment or as immunity is acquired, the borderline type. Skin lesions are more numerous than in tuberculoid leprosy and are frequently seen around the eyes, nose and mouth. In pure borderline leprosy there is no involvement of the mucous membranes of the nose, mouth, pharynx or larynx. A conversion to the lepromatous type is indicated by the appearance of mucosal involvement.

Clinical picture

With lepromatous leprosy the earliest sign is a nodular thickening of the nasal mucosa which appears paler than normal and often has a yellowish tinge. These isolated nodules first involve most commonly the anterior end of the inferior turbinate. The disease progresses to gross inflammation of the nasal mucosa and severe obstruction and is out of proportion to the almost imperceptible clinical changes of lepromatous leprosy elsewhere in the body. Perforation of the cartilaginous portion of the nasal septum is followed by perichondritis and periostitis of the nasal cartilages, inferior turbinates and anterior nasal spine which leads to the typical nasal deformity. Atrophic rhinitis, fibrotic atresia or stenosis of the airway are typical sequelae (*Figure 9.7*).

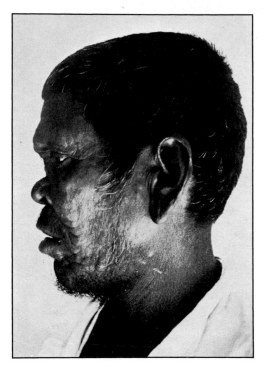

Figure 9.7 Advanced lepromatous leprosy: nasal deformity. (Reproduced by courtesy of Mr. R. P. E. Barton, FRCS and the Editor, *The Journal of Laryngology and Otology*)

McDougall *et al.* (1974) have made an extensive histological study of biopsies of nasal mucosa in patients suffering from leprosy. They found no bacilli or evidence of leprosy infection in the septum and turbinates of borderline cases. However in lepromatous leprosy bacilli were found in macrophages, fibroblasts, within the cytoplasm of endothelial cells of blood vessels and lymphatics and within the free lumina of secretory gland acini (*Figure 9.8*).

Diagnosis

Diagnosis of early and intermediate changes in the nose, pathognomonic of lepromatous leprosy, can be made often in the absence of other manifestations of the disease. The presence of atrophic rhinitis and septal perforations is indicative of late disease with other systemic manifestations (Barton *et al.*, 1976).

Early diagnosis is essential as the nasal component of the infection results in a highly bacilliferous nasal discharge which is the principal route of transmission of the disease (Davey and Rees, 1974). Confirmation is by microscopy of the nasal discharge for acid-fast bacilli, microscopy of scrapings of the nasal mucosa (the most positive site being the anterior end of the inferior turbinate) for acid-fast bacilli, and histology of the nasal mucosa. Radiographs of the anterior nasal spine frequently show erosion (Møller-Christensen, Bakke and Melsom, 1952).

It should always be borne in mind that, with the current patterns of migration, cases of leprosy may be seen in countries where it is no longer endemic (Barton *et al.*, 1976).

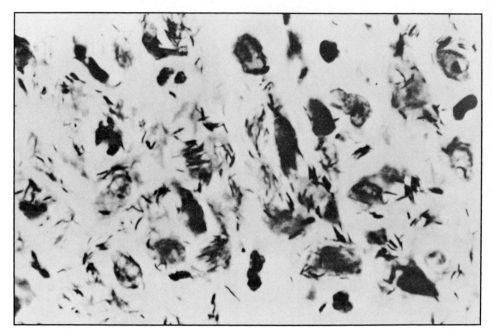

Figure 9.8   From anterior end of middle turbinate. Numerous oil immersion fields show bacilli in the mid-submucosa with a very high percentage of solid staining forms. The host cell is the macrophage (× 3750) (Reproduced by courtesy of Dr. A. C. McDougall and the Editor, *The Journal of Pathology*)

Treatment

Dapsone remains the standard drug in the treatment of leprosy and will reduce the bacterial count of nasal discharge to zero or near zero in two months; however, there are increasing reports of dapsone resistance. The more expensive drugs rifampicin (Rifadin) and clofazimine (Lamprene) act more rapidly and reduce the count to zero in ten days; however, their cost precludes their general usage in developing countries. Local treatment to the nose will help to prevent the external deformity of advanced lepromatous leprosy. Betnovate (1 part) in Unguentum (2 parts) has been used with good results (Barton *et al.*, 1978).

Yaws

Yaws (framboesia) is a disease closely resembling syphilis, if not identical with it, and occurs only in natives of the tropics. It is widespread in Central Africa, Jamaica and the Philippines. The causative organism is the *Treponema pertenue*, which is indistinguishable morphologically from *T. pallidum*. Transmission of the disease is by direct contact, which is usually extragenital; there is a high incidence in infancy and childhood.

Clinical picture

Primary, secondary and tertiary stages occur as in syphilis. Characteristically yaws affects principally the skin and only rarely the mucous membranes, except at the mucocutaneous junctions. Nasal lesions are very rare; in 1500 cases of yaws Turner (1932) saw four cases of active ulceration of the nasal septum and palate, and a few others presented evidence of former active lesions. The nasal lesions do not differ in appearance from those of syphilis. When very extensive and advanced there may be complete destruction of the nose and palate, involving the whole maxilla, face and pharynx. Clinically this is indistinguishable from true gangosa (*Figure 9.9*), but in yaws the serological tests for syphilis are positive, and the lesions respond to anti-syphilitic treatment.

Another special form is designated 'goundou'. In this there is a chronic osteitis, forming bilateral rounded swellings of the nasal processes of the maxillae, which may encroach on the orbits and destroy the eyes. In the early months there is pain and serosanguinous nasal discharge.

The lesions in the nose are indistinguishable from syphilis. Some authorities consider that the two diseases are identical, but that their manifestations differ in natives of certain areas of the tropics. Differentiation from syphilis is made on the country of origin, the onset in childhood by extragenital infection, the gross skin lesions, and the facts that it is never congenital and that it does not cause quaternary lesions in the nervous system.

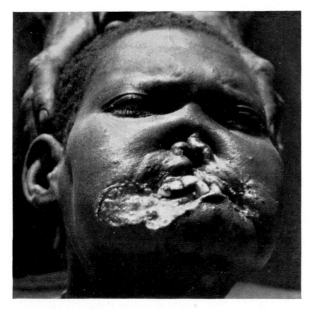

Figure 9.9 A case of gangosa due to yaws. (Reproduced by courtesy of Professor T. F. Hewer)

Treatment

The lesions respond rapidly to treatment with a single large dose of long-acting penicillin. Attention must be paid to general nourishment and hygiene.

Chronic glanders

Glanders is a specific inflammatory disease due to infection with *Loefflerella mallei* which is parasitic in horses, donkeys and mules. The infection is extremely rare in man. It occurs in both acute (*see* p. 174) and chronic forms in grooms and others who handle horses. The infection is transferred directly from the horse to the human through an abrasion of the skin, or occasionally through the nose or mouth. The incubation period may be a few hours, but is usually 2–6 days in the acute form. In the chronic form it may be as long as a year.

Clinical picture

The disease is usually ushered in with an acute febrile attack, and in some cases a rash develops which resembles smallpox. After a variable length of time, up to five years, during which the organisms lie latent, subcutaneous and intramuscular abscesses appear and nodules develop in the skin and in the mucous membrane of the mouth, palate and nose (Robins, 1906). The nodules ulcerate and later heal, and fresh ones appear and pass through the same stages. The ulceration closely resembles that of tertiary syphilis. In the nose there is also a severe generalized rhinitis, with tenacious mucopus and crusts lying on a reddened and scarred mucous membrane.

Throughout the active stages a variable pyrexia of 1 or 2 °C is constant, but periods of complete remission of all signs of the disease are common.

In fatal cases, death is due to toxaemia and pulmonary and intracranial complications. The duration of the disease may be anything from six weeks to 15 years. It has been estimated that 6 per cent of cases recover (Robins, 1906).

It is very difficult to distinguish the lesions from those of tertiary syphilis, but in glanders there is usually a characteristic daily intermittent pyrexia, and in syphilis the serology is positive. In the latter condition there is prompt response to anti-syphilitic treatment, and characteristic papery scars are left after healing.

Any cases diagnosed as tertiary syphilis with a negative serology, and no response to anti-syphilitic treatment, should be suspected as possible cases of chronic glanders. Culture and isolation of *Loefflerella mallei* are often difficult, but intraperitoneal inoculation of the male guinea-pig produces inflammatory changes in the tunica vaginalis of the testis (Straus's reaction). Biopsy may not show any certain points of differentiation.

Treatment

The organism is sensitive to the tetracyclines, streptomycin, chloramphenicol and the sulphonamides.

Pathogenic fungi and yeasts

The classification and pathology of these diseases is complex and the reader is referred to the superb and exhaustive description given by Emmons *et al.* (1977).

Rhinosporidiosis

Rhinosporidiosis is a chronic infestation by the fungus *Rhinosporidium seeberi*, which predominantly affects the mucous membranes of the nose and nasopharynx but occasionally involves the lips, palate, uvula, maxillary antrum, conjunctiva, lacrimal sac, epiglottis, larynx, trachea, bronchus, ear, scalp, skin, penis, vulva and vagina. Osteolytic lesions (*Figure 9.10*) in the bones of the hands and feet have been reported by Chatterjee *et al.* (1977). Rhinosporidiosis is usually limited, though, to surface epithelium but may on occasions be widespread with visceral involvement. The disease, which is chronic and is characterized by the formation of papillomatous and polypoid lesions, tends to affect young males and is endemic in many parts of India and Sri Lanka (Satyanarayana, 1966). Very occasionally the disease has been seen in Europeans who have visited India and Sri Lanka but it is recognized as an exceptional rarity in patients who have never been out of Europe (Friedmann, 1966). The mode of infection is probably by dust from the dung of infected horses and cattle, but this has not been conclusively proved.

The characteristic lesion is a bleeding polypus. Histologically the polypus has a vascular fibromyxomatous structure. Throughout the tissue are seen round or oval cells containing the sporangium. The walls of these are of thick chitin, but are thinned at one point where the cells will burst, sporulation will take place, and the spores will spread through the lymphatics into the connective tissues, where they develop into the trophic stage and complete the life cycle.

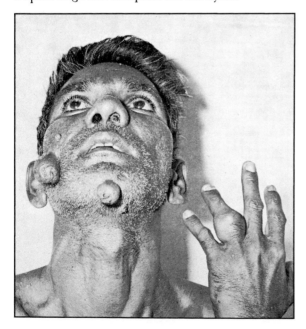

Figure 9.10 Rhinosporidic nodules in the face and nose, and swelling of the finger. (Reproduced by courtesy of Dr. P. K. Chatterjee and the Editor, *The Journal of Laryngology and Otology*)

Epistaxis is often the only symptom, but in the early stages there is a viscid nasal discharge, with irritation and partial obstruction. With the development of the characteristic polypi the obstruction gradually increases until it may interfere with swallowing. Constitutional symptoms are rare, and the disease runs a slow course. The polypi may be present for years before the patient seeks advice.

The lesions are friable, in shape and colour resembling a strawberry, with a greyish under-surface studded with sporangia, showing as white dots. When sessile the polypi appear as multiple nodules, or may assume a leaf shape, with rounded or dentate margins. They arise primarily in the vestibule and are usually attached to the septum, but may spread backwards into the nasopharynx, and even hang down into the oropharynx. The nasal mucosa is generally swollen, hyperaemic and covered with copious viscid secretion, containing spores but no pus cells. The lymphatic glands are not affected.

Microscopical examination of the nasal discharge will show spores. Biopsy and histological examination of the polypi will show the characteristic appearance described above. At first sight carcinoma may be suspected, on account of the friable masses which bleed on contact. The studding of the under-surface with white sporangia should suggest the diagnosis, and this may be confirmed by the special investigations.

Treatment consists of a combination of medical and surgical methods. The former includes the local injection of depot corticosteroids into the polypoidal masses, and in some cases systemic treatment with amphotericin B (Fungizone) can be tried. Growths are removed by wide excision with the cutting diathermy and cautery to the base, as on occasions excessive bleeding may occur.

The phycomycoses

The phycomycoses are a diverse group of mycoses caused by fungi which are traditionally placed in the class, *Phycomycetes*. Although the term is now rejected by the formal taxonomic system it is retained in medical mycology (Emmons *et al.*, 1977). In 1968 Clark recommended a reversion to the name *mucormycosis* for those mycoses caused by fungi belonging to the order *Mucorales* and proposed the name *entomophtharamycosis* for those mycoses caused by the fungi which belong to the order *Entomophtharales*. Certain members of each order can produce nasal disease of which the two major conditions are:

(1) Entomophtharamycosis conidiobolae (rhinophycomycosis)
This disease is caused by *Conidiobolus coronatus* and is manifested as prominent nasal polyps and granulomas in the nasal cavity. Most cases have been seen in Central Africa, India, Brazil and the West Indies. Males are affected more than females. Symptoms consist of nasal obstruction and swelling over the nose and later the cheek and upper lip. Lesions usually begin in the inferior turbinate and spread in the submucosa through the natural ostia to the paranasal sinuses and to the subcutaneous tissues of the face. Histological examination shows a granulomatous reaction with collections of multinucleate giant cells in the centres of which hyphae can be seen. Treatment consists of removal of the tumour masses and systemic amphotericin B (Fungizone).

(2) Orbital and central nervous system mucormycosis (rhinocerebral phycomycosis)

This condition is a short-term and often rapidly lethal fungal disease in the nose and paranasal sinuses (Groote, 1970). The principle causative fungi are the genera *Mucor circinelloides, Absidia corymbitera, Mucor javanicus* of the family Mucoraceae and order Mucorales. Because *Mortierella* (order Mucorales) and *Basidiobolus* (order Entomophtharales) have been also identified as a cause, the use of the term phycomycosis was recommended by Straatsma, Zimmerman and Gass (1962).

Phycomycetes are ordinarily saprophytic organisms existing in soil, manure, fruits and starchy food. They can be cultured from the human nose and gastrointestinal tract. They become pathogenic when the patient's general resistance has been altered by metabolic disorders or chemotherapeutic agents. This is most often associated with diabetic ketosis but can be seen with uraemic acidosis, leukaemia, malnutrition; steroid, antimetabolic or antibiotic therapy; and severe burns. The fungus has a remarkable affinity for arteries and by dissecting the internal elastic lamina from the media leads to extensive endothelial damage and thrombosis. Pathologically there is a mixed picture of inflammatory and necrotic changes. Later the veins and lymphatics are involved.

Mucormycosis appears in cerebral, pulmonary, ocular, superficial and disseminated forms. Orbital and central nervous system mucormycosis is the most common, and usually commences in the nose and extends by direct extension and intravascular propagation to involve the paranasal sinuses, orbit, cribriform plate, meninges and brain. The most characteristic rhinological finding is a black necrotic turbinate resembling a mass of dried clotted blood. Unilateral gangrene and perforation of the hard and soft palates may occur due to involvement of the palatine arteries. Sinus radiographs show thickening of the lining of the sinuses, no fluid levels and spotty destruction of the bony walls.

Early clinical recognition of this potentially fatal disease is essential before irreversible changes occur. The disease is confirmed by biopsy.

Treatment consists of control of the original precipitating condition, heparinization, systemic amphotericin B (Fungizone) and local drainage and débridement.

Aspergillosis

Aspergilloses are infestations, which usually occur in those who handle doves and other small captive birds, in which the *Aspergillus fumigatus* and *A. niger* are common, or as secondary infestations during treatment with antibiotics or corticosteroids.

There is a leucocytic and endothelial-cell infiltration, with patchy necrosis and a few giant cells.

The symptoms are nasal obstruction, sneezing and watery mouldy-smelling discharge. On examination the nasal mucous membrane is covered with a greyish (*fumigatus*) or black (*niger*) false membrane. The infection usually also invades the antrum (Tilley, 1915). The course of the disease resembles that of tuberculosis.

It is most likely to be mistaken for diphtheria, syphilis, tuberculosis or atrophic rhinitis; cultural examination of the membrane should determine the diagnosis.

A few fatalities due to aspergillosis have been reported.

The specific treatment consists of repeated cleaning and the local application of 1 per cent aqueous solution of gentian violet or nystatin. Amphotericin B (Fungizone) may be given systemically. When the sinuses are involved, operative clearance should be performed (Adams, 1933).

Blastomycosis

Blastomycosis is due to an infection by *Blastomyces dermatidis*, an encapsulated yeast-like fungus, which is practically confined to certain parts of America. The disease starts in the skin, though primary inhalational infection of the lungs may occur in some cases. Although the nose is rarely affected, oronasal mucosal involvement is a manifestation of disseminated blastomycosis. The mucosal lesion consists of a papillary hyperplasia with cysts which contain polymorphonuclear leucocytes surrounding the organisms. Regional lymph nodes are not usually affected but dissemination by the blood stream may produce widespread abscesses in the viscera, especially the lungs.

The specific treatment is with amphotericin B (Fungizone).

Cryptococcosis

Cryptococcosis is caused by inhalation or ingestion of *Cryptococcus neoformans*, a yeast-like fungus closely resembling but nevertheless distinct from *Blastomyces dermatidis*. The fungus is found in pigeon or other avian excreta and of the fatal fungal infections in the USA is second only to histoplasmosis (Briggs, Barney and Bahu, 1974). There is, however, a worldwide distribution of the infection, which disseminates after pulmonary infestation to almost any tissue but particularly to the brain and meninges to give a chronic meningitis resembling tuberculous meningitis. Isolated lesions may occur in lymph nodes, skin, bone and eye. Nasal involvement is uncommon but external ulceration, nasopharyngitis and pansinusitis have been described. Briggs, Barney and Bahu (1974) describe a case of ulceration of the nasal vestibule, biopsy of which revealed focal ulceration of the squamous mucosa and oedematous submucosa containing numerous round-to-oval yeast organisms surrounded by a clear 'halo-like' space caused by the capsule.

Treatment with amphotericin B (Fungizone) and flucytosine (Alcobon) can be monitored by a specific slide latex agglutination test. Complete resolution can occur.

Actinomycosis

The genus *Actinomyces* consists of two principle species: *A. bovis*, the cause of actinomycosis or 'lumpy jaw' in cattle; and *A. israelii*, the cause of actinomycosis in man.

The anaerobic fungus, *Actinomyces israelii*, grows in the tissues in the form of colonies composed of branching mycelial threads with clubbed ends—'ray fungus'. The colonies appear in pus as 'sulphur granules'.

Actinomyces israelii is frequently present as a harmless parasite in the mouths of normal individuals where it is found around the teeth and in the tonsillar crypts. Trauma is an important predisposing factor in the development of 'cervico–facial' actinomycosis although the exact conditions necessary to cause an infection are unknown. The infection may originate in a tooth socket and spread to adjacent tissues to produce a large hard, woody mass involving the face, jaw and neck. Softening occurs and multiple sinuses may develop, through which the characteristic pus exudes. The nose is rarely the site of primary infection.

The general symptoms are pyrexia, toxaemia and rarely death. There is extensive tissue destruction and scarring.

Treatment consists of penicillin in large doses for 4–6 weeks and surgical drainage.

Candidiasis (moniliasis)

Candidiasis, commonly known as thrush, is caused by the yeast-like fungus *Candida albicans* which is a common inhabitant of skin and oral cavity.

The infection occurs very commonly in the mouth and occasionally in the nose in neglected and marasmic infants and old people. It may occur in epidemic form in institutions and may be seen as a complication following courses of broad spectrum oral antibiotics and long courses of systemic steroids. These is a predisposition to candidiasis in patients suffering from diabetes or tuberculosis.

Candidiasis presents as small, discrete, pearly or dirty-white patches in the mucous membrane on a red moist surface. The patches are easily removed without bleeding.

The condition responds to simple cleansing and painting with 1 per cent aqueous solution of gentian violet or the local application of nystatin; alternatively amphotericin B (Fungizone) or flucytosine (Alcobon) may be given in severe cases. Any predisposing cause should be sought and corrected.

Histoplasmosis

Histoplasmosis is an infestation due to a yeast-like fungus, *Histoplasma capsulatum*. It is most commonly found in central regions of the USA but cases have been described throughout the world. Histoplasmosis is a diffuse disease of the reticulo–endothelial system and is usually manifest by enlarged spleen, liver and lymph nodes with intestinal ulceration and anaemia. Nasal lesions are rare and may be nodular or infective. Secondary lymphadenitis develops.

The diagnosis is made by biopsy and the Histoplasmin Skin Test which helps to differentiate pulmonary lesions from tuberculosis.

Treatment is with amphotericin B (Fungizone).

Sporotrichosis

Primarily an infection of the skin, usually of the hand, due to *Sporothrix schenckii*. It very rarely affects the nasal mucous membrane but could be transposed there either directly from a lesion on the hand or by haemotogenous spread. Infection follows a prick with a thorn. After a few days a nodule develops which becomes red and tender, finally bursting to discharge viscid yellow mucopus in which organisms may be found. Spread is also by the lymphatics along which secondary nodules develop.

Treatment is with iodides or amphotericin B (Fungizone).

Nasopharyngeal leishmaniasis

This condition, sometimes known as American Leishmaniasis or espundia, is caused by *Leishmania braziliensis* as distinct from *L. donovani*—the cause of visceral leishmaniasis or *L. tropica*—cutaneous leishmaniasis. It is found chiefly in South and Central America and is transmitted by the sandfly (Phlebotomus).

The Leishman–Donovan bodies, which in the mammalian host do not occur in flagellated form, are approximately oval in shape and 2–6 μm in length with an eccentrically placed vesicular nucleus. They may be demonstrated in the discharge from the ulcers and in the reticulo–endothelial cells in the granulomatous tissue.

The site of inoculation is usually on the exposed parts where a papule resembling a chancre develops and ulcerates, later healing and leaving a scar. Polypoid growths may form and there may be extensive destructive lesions involving the soft tissues or cartilage of the nasal septum, mouth, pharynx and larynx. Bone is generally not involved. There may be regional lymphadenitis and in untreated cases death follows from exhaustion.

Treatment consists of local cleansing and curettage. Specific treatment is with systemic pentavalent antimony in the form of sodium stibogluconate BP (Pentostam). Amphotericin B (Fungizone) may be helpful but is not the primary drug of choice.

Myiasis

Nasal myiasis, which is not uncommon in hot and humid climates, particularly in India where it is known as peenash, is a demoralizing condition of infestation of the nasal cavities by maggots, the larvae of a fly (Genus *Chrysomyia*).

Myiasis can also affect the ear, mouth or larynx and reaches a peak in the months of September to November. It can affect any age, and both sexes equally. The majority of sufferers live in bad hygienic conditions and have a source of offensive decaying material, for example atrophic rhinitis, chronic sinusitis or CSOM, which provides a suitable environment for the eggs of the fly to hatch into larvae no less than 1.5 cm in length. The eggs may also be deposited in a slight abrasion or crack in mucous membrane.

The entomological aspects of myiasis are well described by Sood, Kakar and Watlal (1976). The patient complains of a diffuse swelling around the nose and eyes, nasal obstruction, epistaxis or the presence of maggots coming out of the nose. Rhinoscopy reveals a congested oedematous mucosa, necrotic material with embedded maggots, ulcerated mucosa or septal perforations. The disease can spread to the paranasal sinuses and via the naso–lacrimal duct to the lacrimal sac. In the later stages the nasal bones may be destroyed and death may result from sepsis, meningitis or suicide.

Treatment is general, with antibiotics and supportive therapy, and local, with olive oil or liquid paraffin which stifle the larvae. Maggots are removed piecemeal and the nasal cavity is douched. To prevent further infestation the predisposing conditions of poor hygiene and a source of chronic infection must be removed.

References

Abel, P. (1895). 'Die aetiologie der ozaena', *Zeitschrift für Hygiene und Infektionskrankheiten*, **21**, 89

Adams, N. F. (1933). 'Infections involving the ethmoid, maxillary and sphenoid sinuses and the orbit due to *Aspergillus fumigatus*', *Archives of Surgery*, **26**, 999

Anderson, T. B. (1969). 'Virus infections of the upper respiratory tract', *Proceedings of the Royal Society of Medicine*, **62**, 2

Andrewes, C. H. (1947). 'Common cold research unit interim report on a transmission experiment', *British Medical Journal*, **1**, 650

Andrewes, C. H. (1950). 'Adventures among viruses 111. The puzzle of the common cold', *New England Journal of Medicine*, **242**, 235

Andrewes, C. H., Burnet, F. M., Enders, J. F., Gard, S., Hirst, G. K., Kaplan, M. M. and Zhdanor, V. M. (1961). 'Taxonomy of viruses infecting vertebrates: Present knowledge and ignorance', *Virology*, **15**, 52

Andrewes, C. H. and Tyrell, D. A. J. (1965). In *Viral and Rikettsial Infections of man*, pp. 546–558. Ed. by Horsfall and Tanm. Philadelphia; Lippincott

Arrowsmith, H. (1921). 'Gangosa', *Laryngoscope*, **31**, 843

Badraway, R. (1962). 'Dacryoscleroma', *Annals of Otology, St. Louis*, **71**, 247

Badraway, R. (1966). 'Affection of bone in Rhinoscleroma', *Journal of Laryngology*, **80**, 160

Badraway, R. (1966). 'Affection of bone in Rhinoscleroma', *Journal of Laryngology and Otology*, **80**, 160

Badraway, R. and El Shennawy, M. (1974). 'Affection of cervical lymph nodes in Rhinoscleroma', *Journal of Laryngology and Otology*, **88**, 261

Barton, R. P. E. (1974). 'Olfaction in leprosy', *Journal of Laryngology and Otology*, **88**, 355

Barton, R. P. E. (1976). 'Clinical manifestations of leprous rhinitis', *Annals of Otology, St. Louis*, **85**, 74

Barton, R. P. E. (1978) Personal communication

Barton, R. P. E., Davey, T. F., McDougall, A. C., Rees, R. J. W. and Weddell, A. G. M. (1973). Paper 6/47, Tenth International Leprosy Congress, Bergen.

Barton, R. P. E., Davey, T. F., McDougall, A. C., Rees, R. J. W., Weddell, A. G. M. and Davey, T. F. (1976). 'Early leprosy of the nose and throat', *Journal of Laryngology and Otology*, **90**, 953

Bernát, I. (1965). *Ozaena, A manifestation of Iron deficiency*. Oxford; Pergamon Press

Black, J. I. Munro, (1966). 'Sarcoidosis of the nose', *Journal of Laryngology and Otology*, **80**, 1065

Boeck, C. (1905). 'Fortgesetzte untersuchungen über das multiple benigne sarkoid', *Archiv für Dermatologie und Syphilis*, **73**, 301

Briggs, D. R., Barney, P. L. and Bahu, R. M. (1974). 'Nasal Cryptococcosis', *Archives of Otolaryngology*, **100**, 390

Bulkley, L. D. (1894). *Syphilis in the Innocent*. New York; Bailey and Fairchild

Chatterjee, P. K., Katua, C. R., Chatterjee, S. N. and Dastidar, N. (1977). 'Recurrent multiple Rhinasporidiosus with osteolytic lesions in hand and foot', *Journal of Laryngology and Otology*, **91**, 729

Clifford, R. E., Smith, J. W. G., Tillett, H. E. and Wherry, P. J. (1977). 'Excess mortality associated with Influenza in England and Wales', *International Journal of Epidemiology*, **6**, 115

Council on Pharmacy and Chemistry, and Council on Industrial Health (1944). 'The use of vaccines for the common cold', *Journal of the American Medical Association*, **126**, 895

Cruickshank, R. (1942). In *Control of the Common Fevers*. London; Lancet Publications

Curtis, G. T. (1964). 'Sarcoidosis of nasal bones', *British Journal of Radiology*, **37**, 68

Davey, T. F. and Rees, R. J. W. (1974). 'The nasal discharge in leprosy: Clinical and Bacteriological aspects', *Leprosy Review*, **45**, 121

Dochez, A. R., Shibley, G. S. and Mills, K. C. (1930). 'Studies in the common cold. IV', *Journal of Experimental Medicine*, **52**, 701

Dochez, A. R., Mills, K. C. and Kneeland, Y. Jnr. (1936). 'Studies on the common cold. VI.', *Journal of Experimental Medicine*, **63**, 559

Dudgeon, J. A. (1969). 'Virus infections of the upper respiratory tract', *Proceedings of the Royal Society of Medicine*, **62**, 1

Dumbell, K. R., Lovelock, J. R. and Lowbury, E. J. (1948). 'Handkerchiefs in the transfer of respiratory infection', *Lancet*, **2**, 183

Emmons, C. W., Binford, C. H., Utz, J. P. and Kwow-Chung, K. J. (1977). In *Medical Mycology*, 3rd Edn, Chapter 18. Philadelphia; Lea and Febiger

Fabricant, N. D. (1941). 'Significance of pH of nasal secretions *in situ*', *Archives of Otolaryngology*, **34**, 150

Fisher, E. R. and Dimling, C. S. (1964). 'Rhinoscleroma', *Archives of Pathology*, **78**, 501

Fleming, A. (1929). 'Arris and Gale Lecture on Lysozyme', *Lancet*, **1**, 217

Friedmann, I. (1963). 'Electron microscopy of rare diseases of the nose', *Transactions of the American Academy of Ophthalmology and Otolaryngology*, **67**, 261

Friedmann, I. (1966). In *Systemic Pathology*, Vol. 1, pp. 295 and 297. Ed. by G. Payling Wright and W. St. Clair Symmers. London; Longmans

Gonzalez-Augulo, A., Marques-Montes, H., Greenberg, S. D. and Cerbon, J. (1965). 'Ultrastructure of nasal scleroma', *Annals of Otology, St. Louis*, **74**, 1022

Gordon, W. W., Cohn, A. M., Greenberg, S. D. and Komorn, R. M. (1976). 'Nasal sarcoidosis', *Archives of Otolaryngology*, **102**, 11

Groote, C. A. (1970). 'Rhinocerebral phycomycosis', *Archives of Otolaryngology*, **92**, 288

Harkness, G. F. (1937). 'Endocrine imbalances and their relations to upper respiratory tract infections', *Annals of Otology, St. Louis*, **46**, 488

Harrison, D. F. N. (1957). 'Familial haemorrhagic telangectases, a survey of a series of cases treated by oestrogen therapy', *Journal of Laryngology and Otology*, **71**, 577

Havens, F. Z. (1931). 'Tuberculosis of nasal mucous membrane', *Archives of Otolaryngology*, **14**, 181

Henriksen, S. D. and Gundersen, W. B. (1959). 'The aetiology of ozaena', *Acta pathologica et microbiologica scandinavica*, **47**, 380

Hilding, A. (1934). 'Changes in the lysozyme content of nasal mucus during colds', *Archives of Otolaryngology*, **20**, 38

Isaacs, A., Cox, R. A. and Rotem, Z. (1963). 'Foreign nucleic acids as the stimulus to make interferon', *Lancet*, **2**, 113

Israel, M. S. (1962). 'The viral flora of enlarged tonsils and adenoids', *Journal of Pathology*, **84**, 169

James, D. G. (1959). 'Dermatological aspects of sarcoidosis', *Quarterly Journal of Medicine*, **28**, 109

Jarvis, D. C. (1938). 'The relation of clinical conditions of the upper respiratory tract to oxygen metabolism', *Laryngoscope*, **48**, 255

Kerr, W. J. and Lagen, J. B. (1933–34). 'Transmissibility of the common cold', *Proceedings of the Society of Experimental Biology, New York*, **31**, 713

Ketler, A., Hamparian, V. V. and Hilleman, M. R. (1962). 'Characterization and classification of ECHO 28-rhinovirus-coryzavirus agents', *Proceedings of the Society of Experimental Biology and Medicine*, **110**, 821

Kistner, F. B. and Robertson, T. D. (1938). 'Benign granuloma of the nose', *Journal of the American Medical Association*, **111**, 2003

Locke, A. (1937). 'Lack of fitness as the predisposing factor in infections of the type encountered in pneumonia and the common cold', *Journal of Infectious Diseases*, **60**, 106

Loewenberg, B. (1894). 'Le microbe de l'ozène', *Annales de l'Institut Pasteur*, **8**, 292

Long, P., Bliss, E. A. and Carpenter, H. M. (1932). 'A note on the communicability of colds', *Bulletin of the Johns Hopkins Hospital*, **51**, 278

Macbeth, R. G. (1943). 'Vitamin C levels in the blood', *Proceedings of the Royal Society of Medicine*, **36**, 625

McDougall, A. C., Rees, R. J. W., Weddell, A. G. M. and Wadji Kanan, M. (1974). 'The histopathology of lepromatous leprosy in the nose', *Journal of Pathology*, **115**, 215

McGibbon, J. E. and Hall, W. (1947). 'Discussion on the association of otitis media with acute non-specific gastro-enteritis of infants', *Proceedings of the Royal Society of Medicine*, **41**, 1

McKelvie, P., Gresson, C. and Pokhrel, R. P. (1968). 'Sarcoidosis of the upper air passages', *British Journal of Diseases of the Chest*, **62**, 200

Mawson, S. R., Adlington, P. and Evans, M. (1967). 'Controlled study evaluation of adenotonsillectomy in children', *Journal of Laryngology and Otology*, **81**, 777

Mawson, S. R., Adlington, P. and Evans, M. (1968). 'A controlled study evaluation of adenotonsillectomy in children', *Journal of Laryngology and Otology*, **82**, 963

Meyersburg, H., Bernstein, P. and Mezz, D. (1936). 'Rhinitis caseosa', *Archives of Otolaryngology*, **23**, 449

Møller-Christensen, V., Bakke, S. N. and Melsom, R. S. (1952). 'Changes in the anterior nasal spine and alveolar process of the maxillary bone in leprosy', *International Journal of Leprosy*, **20**, 335

Mossallam, I. and Attia, D. M. (1956). 'Primary scleroma of the maxillary sinus', *Journal of the Egyptian Medical Association*, **39**, 512

Mudd, S., Goldman, A. and Grant, S. B. (1921). 'Reactions of the nasal cavity and postnasal space to chilling of the body surface', *Journal of Experimental Medicine*, **34**, 11

Myerson, M. C. (1933). 'Gangosa—occurrence in a white man', *Laryngoscope*, **43**, 394

Paul, H. H. and Freese, H. L. (1933). 'An epidemiological and bacteriological study of the common cold in an isolated arctic community (Spitsbergen)', *American Journal of Hygiene*, **17**, 517

Rees, R. J. W. (1966). 'Enhanced susceptibility of thymectomized and irradiated mice to infection with *M. Leprae*', *Nature*, **211**, 657

Ritchie, J. M. (1958). 'Autogenous vaccine in prophylaxis of the common cold', *Lancet*, **1**, 615

Robins, G. D. (1906). 'A study of chronic Glanders in man', *Studies of the Royal Victorian Hospital, Montreal*, **2**, 1

Ruskin, S. L. (1938). 'Calcium cevitamate in the treatment of acute rhinitis', *Annals of Otology, St. Louis*, **47**, 502

Ruskin, S. L. (1942). 'Rationale of oestrogen therapy of primary atrophic rhinitis (ozaena)', *Archives of Otolaryngology*, **36**, 632

Satyanarayana, C. (1966). In *Clinical Surgery—Ear, Nose and Throat*, p. 143. Ed. by Maxwell Ellis. London; Butterworths

Sharma, A. N. and Sardana, D. S. (1966). 'Stellate ganglion block in atrophic rhinitis', *Journal of Laryngology and Otology*, **80**, 184

Sherman, J. B. (1938). 'Prophylaxis of the common cold', *British medical Journal*, **2**, 903

Simpson, R. E. Hope (1958). 'Symposium on the epidemiology of non-infectious diseases. (a). Common upper respiratory diseases', *Royal Society of Health Journal*, **78**, 593

Simpson, R. E. Hope (1958). 'Discussion on the common cold', *Proceedings of the Royal Society of Medicine*, **51**, 267

Sinha, A., Pandhi, S. C. and Prakash, O. M. (1969). 'Aetiopathogenesis of scleroma', *Journal of Laryngology and Otology*, **83**, 133

Sinha, S. M., Sardana, D. S. and Rjvanshi, V. S. (1977). 'A nine years' review of 273 cases of atrophic rhinitis and its management', *Journal of Laryngology and Otology*, **91**, 591

Smiley, D. F. (1924). 'A study of the acute infections of the throat and respiratory system', *Journal of the American Medical Association*, **82**, 540

Sood, V. P., Kakar, P. K. and Watlal, B. L. (1976). 'Myiasis in otolaryngology with entomological aspects', *Journal of Laryngology and Otology*, **90**, 393

Spencer, H. (1968). *Pathology of the lung.* 2nd Edn. Oxford; Pergamon Press

Ssali, C. L. K. (1975). 'The management of rhinoscleroma', *Journal of Laryngology and Otology*, **89**, 91

Steffen, T. N. and Smith, I. M. (1961). 'Scleroma, *Klebsiella rhinosleromatis* and its effect on mice', *Annals of Otology, St. Louis*, **70**, 935

Straatsma, B. R., Zimmerman, L. E. and Gass, J. D. (1962). 'Phycomycosis', *Laboratory Investigations*, **11**, 963

Stuart-Harris, C. H. (1963). 'Acute respiratory virus infections in childhood', *Journal of Laryngology and Otology*, **77**, 981

Taylor, M. and Young, A. (1961). 'Studies on atrophic rhinitis', *Journal of Laryngology and Otology*, **75**, 574

Thomson, D., Thomson, R. and Morrison, J. T. (1948). *Oral Vaccines.* London; Livingstone

Tilley, H. (1915). 'Aspergillosis of nasal accessory sinuses', *Journal of Laryngology and Otology*, **30**, 145

Tweedie, A. R. (1934). 'Nasal flora and reaction of nasal mucus', *Journal of Laryngology and Otology*, **46**, 586

Tyrell, D. A. J. and Bynde, M. L. (1961). 'Some further virus isolations from common colds', *British medical Journal*, **1**, 393

US Public Health Services Report (1927). **42**, 97

Walsh, T. E. and Cannon, P. R. (1938). 'Studies of immunization of the upper part of the respiratory tract', *Archives of Otolaryngology*, **27**, 655

Weiss, J. A. (1960). 'Sarcoidosis in otolaryngology', *Laryngoscope*, **70**, 1351

Wells, W. F. and Wells, M. W. (1936). 'Air-borne infection', *Journal of the American Medical Association*, **107**, 1698; 1805

Wilson, T. G. (1964). 'Teflon in glycerine paste in rhinology', *Journal of Laryngology and Otology*, **78**, 953

Yassin, A. and Safwat, F. (1966). 'Unusual features of scleroma', *Journal of Laryngology*, **80**, 524

Young, A. (1967). 'Closure of the nostrils in atrophic rhinitis', *Journal of Laryngology and Otology*, **80**, 524

Zaiman, E., Balducci, D. and Tyrell, D. A. J. (1955). 'A.P.C. Viruses and respiratory disease in Northern England', *Lancet*, **2**, 595

10 Vasomotor rhinitis—allergic and non-allergic
Neil Weir

Rhinitis may be defined as that condition giving rise to one or more of the symptoms of nasal obstruction, increased secretion of mucus and sneezing.

Any symptom of rhinitis can arise from tissue-damaging allergic hypersensitivity and from unknown causes, among which may be autonomic nervous disorder.

Some vasomotor disturbance is common to all forms of rhinitis, but the term 'vasomotor rhinitis' is used in the present chapter to distinguish non-infective from infective rhinitis, the latter having been discussed in the previous chapter. Hence the classification adopted here is as follows:

Vasomotor rhinitis
- Allergic (Extrinsic) → Seasonal / Perennial
- Non-allergic (Intrinsic) — Perennial

Allergic rhinitis (extrinsic)

Allergic rhinitis arises from altered reactivity to an exogenous antigen (allergen). It is one of the diseases originally included by Coca and Cooke (1923) as part of the atopic state. For clinical purposes, atopic individuals may be identified as those who react to more than one group of allergens in a standard range of allergens used for skin prick tests. Atopy tends to run in families. The risk that the atopy will be associated with clinical disorder, according to different investigators, is shown in *Table 10.1*.

Table 10.1 Proportional risks of children becoming allergic, with allergy in both, one or no parents respectively, and probable age of onset

PARENTAL ALLERGY			
Bilateral	*Unilateral*	*None*	*Reference*
75	50	10–20	(Spain and Cooke, 1924)
60	40	10–20	(Van Arsdel and Motulsky, 1959)
30–40	30	10–20	(Lubs, 1971)
AGE OF ONSET			
5 years	10–12 years	30 years	(Spain and Cooke, 1924)

The age of onset of symptoms can be a guide to the degree of atopy. In one study the proportion of positive skin prick tests was greater in those developing symptoms before the age of ten years (about 91 per cent) than in those developing symptoms later (about 75 per cent between ages 11–30 years, and 30 per cent after the age of 30 years). The individual with an earlier age of onset tended to be hypersensitive to a greater number of allergens than those of late onset (Pepys, 1969).

The major immunoglobulin class responsible for Type 1 (anaphylactic) reactions in man is IgE which is produced in large amounts by allergic (atopic) individuals on exposure to common allergens. IgE attaches firmly to the cell membranes, thus 'sensitizing' the cell. Union of allergens with IgE in its most cell-bound state triggers a series of events which result in mast-cell degranulation. The significant correlation between the concentration of circulating IgE and the number of positive skin reactions to common allergens can be used as an index of 'atopic status'.

Predisposing factors

The airway of subjects with allergic rhinitis is seen often to be hyper-reactive to a series of non-specific stimuli which include ambient air temperature, humidity and pollution. Cold air inhalation stimulates nasal glands and reduces nasal patency. Low indoor humidity is an important cause of nasal symptoms. Sulphur dioxide is a common outdoor air pollutant which not only acts as an irritant but also impairs the mucociliary function of the nose. Inert dust will regularly provoke symptoms in a hyper-reactive mucous membrane as will smoke, fumes and irritant smells.

Allergic inflammatory reactions in the nose will not apparently increase the frequency of acute viral infections, such as common cold and influenza, but marked nasal obstruction will alter the course of the infection and may lead to a sustained purulent rhino-sinusitis. Airway infections, too, may initiate and precipitate perennial rhinitis. The mechanism is unknown, but direct tissue damage, altered receptor responsiveness and immune mechanisms may play a part.

Acetylsalicylic acid can produce severe reactions, probably via a non-immunological mechanism currently thought to be due to an inhibition of prostaglandin E biosynthesis (Szczeklik *et al.*, 1976). Often analgesics, dyes and preservatives in food have a similar effect.

Psychological factors have been thought to play a part in allergic subjects and may act as predisposing factors or exciting factors, or may be the result of the allergic disease, brought on by the long and incapacitating nature of the condition.

Seasonal allergic rhinitis

Seasonal rhinitis is allergy to the pollens of grasses, flowers, trees and shrubs. It affects the nasal mucous membranes. The pharyngeal, conjunctival and bronchial mucous membranes may also be involved.

It commences, as a rule, during the first half of life. On average about 10 per cent of the population suffer from hay fever. Ocular and nasal symptoms are closely associated and in some cases, when these symptoms alone have been troublesome for several years, the picture is further complicated by the development of bronchial symptoms (pollen asthma). For the whole hay fever population, the risk of developing asthma is increased two- to three-fold.

The earliest pollens are the tree pollens in March, April and May and the latest are the weed pollens in August and September. In England, the hay-fever season usually begins about the third week in May and continues until the middle of July. Attacks are most severe on bright still days and least severe in rainy weather when the pollen production is diminished and the grains are washed down from the atmosphere. In the USA, ragweed is the commonest allergen whereas in the British Isles and Northern Europe, it is uncommon.

Clinical features of hay fever

When the allergic subject is exposed to the appropriate pollen, the symptoms of hay fever include nasal irritation and itching, recurrent attacks of paroxysmal sneezing, nasal obstruction and copious watery rhinorrhoea. Frequently there is intense conjunctival irritation and consequently increased lacrimation. Some patients are troubled by itching of the soft palate and others experience 'referred pain' (via the glossopharyngeal nerve) resulting in itching in the ears.

The conjunctivae are red and the eyelids may be swollen. The nasal passages contain clear mucoid secretion and the nasal mucous membrane is congested and varies in colour from exceeding pallor to dull red. Most commonly, it is pale heliotrope or pale purple. The most gentle probing will cause sneezing and further secretion.

Perennial nasal allergy

The causes of perennial allergy are house dust, house-dust mite and moulds. Food allergens, which are often not discovered, are important. The common food allergens are cows' milk proteins, eggs, fermented drinks and citrus fruits. How far food additives, such as trace antibiotics in milk are important, is unknown.

Clinical features of perennial allergy

The diagnosis of perennial allergic rhinitis is commonly made by inference when the perennial rhinitis is found in an atopic subject.

Investigation and management

Case history   In all cases of allergic rhinitis, a careful history must be taken which should include an enquiry about diet, pets, especially cats, fumes and dusts at home and at work, cosmetics and soap powders. Any seasonal influence or association with specific locale, family history of rhinitis, hay fever, asthma or eczema may be relevant.

An assessment of the nature and severity of symptoms is extremely important. Many patients with mild symptoms which interfere neither with work nor play, need no more help than reassurance that there is no serious underlying disease and that spontaneous improvement can occur.

Examination

In addition to the characteristic appearance of the nasal mucosa referred to above, care must be taken to note the presence or absence of ethmoidal polypi, antrochoanal polypi, septal deviations and spurs, pus and hypertrophic mucous membrane.

Special tests
Radiological examination of the sinuses will reveal any thickening of the sinus mucosa or the presence of polyps. These do not as a rule call for special treatment and only rarely require sinus surgery. On the other hand, marked sinus opacity or fluid levels may denote the presence of infection and proof-puncture is advisable in such cases, particularly if purulent secretion is present in the nose.

Specific tests for allergy
(1) Nasal secretions   Eosinophils may constitute 90–100 per cent of the pus cells. Nasal eosinophilia is consistent for patients recently exposed to an actual allergen and is also present in those suffering from nasal polyposis without demonstrable allergy

(2) Blood tests   (a) Peripheral blood eosinophil counts can give information about the size of the 'shock-organ'. If the nose is the only organ affected, the eosinophil count will usually be within normal limits.

(b) Serum IgE concentrations can be measured and used as a research tool but are not necessary in the diagnosis and management of allergic rhinitis. High levels are associated with multiple positive skin tests but again the individual case of allergic rhinitis may have levels within normal limits, particularly if there is no associated asthma.

(3) Skin tests   Because allergens causing skin-test hypersensitivity are not necessarily those causing symptoms and skin hypersensitivity to test allergens is found in symptom-free people, skin tests alone do not play a major role in the management of allergic rhinitis. They do, however, help to confirm the presence of an allergen suspected from the history, and positive tests indicate an atopic subject.

The skin prick test (*Figure 10.1*) is now most commonly used and involves gently raising the skin of the forearm with the point of a disposable needle dipped through solutions of the test allergen and control. The skin should not be prepared with a spirit of cleansing fluid beforehand. The allergens should include grass pollens, house dust, house-dust mite and *A. fumigatus*. Results from food test allergens are generally unhelpful.

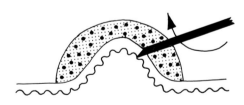

Figure 10.1   The skin prick test is performed by placing a drop of the test extract solution on the unprepared skin and pricking with a slight lifting motion through the drop into the epidermis. (From *Nasal Allergy* by Niels Mygind, by courtesy of the author and Blackwell Scientific Publications)

The immediate positive weal and flare reaction is indicative of a reaction between allergen and IgE-sensitized mast cells. In an early phase of sensitization it is possible to find highly sensitive mucous membranes of the upper and lower respiratory tracts without positive skin tests. It is also not uncommon to find the reverse situation of a patient with positive skin tests in the absence of nasal sensitivity. There is no quantitative correlation between the degree of skin and nasal sensitivities (Taylor and Shivalkar, 1971).

(4) Nasal provocation or nasal challenge tests These tests, which may be either qualitative or quantitative, are of some value in the identification of allergens. Qualitative techniques require application of an aqueous extract of allergen to the nasal mucosa by either glass pipette or aerosol and observation of the reaction by the appearance of the nasal mucous membrane and by the degree of sneezing, nasal irritation, discharge and obstruction. The concentration of test allergen is judged by the severity of the patient's rhinitis prior to nasal challenge testing. Quantitative methods which involve measuring changes in nasal airflow following challenge are purely experimental.

Three different types of response to nasal challenge are recognized. The 'early' response commences within minutes of challenge, lasts approximately 30 min and consists of nasal irritation, sneezing, nasal discharge and obstruction. The 'late' Type III reaction may follow an early reaction ('early' + 'late') or may occur as the sole response. It commences about 4–6 h after challenge and consists of nasal obstruction with minimal irritation and slight nasal discharge which persist for 24 h or longer. Late nasal reactivity is common in patients with allergic rhinitis, particularly in young adults with grass pollen sensitivity and in patients sensitive to house-dust mite.

Because of the possibility of a later reaction only one allergen can be tested at a time and an interval of at least 48 h should elapse between tests. This makes challenge testing difficult and therefore not suitable for routine clinical use.

(5) The radioallergosorbent test (RAST) This is a sensitive *in vitro* method for the assay of reaginic (IgE) antibodies to particular allergens (Wide, Bennick and Johansson, 1967). Reaginic (IgE) antibodies in a serum react with the allergen which is chemically coupled to a solid phase like cellulose which may either be in the form of fine particles or as a paper disc (Wide *et al.*, 1971). The bound reagins are then detected by their ability to bind 125 I-labelled antibodies directed against IgE, and the uptake of labelled antibodies measured in terms of radioactivity on the solid phase is directly correlated with the level of specific reaginic (IgE) antibodies to that particular allergen. The result of RAST can be expressed semiquantitatively in arbitrary units, e.g. sorbent units (SU) or/ml of activity of a laboratory standard serum tested against a particular allergen extract.

Studies on the clinical significance of RAST for diagnosis of atopic or immediate type of hypersensitivity have shown highly significant correlations between RAST and skin tests and nasal provocation tests.

The RAST is a valuable tool in the diagnosis of IgE-mediated allergy but its use is still very much restricted to research projects.

Treatment
Allergy rhinitis may be managed by:

(1) Avoidance Certain allergens can be avoided, for example: pets, feather pillows, and soap powders. The decision must always rest with the patient when the need to remove a favourite pet arises. Young girls keen on riding who develop an allergy to horse dander must make up their own minds. Exclusion from the house-dust allergen is impossible but control of house dust, particularly in the bedroom, may reduce the intensity of exposure to the allergen.

(2) Hyposensitization In the British Isles hyposensitization is accepted for the

management of troublesome hay fever in patients with skin tests confirming grass pollen hypersensitivity. It is unlikely to help in those with perennial symptoms or in those in whom a previous course of injections has failed. No good evidence supports the routine use of hyposensitization in rhinitis due to other allergens. In particular vaccines made up of bacterial flora from the respiratory tract have no place in the treatment of rhinitis.

In practice the methods of hyposensitization using long courses of soluble extracts or slow-release preparations have been largely superseded by alum-precipitated preparations (Alavac-P, Allpyral-G), which necessitate 7–9 injections at weekly or fortnightly intervals.

Hyposensitization is best completed before the end of March or early April and is not recommended for children under the age of six. With all forms of hyposensitization, the possibility of an anaphylactic reaction must be anticipated; therefore, adrenaline 1:1000 intramuscularly, hydrocortisone acetate 100 mg intravenously and an antihistamine intravenously should always be at hand. An antihistamine tablet may be given half an hour before an injection. Reactions to a course of alum-precipitated preparations are not uncommon and are usually in the form of the symptoms of allergic rhinitis which occur within 24 h of injection. Some patients may also experience mild asthma.

Treatment is usually carried out for at least three successive years.

(3) Drugs   (a) Antihistamines. These block the cellular histamine receptors and act as pharmacological histamine antagonists. They are useful in the symptomatic treatment of nasal allergy, particularly in reducing sneezing and rhinorrhoea. Most adults are unable to take enough antihistamine to control severe symptoms without unacceptable drowsiness. Patients should therefore be warned not to drive or operate machinery whilst on antihistamines and to refrain from consuming alcohol which readily potentiates this side effect. Because individuals vary considerably in their susceptibility to the effects of antihistamines it is often worthwhile trying a sequence of drugs, at various dose levels, until a satisfactory regime is achieved.

Antihistamines are often used in association with oral decongestants such as ephedrine, pseudoephedrine and phenylpropanolamine. This combination is justified, as synergism has been demonstrated between antihistamine (pharmacological histamine antagonist) and a sympathomimetic compound (physiological histamine antagonist). The CNS stimulatory effect of the sympathomimetic compound minimizes the sedative effect of the antihistamine in some patients.

(b) Sodium cromoglycate (SCG). Sodium cromoglycate stabilizes the mast cell and blocks the process of degranulation at an early stage following antigen–antibody union at the cell surface. This union is allowed to occur and antibody is used up but without the subsequent mediatory release. It is important, therefore, that SCG is available to the mast cell *at or before* exposure to allergen, as no stabilizing effect can be achieved if it is introduced after degranulation has occurred.

SCG can control both seasonal and perennial allergic rhinitis. Therapy initiated about one week before the start of the pollen season and continued throughout the season in regular dosage is a regime virtually free of side effects and is helpful in about 70 per cent of subjects. SCG is presented either as Rynacrom powder insufflation (10 mg SCG/nostril, four times daily), Rynacrom nasal drops or spray (two drops or two sprays in each nostril six times daily), Lomusol nasal solution in a metered dose nasal spray (one dose in each nostril six times daily) or as 2 per cent eye drops (Opticrom one or two drops in each eye four times daily). Where nasal blockage is the predominant symptom an aqueous spray gives a better distribution of the drug than powder insufflation. For all cases therapy should be continuous and evenly spread in order to achieve full protection.

(c) Corticosteroids. Systemic corticosteroids, given either as oral prednisolone tablets or by depot injections, have been largely replaced by topical corticosteroid preparations in the treatment of allergic rhinitis. There are occasional instances (for example, in patients with seasonal allergic rhinitis who are sitting examinations) where systemic therapy may be justifiable.

Where symptoms of allergic rhinitis are troublesome a *topical* corticosteroid may be used either as the first choice of drug or where sodium cromoglycate has failed.

Beclomethasone dipropionate (Beconase) is a synthetic steroid with a high anti-inflammatory activity 5000 times stronger than hydrocortisone. *In vivo* there is a rapid enzymatic degradation to the less active beclomethasone monopropionate and inactive beclomethasone. The drug is administered by a standard metered aerosol which delivers 50 µg of beclomethasone/puff. Delivery of the drug should be synchronized with a powerful sniff. To achieve an even distribution of the material it is recommended that the canister is held in the sagittal plane and that one puff is applied to the upper and another to the lower part of the nose.

Brown, Storey and Jackson (1977), reviewing five years' experience of beclomethasone dipropionate in the treatment of perennial and seasonal allergic rhinitis, found no evidence of side effects (with the exception of occasional slight nasal bleeding) either clinically or on nasal biopsy. Bacterial infection was not enhanced and there was no evidence of nasal candidiasis. Nasal mucosal biopsies taken from patients treated with beclomethasone dipropionate for one year and examined by scanning electron microscope (Mygind, 1977) showed no evidence of squamous cell metaplasia or atrophic rhinitis (*Figure 10.2*).

Nasal hay fever symptoms can be controlled in most patients, adults as well as children over the age of eight years, by 200–400 µg beclomethasone dipropionate in divided doses daily. Simultaneous treatment of eye symptoms and pollen asthma is necessary. At least two-thirds of patients with perennial allergic rhinitis will benefit from treatment. Beclomethasone dipropionate aerosol does not act immediately and must be used regularly throughout the day to achieve 24 h of relief of symptoms.

Non-allergic rhinitis (intrinsic)

The term 'vasomotor rhinitis' has been applied to forms of non-allergic rhinitis but as all rhinitis is a vasomotor disturbance, the term is not particularly helpful. Non-allergic rhinitis may be diagnosed if an allergic cause for the patient's symptoms cannot be found by skin or nasal challenge tests.

A review of the vascularization and innervation of the nasal mucosa and the mechanism of the nasal cycle is helpful at this stage in the description of non-allergic rhinitis.

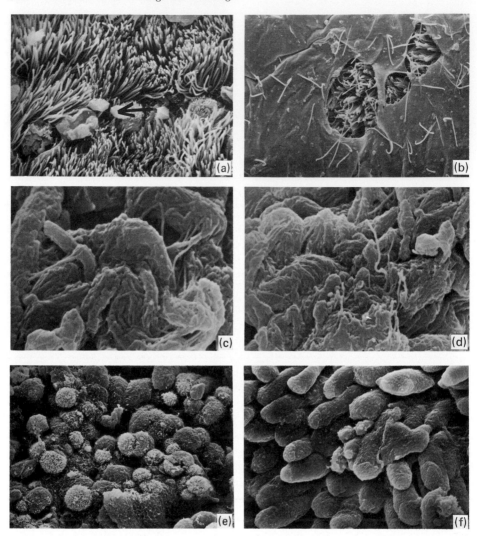

Figure 10.2   Scanning electron microscopy of nasal mucosa. (a) × 4000—Normal mucosa showing a confluent cilial field with mucus emerging from gland mouths. Note (arrowed) cocaine crystals used incidentally in preparation of the nose. (b) × 4000—Normal mucous blanket with cilia seen beneath. (c) and (d) × 5000—Allergic rhinitis showing tangled and matted cilia. (e) × 4000—Atrophic rhinitis. Epithelial cells without cilia showing microcilli and cell disintegration. (f) × 5000—Atrophic rhinitis. Individual cells being shed from closed packed array of cells. (Scanning micrographs by courtesy of Professor Noel Dilly, St. George's Medical School, and Mr Roger Gray, FRCS, St. Mary's Hospital, London)

Vascularization and innervation of nasal mucosa

The principal arterial supply to the nose is from the spheno–palatine artery (which arises from the maxillary artery) and the anterior and posterior ethmoid arteries which supply the top part of the nose including the olfactory region. Venous drainage is by means of veins following the arteries. Electron microscopic studies of nasal mucosa taken from the turbinates show pronounced fenestration of the endothelial layers of the capillaries and corresponding porosity of the surrounding basal membrane which is adjacent to the ciliated mucous membrane (Stoksted and Khan, 1976). It is thought that this vast network of fenestrated capilliaries provides the moisture of the nose. Most of the blood in the capillary area flows from the arterial to the venous side through the metarteriole which acts as a bypass and feeds the capillary bed only when humoral effects (e.g. by the influence of histamine) cause relaxation of the pre-capillary sphincter, resulting in flooding of the capillary bed, slowing of circulation, hypoxia and accumulation of oedema fluid. This control is normally autonomous and depends upon local metabolic requirements. The transitional erectile cavernous tissue in the turbinates allows combinations of changes in the mucosal temperature and its volume.

Sensation of the nasal mucous membrane is derived from the trigeminal nerve via the ophthalmic and maxillary nerves. The anterior ethmoidal nerve arises from the former and the spheno–palatine nerves from the latter.

The vasomotor nerve supply is derived from the autonomic nervous system. The sympathetic pre-ganglionic branches arise from the first and second thoracic segments of the spinal cord. Post-ganglionic fibres pass from the superior cervical ganglion to the plexus around the internal carotid artery and then via the deep petrosal nerve and the nerve to the pterygoid canal (Vidian nerve) to the spheno–palatine ganglion where they continue without synapsing to the turbinates. Pre-ganglionic parasym-pathetic fibres from the superior salivatory nucleus pass in the facial nerve through the geniculate ganglion and along the greater superficial petrosal nerve where they join the deep petrosal nerve and continue, as the nerve of the pterygoid canal, to the spheno–palatine ganglion where they synapse. Post-ganglionic secreto–motor fibres continue to the nasal mucosa.

Resection or local anaesthetic block of the cervical sympathetic ganglion is followed by ipsilateral hyperaemia, swelling and hypersecretion of the nasal mucosa. Resection of the parasympathetic innervation results in a shrunken, pale mucous membrane and excessive drying followed by crusting. Resection of the nerve of the pterygoid canal, containing both sympathetic and parasympathetic fibres results in a predominant reduction of parasympathetic activity. The exact termination of the nerve fibres is not completely known. The erectile vessels have a very rich innervation, such that each smooth muscle fibre would seem to receive its own innervation.

How the autonomic outflow is regulated is not known with certainty, though it is probable that the hypothalamus may act as an integrating centre receiving numerous afferent impulses including emotional stimuli from higher centres. Normally, the vasomotor balance may be temporarily disturbed by such factors as circulating catecholamines, emotion, posture, exercise and change of external temperature or humidity but as a rule without any feeling of discomfort. It is probable, however, that in some individuals suffering from non-allergic rhinitis the mechanism of control is hyperactive and the balance tends to be disturbed in favour of increased parasympathetic activity. Psychogenic stimuli, endocrine factors and some drugs may influence the balance in quantities which induce only small changes in unaffected subjects.

The nasal cycle

The alternating changes in patency of the two nasal cavities whereby the ability to breathe through the nose remains normal is called the nasal cycle. Each cycle varies from 30 min to about 5 h and is present in 80 per cent of normal people whilst in an upright position. The effect of posture is to cause an alteration in swelling of the erectile tissues of the nasal chambers due to changes in gravity. Damp and cold atmospheres bring about the greatest swelling of the turbinates, dry warm air a little less, while optimal atmospheric conditions (humidity 50–60 per cent, temperature 13–18 °C) cause cycles of the least degree. The cycle's activity is maximal during adolescence (due to hormonal activity) and decreases with increasing age. Vasoconstriction of sympathetic reaction occurs in sudden fright situations (emotional influences), and vasodilatation of parasympathetic reaction in anxiety situations.

Vasoconstrictive drops may cause the nasal cycle to stop and to resume again when the drops are withdrawn. The rebound effect of nose drops, a period of nasal stuffiness after the vasoconstriction phase, is due to the resumption of cyclic activity.

Factors contributing to non-allergic rhinitis

Drugs
(1) Drugs acting on the sympathetic nervous system   Nasal stuffiness can result from antihypertensives such as guanethidine (Ismelin) and bretylium tosylate (Bretylate) acting as alpha adrenergic blocking agents, and from antihypertensives such as reserpine (Serpasil) and methyldopa (Aldomet) which deplete sympathetic nerve endings of their catecholamine stores (Ariens, 1967). If the blood pressure, however, is to be satisfactorily controlled nasal stuffiness may be a small price to pay. Sympathomimetic agents, such as ephedrine, which act by releasing noradrenaline from sympathetic nerve endings will be less effective than usual in the presence of antihypertensive drugs.

Sympathetic blocking agents causing peripheral vasodilatation which may be used in the treatment of peripheral vascular disease and migraine, such as the ergot alkaloids, e.g. dihydroergotamine mesylate (Dihydergot), can cause nasal stuffiness.

(2) Topical vasoconstrictors   Disturbance of the normal vasomotor response in nasal mucous membrane is aggravated by frequent and continued use of vasoconstrictor preparations locally in the form of drops or sprays. The most notorious preparation is naphazoline (Nomaze, Antistin–Privine) a potent sympathomimetic vasoconstrictor. They all cause after-congestion by rebound vasodilatation which, with the attendant return of obstruction, results in the drug being taken again, thus perpetrating the symptom and eventually leading to irreversible changes in the vasomotor structure and mucous membranes. This state is called '*rhinitis medicamentosa*'.

The long-term use of these potent vasoconstrictor drugs is therefore not recommended. Care should also be taken to ensure that they are not used in patients who are receiving monoamine oxidase inhibitors (MAOIs) concurrently.

(3) Anticholinesterases   Drugs such as neostigmine, used in the treatment of myasthenia gravis, which inhibit cholinesterase and potentiate the action of acetylcholine, produce nasal obstruction.

Physical
Certain physical agents such as draughts of cold air, irritating smokes and vapours, and extremes of temperature and humidity can evoke a non-allergic rhinitis. Most

individuals would consider this response to be a normal transient physiological mechanism; however in susceptible subjects with hypersensitive noses the disturbance may be profound and lasting.

Endocrine
Nasal stuffiness may be a consequence of pregnancy or of some of the earlier types of high oestrogen contraceptive pill.

Psychogenic   The relationship between stress and the onset and course of non-allergic rhinitis has been instigated and proposed by many workers (O'Neill and Malcomson, 1954; Linford Rees, 1964; Holmes *et al.*, 1950). Precipitating causes may include emotional factors such as anxiety, tension, anger, hostility, humiliation, resentment, indignation, grief or even pleasurable excitement. However, there is a large subjective element involved in the assessment of this contributory factor and often insufficient controlled evidence.

Clinical picture

The variety of symptomology in this condition is legion. Patients tend to fall into one of two categories: those whose main complaint is that of nasal obstruction and those whose main troublesome symptom is excessive rhinorrhoea. However, these symptoms may alternate or coexist. The condition is usually perennial and can, like allergic rhinitis, make life extremely uncomfortable.

Nasal obstruction in some patients may be worse when they wake up and clear as the day proceeds and in others may prevent sleep by being worse at night.

Climate has a variable effect. The majority of patients respond well to low humidity and high altitude, the alpine climate being ideal. On the other hand some patients seem to prefer a maritime environment and high humidity. Many noses become blocked in stuffy, centrally heated rooms and some respond badly to cold.

Patients frequently complain that their nasal obstruction alternates from side to side. This is because the normal physiological cycle of alternating vasoconstriction and dilatation is now superimposed on a basically inadequate airway and has therefore become apparent to them.

Excessive rhinorrhoea often associated with paroxysmal sneezing is a manifestation of nasal vasomotor instability which occurs much more commonly in females in the second, third and fourth decades. The symptoms may be constant or liable to exacerbations which are almost indistinguishable from allergic attacks. However, the conjunctivae are seldom affected as in allergy, and provided a full history is taken and careful investigations made, allergy can be excluded. As a rule the patients with excessive watery rhinorrhoea are psychologically unstable and are undoubtedly more resistant to treatment than those whose main complaint is obstruction and in whom rhinorrhoea does not largely figure. They often carry with them a box of tissues, one of which is applied to the nose at frequent intervals throughout the history-taking and examination.

Post-nasal drip is a common complaint and examination only too often reveals a perfect nasopharynx apparently completely devoid of excessive secretion.

Atypical facial neuralgias, headaches, malaise and undue fatigue are not uncommon and occur frequently in association with migraine, migrainous neuralgia and non-allergic rhinitis. Migraine may be misinterpreted as 'sinusitis'.

Examination

On clinical examination the findings are variable. In the predominantly obstructive cases the turbinates are usually enlarged, sometimes enormously. They vary in colour from very pale pink to deep dusky red and their surface contour may be smooth or morulated.

In longstanding cases the condition of *chronic hypertrophic rhinitis* may be present. In this condition, which may also result from chronic nasal allergy or infection, the mucosa of the turbinates is commonly mulberry-like in appearance. A time-honoured diagnostic test is to apply local vasoconstrictors, when minimal shrinkage denotes the presence of excessive fibrous tissue. Good shrinkage suggests a pseudo-hypertrophy due to chronic vascular engorgement and often indicates that a good result may be achieved with submucous diathermy.

Attention must be drawn to that variety of hypertrophic change which affects only the posterior ends of the inferior turbinates. This is often seen in young people and may in fact be entirely responsible for their complaint of nasal obstruction. No abnormality may be obvious on anterior rhinoscopy but careful posterior rhinoscopy is called for and may reveal in each choana a huge whitish mass resembling a pale mulberry. If clinical posterior rhinoscopy is unrewarding, examination of the nasopharynx under general anaesthetic using a large post-nasal or laryngeal mirror and a palate retractor is advocated. The patient is examined thus in the 'tonsil position' and an excellent view of the nasopharynx and posterior ends of the turbinates can be guaranteed. These cases are often missed on account of inadequate examination and unrewarding nasal surgery has been performed.

Nasal polypi may be present and add to the general picture of obstruction and increased nasal secretion.

In the cases whose predominant symptom is excessive watery rhinorrhoea the clinical appearances are often distinctive. There may be no hypertrophy of the turbinates; indeed in some cases the airways may be so unobstructed that the posterior nasopharyngeal wall may be seen via the anterior nares. The mucous membrane is usually pale and fairly smooth but invariably thoroughly wet, and in the worst cases excessive secretion may be seen in the nose and nasopharynx.

Differential diagnosis

Nasal allergy must be excluded in all cases by a careful history, skin sensitivity testing and if necessary nasal challenge tests.

Sinus infection has also to be excluded by examination of the nasal passages for purulent material, by radiological examination of the sinuses and, if necessary, by antral lavage.

A word of warning is necessary in connection with the radiological appearances of the sinuses in non-allergic rhinitis. Thickening (sometimes polypoidal) of the lining mucosa of the maxillary antra is frequently present, and is often taken by the inexperienced to indicate the presence of infection. If there is any doubt proof-puncture should be carried out but in the great majority of these cases the effluent is clear.

Management

The management of any case of non-allergic rhinitis depends on a number of factors and will vary from case to case according to the pattern and severity of symptoms. It is therefore advisable to make an attempt to classify each case by selecting the predominant symptoms, and by assessing the degree of incapacity or discomfort caused, and treating accordingly. As a general rule, medical management with drugs is preferred in the first instance.

Medical
Antihistamines are valuable in the treatment of non-allergic rhinitis but the side effect of sedation is often severe enough to warrant withdrawal of the drug. Therefore they are often used in association with *oral decongestants* such as ephedrine, pseudoephedrine and phenylpropanolamine in patients with sneezing, rhinorrhoea and nasal blockage. This constitutes a combination of an antihistamine (pharmacological histamine antagonist) and a sympathomimetic compound (physiological histamine antagonist), but the prolonged use of such combinations in a chronic condition should be avoided.

Severe rhinorrhoea may be treated with antihistamines acting by virtue of their anticholinergic side effects such as deptropine (Brontina) or by imipramine (Tofranil).

Intranasal *topical corticosteroids* such as beclomethasone dipropionate (Beconase) applied as an aerosol twice daily in doses between 100–200 µg/day have been shown to be of value in non-allergic rhinitis. The dose may need to be increased to 400 µg/day but the results of treatment should not be assessed until a whole aerosol (four weeks) has been used as the full effect of beclomethasone dipropionate is not apparent in less than two weeks.

Surgical
Those cases not responding to medical management may be offered surgery. Although the surgical procedures to be described below may have good results in selected cases, there is, as yet, insufficient controlled evidence with follow-up to hold promise that they are necessarily helpful in the long run.

Each case must be treated on its own merits and it is often found that attention to both septum and turbinates is necessary to produce a satisfactory result.

Submucosal diathermy of the inferior turbinates has been described in detail by Simpson and Groves (1958) who use a unipolar electrode with a tip resembling a rather large myringotome: the shank and handle of the instrument are encased in insulating material. An indifferent electrode is applied to the patient's leg and the electrode tip is pushed into the most prominent part of the anterior end of the inferior turbinate. It is then passed along almost the entire length of the turbinate submucosally keeping close to the medial surface of the bone. Withdrawal takes 10–20 s and it is during this phase that the circuit is closed and the coagulating current applied.

Some surgeons prefer to apply the diathermy needle to the surface of the turbinates but this is clearly more damaging to the mucosal epithelium and results in excessive and prolonged crusting.

Cryosurgery to the inferior turbinates has been found to give a sharply circumscribed fibrosis with little or no inflammatory reaction of surrounding tissues over a period of four to eight weeks. There is an improvement in nasal obstruction but often no change in rhinorrhoea and sneezing (Ozenberger, 1970 and 1973).

Surgical reduction of the turbinates is necessary when chronic hypertrophy is present and is particularly relevant to those cases in which obstruction is caused by enormously enlarged, morular posterior ends of the inferior turbinates. In such cases it is usually necessary to use Struycken's turbinectomy scissors which are applied to the lower border of the inferior turbinate about two-thirds of the distance from the anterior to the posterior extremities. They are then used to divide the turbinate along a postero–superior line (at 30–45 degrees to the horizontal) as far as its attachment, the severance of the posterior mulberry-like portion being completed with the aid of a cutting nasal polypectomy snare. In other cases fibrous polypoidal fringes must be removed by turbinectomy scissors from both inferior and middle turbinates, or simple ethmoidal polypi may require attention. Lateral fracture of the inferior turbinates is often a useful procedure and on some occasions this manoeuvre together with minimal diathermy may be all that is required to restore a satisfactory airway.

Care should be taken not to remove too much of the mucosal covering of the turbinates or an atrophic condition of the remaining mucosa with continued crusting may result. Knowing exactly how much to remove is largely a matter of experience but it is wise to err on the side of conservation. Further surgical attention at a later date is a lesser evil than atrophic rhinitis.

When multiple procedures such as submucous resection of the septum, or septoplasty, diathermy and trimming of the turbinates and polypectomy are carried out, the problem of the post-operative formation of adhesions is ever present. It is undeniable that if gentleness and skill are exercised in handling the intranasal structures the danger of adhesion formation is reduced to a minimum; nevertheless adhesions do form in some cases however much care is taken. They may be prevented by inserting nasal splints at the end of the operation between the turbinates and the nasal septum. The author favours splints made of 'Dacron Silastic' (*Figure 10.3*) which can be removed simply and painlessly some 6–8 days post-operatively. Nasal packing with tulle gras or glove fingers may be inserted between the turbinates and the splints, and removed in 24 h.

Submucosal diathermy, though of great value in cases where the predominant symptom is nasal obstruction, is likely to be extremely disappointing in cases of excessive watery rhinorrhoea. The patients, if psychiatrically stable and uncontrolled by medical means, are the most suitable candidates for division of the nerve of the pterygoid canal (Vidian neurectomy). The nerve contains predominantly parasympathetic fibres but is not the only source of these fibres to the nose. Access to the nerve by the trans-maxillary approach was described by Golding-Wood in 1961. Variations of the approach which have since been recommended are the transpalatal (Ranger, 1970), and the trans-septal (Minnis and Morrison, 1971).

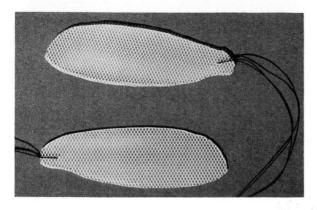

Figure   10.3   Dacron-Silastic
nasal splints

The maxillary antrum is opened as for a Caldwell–Luc operation, and its posterior wall removed. The operating microscope is then employed and the internal maxillary artery and its branches are secured by extra large Cushing type clips. The maxillary nerve is defined and traced to the foramen rotundum—the *essential landmark* of the operation. A more or less vertical bony ridge is found several millimetres medially and the medial face of this ridge leads backward to the anterior funnelled mouth of the pterygoid (Vidian) canal. After severance of the Vidian nerve and careful retraction of the spheno–palatine fibres a guarded flexible probe is inserted into the opening of the pterygoid canal and coagulation diathermy is applied.

Complications of Vidian neurectomy include recurrence of symptoms after initial improvement, diplopia, anaesthesia of the palate or infraorbital regions, impairment of lacrimation, blindness, infraorbital neuralgia and sinusitis.

Golding-Wood (1973) claims that up to 90 per cent of patients are completely relieved by the operation and that this effect is maintained in 95 per cent of these for 5–12 years. However, no controlled long-term studies exist, and the operation is best left to those few surgeons who have special experience of it. Until long-term controlled studies have been carried out, and its safety and efficacy established, it should be avoided by others.

References

For an extensive review of the subject matter of this chapter the following book is highly recommended:
Mygind, N. (1978). *Nasal Allergy.* Oxford: Blackwell Scientific Publications

Ariens, E. J. (1967). 'Drugs and rhinitis', *International Rhinology*, **5**, 138
Brown, H. Morrow, Story, G. and Jackson, F. A. (1977). 'Beclomethasone dipropionate aerosol in treatment of perennial and seasonal rhinitis: a review of five years' experience', *British Journal of Clinical Pharmacology*, **4** (Suppl. 3) 283
Coca, A. F. and Cooke, R. A. (1923). 'On the classification of the phenomenon of hypersensitiveness', *Journal of Immunology*, **8**, 163

Golding-Wood, P. H. (1961). 'Observations on petrosal and Vidian neurectomy in chronic vasomotor rhinitis', *Journal of Laryngology*, **75**, 232
Golding-Wood, P. H. (1973). 'Vidian neurectomy: its results and complications', *Laryngoscope (St. Louis)*, **83**, 1673
Holmes, T. H., Goodell, H., Wolf, S. and Wolff, H. G. (1950). *The nose.* Springfield. Ill.; Thomas
Lubs, M. L. E. (1971). 'Allergy in 7000 twin pairs', *Acta allergica, (Kbh)*, **26**, 249
Minnis, N. L. and Morrison, A. W. (1971). 'Transseptal approach for Vidian neurectomy', *Journal of Laryngology*, **85**, 255
Mygind, N. (1977). 'Effects of beclomethasone dipropionate aerosol on nasal mucosa', *British Journal of clinical Pharmacology*, **4** (Suppl. 3), 287
O'Neill, D. and Malcomson, K. (1954). 'Results of

treatment of chronic vasomotor rhinitis', *British medical Journal*, **1**, 554

Ozenberger, J. M. (1970). 'Cryosurgery in chronic rhinitis', *Laryngoscope (St. Louis)*, **80**, 723

Ozenberger, J. M. (1973). 'Cryosurgery for the treatment of chronic rhinitis', *Laryngoscope (St. Louis)*, **83**, 508

Pepys, J. (1969). *Hypersensitivity diseases of the lungs due to fungi and organic dusts*. Basel; Karger

Ranger, D. (1970). Personal communication

Rees, L. (1964). 'Physiogenic and psychogenic factors in vasomotor rhinitis', *Journal of psychosomatic Research*, **8**, 101

Simpson, J. F. and Groves, J. (1958). 'Submucosal diathermy of the inferior turbinate', *Journal of Laryngology*, **72**, 292

Spain, W. C and Cooke, R. A. (1924). 'Studies in specific hypersensitiveness', *Journal of Immunology*, **9**, 521

Stoksted, P. and Khan, M. A. (1976). 'Air conditioning function'. Chapter 36 in *Scientific Foundations of Otolaryngology*. Ed. by Ronald Hinchcliffe and Donald Harrison. London; William Heinemann Medical Books

Szczeklik, A., Gryglewski, R. J., Czerniawska-Mysik, G and Zmuda, A. (1976). 'Aspirin-induced asthma', *Journal of Allergy and Clinical Immunology*, **58**, 10

Taylor, G. and Shivalkar, P. R. (1971). 'Disodium cromoglycate: laboratory studies and clinical trial in allergic rhinitis' *Clinical Allergy*, **1**, 189

Van Arsdel, P. P. and Motulsky, A. G. (1959). 'Frequency and hereditability of asthma and allergic rhinitis in college students', *Acta genetica (Basel)*, **9**, 101

Wide, L., Bennick, H. and Johansson, S. G. O. (1967). 'Diagnosis of allergy by an *in vitro* test for allergen antibodies', *Lancet*, **2**, 1105

Wide, L. Aronsson, T., Fagerberg, E. and Zetterström, O. (1971). 'Radioimmunoassay of allergen specific IgE'. (Proceedings of the VIII European Congress of Allergology.) *Excerpta medica*, **235**, 85

11 Nasal polyposis

John Ballantyne

Simple nasal polypi—and the vast majority of nasal polypi *are* 'simple'—are pedunculated pieces of oedematous upper respiratory mucosa. They can arise from any part of the nasal and/or sinus mucosa, and very often they are bilateral; their commonest site of origin is in the ethmoidal labyrinths, and they tend also to be multiple. Much less commonly they begin in one or other antrum, entering the nasal cavity posteriorly through its ostium, and passing backwards through the posterior choana on the affected side (for these are usually unilateral) to become an antro–choanal polypus.

In either event, the mechanism of formation is essentially the same.

Pathogenesis of polyposis

Polyposis of the respiratory mucosa may result either from vascular derangements in the mucosa or, less commonly, from mechanical obstruction.

Vascular changes are induced by vasomotor instability and most commonly they affect the region of the middle meatus (*Figure 11.1 a*). At first there appears to be an area of simple oedema (*Figure 11.1b*); then, as the stroma becomes filled with intercellular fluid, the oedematous mucosa becomes polypoid (*Figure 11.1c*); and if not arrested at this stage, it enlarges to come down into the nasal cavity, at the same time acquiring a pedicle (*Figure 11.1d*). This is now a polypus.

Lindsay Gray (1967) believes that Bernouilli's phenomenon may also play a part in the production of nasal polypi. Bernouilli's theorem postulates that, when gases or fluids pass through a constricted area, a negative pressure may develop in the vicinity of the constriction; and Gray contends that the lowered pressure at the constriction may reduce the extravascular fluid pressure in the surrounding tissues, thus leading to an increased formation of tissue fluid.

Chandra and Abrol (1974) studied the concentrations of various immunoglobulins, in both serum and nasal polypus fluid, in patients with nasal polypi; and they calculated the amounts which may have been produced locally. There was a significant elevation of all serum immunoglobulins, and IgA and IgE were present in

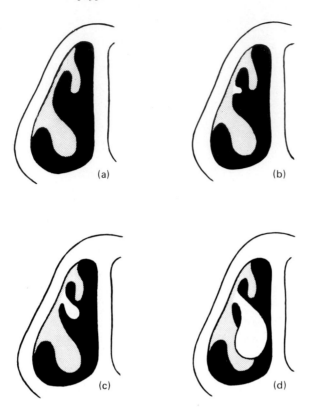

Figure 11.1   Pathogenesis of polyposis (see text)

greater amounts in the polypus fluids than would have been expected from passive infiltration due to increased vascular permeability. They concluded that 'allergic' processes acting locally on the nasal mucosa, combined or associated with infection, were probably significant factors in the genesis of nasal polypi.

The precise role of infection in the development of nasal polypi is uncertain, but there is no doubt that infection in the nose and/or sinuses commonly co-exists with polyposis.

Pathology of nasal polypi

To the naked eye simple nasal polypi appear as soft, smooth masses, varying somewhat in colour—sometimes translucent, sometimes white and opaque, at other times yellowish or pink, and occasionally fleshy.

Microscopically there is an oedematous hypertrophy of the submucosa, with intercellular serous fluid spaces in a fibrillar stroma, and infiltration with eosinophils and round cells (*Figure 11.2*). Chandra and Abrol (1974) found a significant relationship between the eosinophilic infiltration of nasal polypi and local IgE production.

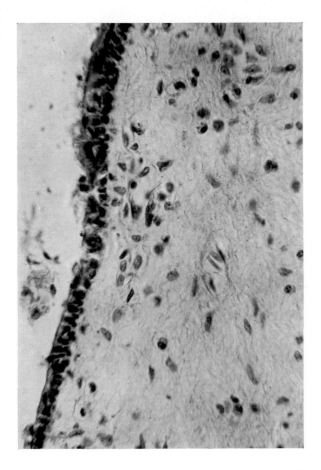

Figure 11.2 Nasal polypus, showing oedema with eosinophil and round cell infiltration. (× 400)

In its early stages, the surface of a simple nasal polypus is covered with ciliated columnar epithelium, but exposure to air currents may lead to transitional, or later to squamous, metaplasia.

Nasal polyposis may occur in mucoviscidosis (cystic fibrosis), and Schwachman and his colleagues (1962) reported 50 cases of polyposis in 742 cases of cystic fibrosis. Despons and Stoller (1965) suggested that there may be some enhancement of the allergic response in this condition, which should be suspected in any case of nasal polyposis in childhood (Toma and Stein, 1968).

Rhinosporidiosis, an infection due to a sporozoon, *Rh. kinealyi* or *Rh. seeberi*, may present as a friable bleeding polypus resembling a strawberry; but the so-called 'bleeding polypus of the septum' is in fact not a polypus, but rather a benign capillary fibroangioma, with grossly distended cavernous vessels and varying amounts of connective tissue. These are probably hamartomas.

Meningocoeles and a wide variety of neoplasms, both benign and malignant, may present as polypoid masses, and they must always be borne in mind when undertaking the surgical removal of nasal 'polypi'.

Polypoid tumours include gliomas, especially in infants, as well as fibromas, neurofibromas, meningiomas, transitional-cell or squamous-cell papillomas, and a variety of malignant tumours—carcinomatous, sarcomatous or (very rarely) melanotic.

There is no characteristic macroscopic appearance to any of these tumours, and diagnosis depends upon histopathological examination.

Clinical features of nasal polyposis

The predominant symptom of nasal polyposis is obstruction, and characteristically it is 'valvular' in nature; in the early stages at least the patient finds it less difficult to breathe in than to breathe out, expiration closing the 'flap valve'.

Hyposmia and anosmia are common, but these may occur in cases of vasomotor rhinitis without obstruction, and they are probably caused by the underlying 'allergic' diathesis as much as by the obstruction.

Rhinorrhoea is often, surprisingly, minimal or absent, and sneezing is not generally troublesome.

The obstruction tends to progress gradually, but it may be suddenly exacerbated by a head cold or by an acute 'allergic' episode. Asthma is not uncommon in patients with nasal polypi, and the condition is often made worse by their development. Chronic infection in the antra and other sinuses frequently accompanies or complicates polyposis, and severe headaches may occur with acute upper respiratory infections.

Epistaxis and orbital symptoms should always arouse suspicions of neoplasia.

When polypi arise from the ethmoidal air-cells, as most of them do, varying numbers of them will be seen on anterior rhinoscopy. Most commonly they are seen in the middle meatus, but they occur also on the medial surface of the middle turbinate, and occasionally they protrude through the anterior nares, with general broadening of the nose (*Figure 11.3*). After being exposed to the continual drying action of air, the presenting surface darkens as a result of metaplastic change.

Ethmoidal polypi can occur at any age, but antro–choanal polypi occur most commonly in the second decade of life. Again the presenting symptom is obstruction, but no abnormality may be seen on anterior rhinoscopy.

Posterior rhinoscopy, however, will reveal a single polypus, which is sometimes so large that it can be seen through the open mouth, hanging down behind the soft palate or pushing it forwards. Reynolds and Groves (1956) have classified choanal polypi into three types: a solitary polypus arising from the antrum; a solitary polypus arising from other sinuses; and a choanal polypus which is merely the hindmost of multiple ethmoidal polypi.

When purulent sinusitis complicates or co-exists with nasal polypi, mucopus will usually be seen in the nose or nasopharynx.

In older patients, the rhinologist must ever be mindful of the possibility of a malignant neoplasm, especially when the 'polypus' is red and fleshy, and bleeds readily on touch; in children or other young patients, a single 'polypus' must be treated with great circumspection, for a meningocoele may enter the nasal cavity through the cribriform plate and thus be mistaken for a simple polypus. Before attempting to remove such a swelling, the surgeon is well advised to puncture it with a needle under sterile conditions, and to submit any clear fluid aspirated to analysis for possible cerebrospinal fluid content.

Any suspicious-looking polypus, especially when unilateral, should be submitted to histopathological examination.

Radiological findings

In the occipito–frontal sinus view, there may be a well-defined soft-tissue shadow in the affected nasal cavity or cavities; in the occipito–mental view, there is nearly always a thickening of the lining mucosa of the antra and, if infection is present, there will be a fluid level or total opacity in the affected antrum. Bony thinning, expansion or erosion is, of course, always suggestive of neoplasia.

With an antro–choanal polypus, the affected antrum is usually opaque, and in the lateral soft-tissue view there is often a radiolucent curvilinear zone between the roof of the nasopharynx and the nasopharyngeal aspect of the polypus (Dodd and Jing, 1977); this radiolucent area is absent in choanal polypi not of antral origin (Reynolds and Groves, 1956).

The treatment of nasal polypi

Several years ago a rotund middle-aged woman was admitted to hospital for the removal of polypi which completely obliterated both nasal cavities, but a severe

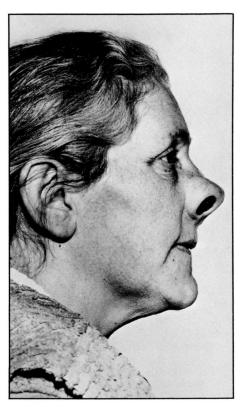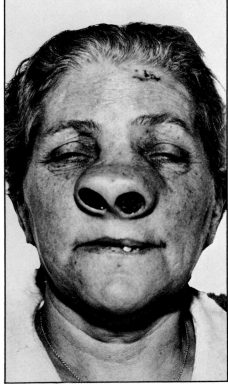

Figure 11.3 Polypi projecting from anterior nares, with metaplastic change and general broadening of nose. (Case of Mr John Groves)

exacerbation of asthma made her unfit for general anaesthesia. In order to prepare her for surgery, a chest physician treated her asthma with systemic steroids. Two weeks later, when she was deemed to be fit, the polypi had totally disappeared.

This brief history is related to emphasize two important points: in the first place, it confirms the nature of simple 'mucous' polypi; secondly it underlines the fact that, although surgery is necessary in most cases, conservative treatment plays an essential part in the management of any patient with nasal polypi, and on occasion may alone suffice.

In the early stages in the pathogenesis of polyposis, when the mucosa is simply oedematous or 'polypoid' (*see Figure 11.1b* and *c*), but before there are any fully-formed polypi with pedicles, the process may be reversed by the regular use of antihistamines; and in many instances these will also restore the sense of smell, so often diminished in such cases even in the absence of gross mechanical obstruction.

When the antihistamines fail to arrest progression, one may sometimes be justified in prescribing a short course of systemic steroid, in small and gradually diminishing dosage. Such a course of treatment is never to be embarked upon lightly, for no steroid is without potential hazard, and it is essential in all cases to exclude any of the recognized contraindications—in particular, hypertension and coronary artery disease; diabetes; pulmonary tuberculosis; pregnancy; and peptic ulceration. Nevertheless, provided that due caution is exercised, systemic steroids in low dosage may be extremely helpful in selected cases, especially when polypi have already been removed on one or more occasions and recurrence threatens once again. It is, not suggested that steroids should be used as a first line of treatment, save on those rare occasions when they are indicated for such co-existing conditions as severe asthma, or for those patients who are exceptionally intolerant of the undesirable side effects of antihistamines.

Betamethasone (Betnesol) has proved to be a useful preparation, and the following oral regime is recommended: 0.5 mg thrice daily for three days; followed by 0.25 mg thrice daily for three days; followed by 0.25 mg twice daily for three days; and finally 0.25 mg daily for three days. During the last three days, the steroid is supplemented by an antihistamine, which should then be continued indefinitely.

The topical use of antihistamines and steroids—by drops, sprays, or injection into the polypi—is not generally successful; and when simple treatment with systemic antihistamines or (rarely) steroids has failed, or when polypi are so large or so numerous as to make it extremely unlikely that relief will be obtained from such conservative measures, then surgery is indicated.

If there are only one or two polypi, and if they are large and have well-developed pedicles, they may be removed with a cold-wire snare, under local or general anaesthesia. Two types (*Figure 11.4*) are in common use: Krause's snare, in which the wire retracts fully into the sheath and therefore cuts across the pedicle; and Glegg's snare, in which the wire is pulled back on to the solid distal extremity of the snare, thus allowing the polypus to be grasped and avulsed.

However, nasal polypi are usually multiple, and in the great majority of cases satisfactory results can only be obtained by removing, through the nose, every polypus and every visible trace of polypoid mucosa, quite meticulously, under general anaesthesia, after careful preparation of the nose. This pre-operative preparation is preferably done on the operating table, after the patient has been anaesthetized, by applying a cocaine–adrenaline 'paste' on a pledget of cotton wool, thoroughly but

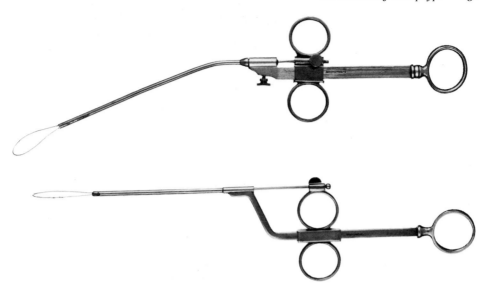

Figure 11.4   Nasal snares: above, Krause's; below, Glegg's

gently, to every accessible area in the nose (Ballantyne, 1973). This is a vitally important part of the operation and, if it is done carefully, it makes all the difference between, on the one hand, a semi-blind operation performed through a pool of blood, and on the other hand, a planned procedure in an almost bloodless field in which every manoeuvre is under direct visual control.

The essential instruments for this intranasal procedure (*Figure 11.5*) are: a Killian's long-bladed speculum, which allows the middle turbinate to be displaced medially and thus permits direct access to the middle meatus; a wide-bore, blunt-ended sucker, which prevents undue trauma to the mucosa and hence discourages the formation of adhesions; Henckel's forceps, for removal of the main polypoid masses; and Citelli's upturned forceps—for the removal of smaller polypoid tags, for uncapping the bulla ethmoidalis, and for removing polypoid mucosa from the cells of the agger nasi.

It is essential to remove all the polypoid mucosa, but nothing should be removed which is not clearly visible, and definable as polypoid mucosa.

In performing these intranasal procedures, it is essential to remember (*Figure 11.6*) that: the roof of the ethmoidal labyrinth is above the level of the cribriform plate; the paper-thin lateral wall of the labyrinth (the *lamina papyracea*) separates it from the orbital periosteum and contents; and the posterior extremity of the lamina papyracea extends almost as far back as the optic foramen.

If instruments are advanced too high, they may penetrate the cribriform plate and thus cause meningitis and other intracranial complications; if they penetrate the lamina papyracea, they may perforate the orbital periosteum, with the possible development of orbital haematoma or abscess; and if they penetrate too far back through the lateral wall, they may injure the optic nerve, with subsequent blindness.

Hence, when working in the ethmoidal labyrinth, all instruments must be kept below the cribriform plate; medial to the lamina papyracea (or at least to the orbital periosteum); and in front of the optic foramen, which lies immediately behind the foramen for the posterior ethmoidal artery.

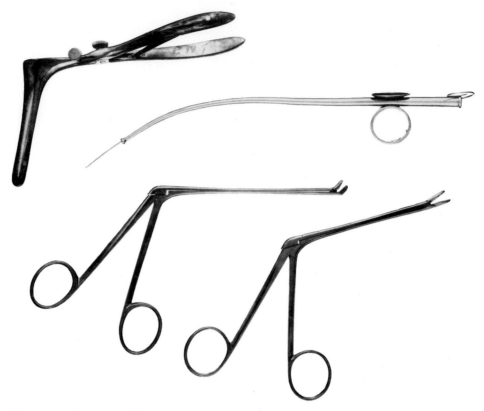

Figure 11.5   Instruments for per-nasal polypectomy: top left, Killian's speculum; top right, blunt-ended sucker; bottom left, Citelli's forceps; bottom right, Henckel's forceps

The middle turbinate itself should always be preserved in its entirety and, in removing polypoid mucosa anteriorly, it is essential to keep close to and behind the attachment of the anterior end of the middle turbinate; if this rule is adhered to, there should be no danger to the cribriform plate. If all the anterior cells have been properly removed, then a fine frontal sinus probe will slip easily, without any force at all, into the frontal sinus; if it does not slip in, then there must be more anterior ethmoidal cells (Scott-Brown, 1978).

Careful study of human skulls is recommended before this type of surgery is undertaken, and provided it is done skilfully, more radical surgical procedures should rarely be necessary. However, in the presence of superadded sinus sepsis, or when extensive recurrences occur with unacceptable frequency, radical measures may be indicated (Hughes, 1973).

The standard operation for ethmoidal polypi, when associated with antro–ethmoidal sepsis, is the Jansen–Horgan operation, in which a transantral ethmoidectomy (via a sublabial approach) is combined with per-nasal surgery. In this operation, the posterior ethmoidal cells are opened (through the antrum) by advancing a closed Henckel forceps in an upward, medial and posterior direction through the upper/inner angle of the antrum, the forceps being pointed in the direction of the opposite parietal eminence.

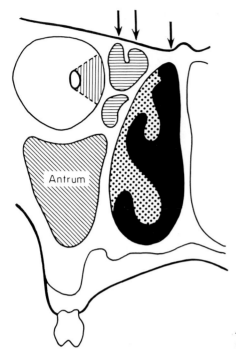

Figure 11.6   Relations of ethmoidal labyrinth (vertical and horizontal stripes). (See text)

External operations on the ethmoidal sinus are performed either through an incision which is medial to (and concave towards) the medial canthus of the eye (Howarth's operation), or through an incision in the natural crease-line below the inferior orbital margin (Patterson's operation). The former operation is more widely practised than the latter, but it is claimed for the Patterson operation (Hughes, 1976) that identification and mobilization of the upper end of the naso–lacrimal duct provide wider exposure of the anterior labyrinth, and permit exenteration of those cells which lie behind and lateral to the duct.

These external procedures require the same caution and precautions as are needed in per-nasal operations, and the same complications can arise.

There is controversy about the best way to deal with an antro–choanal polypus, and some surgeons aver that they should always be removed by a Caldwell–Luc approach; but this is certainly not always necessary, and indeed the mass of such a polypus may be so great as to make it impossible to withdraw it through the antrum. With the help of Killian's long-bladed speculum, it is usually possible to retract the middle turbinate medially and, grasping its 'neck' just as it leaves the antral ostium, to avulse the polypus backwards, and then forwards through the nose. With a very large polypus occupying much of the nasopharynx, removal may best be achieved with the patient in the standard position for tonsillectomy by dissection. With a Boyle–Davis gag in place, the palate is retracted by means of a soft rubber catheter; a long-wired snare is now passed along the affected nasal cavity and the surgeon, holding a small laryngeal mirror in his free hand, can manoeuvre the wire loop around the polypus under indirect vision; then, after avulsing the polypus with the snare, he can deliver it through the mouth.

It should go without saying that the treatment of a neoplastic polypus must be directed to the tumour itself and that all nasal polypi, however removed, must be examined histologically for the rare possibilities of transitional-cell papilloma and malignancy.

References

Ballantyne, J. C. (1973) *Journal of Laryngology and Otology* **87**, 197

Chandra, R. K. and Abrol, B. M. (1974) *Journal of Laryngology and Otology* **88**, 1019

Despons, J. and Stoller, F. M. (1965) *Laryngoscope* **75**, 475

Dodd, G. D. and Jing, B. S. (1977) In *Radiology of the Nose, Paranasal Sinuses and Nasopharynx.* p.121. Baltimore; Williams & Wilkins

Gray, L. (1967) *Journal of Laryngology and Otology* **81**, 953

Hughes, R. G. (1973) *Journal of Laryngology and Otology* **87**, 117

Hughes, R. G. (1976) In *Operative Surgery*, Vol. 2, *Nose and Throat*, p. 123. Ed. by Robb, C. and Smith, R. London; Butterworths

Reynolds, D. F. and Groves, J. (1956) *Journal of the Faculty of Radiology* **57**, 278

Schwachman, H., Kulczycki, L. L., Mueller, H. L. and Flake, C. G. (1962) *Pediatrics* **30**, 389

Scott-Brown, W. G. (1978) Personal communication

Toma, G. A. and Stein, G. E. (1968) *Journal of Laryngology and Otology* **82**, 265

12 Abnormalities of smell

Ellis Douek

Complaints from patients who suffer from abnormalities of taste and smell are relatively common but the distress these cause varies from individual to individual. This is never as serious as loss of vision or loss of hearing and on many occasions, such as during common cold attacks or hay fever, there can be severe, if temporary, loss of smell. It is only when symptoms persist for a considerable time that most patients will realize that they have lost a sense.

When faced with loss of smell it is a mistake to give it a name such as 'anosmia' and in doing so to consider it as though it were a disease in itself which may or may not be cured. If it is recognized to be only a symptom there is then a necessity, first to find the cause and, second to decide whether it can or should be treated. The first step in doing this is to classify the symptom and then the possible causes.

Classification of symptoms

The first question we have to ask is whether this is quantitative, in other words whether the patient has 'lost' smell, or whether it has been altered in a qualitative way.

Quantitative changes

(1) Decreased sensitivity to smells.
(2) Increased sensitivity to smells.

Qualitative changes

(1) Peripheral type—local causes
        anosmic zones
        Single Non-Discriminating (SND) response
        essential parosmia

(2) Central type—illusions
                        hallucinations
                        abnormal sense-memory

Causes of these abnormalities

Lesions of the nose

Deviated nasal septum—rarely causes loss of smell
Nasal polyps—decrease in smell
Allergic and vasomotor rhinitis—decrease in smell or parosmia
Infective rhinitis—decrease in smell
Tumours—decrease in smell
Fumes

Lesions of olfactory nerves

Injury—tends to be complete loss
Viral—SND response
General disease—diminution of threshold

Intracranial lesions

Trauma—tends to be complete loss
Anterior fossa tumours—progressive, often unilateral loss
Temporal lobe tumours—fits with olfactory or gustatory aura
Intracerebral tumours—subtle changes in adaptation and fatigue
Epilepsy—bizarre hallucinations and other disturbances

Psychogenic disorders

Can occur in schizophrenia-like psychoses and confusional states as well as depressive illness and a specific olfactory reference syndrome. The symptoms include illusions of smells and hallucinations.

Hysteria and malingering have a place among these disorders.

The relation between these conditions and the sense of smell will be considered in detail after the methods of testing are discussed.

Testing smell

This poses a problem today as objective tests are still in the developmental phase and because we have as yet not enough knowledge to classify smell in a manner comparable to hearing or sight. Generally speaking these tests can be classified in the following manner.

Subjective tests

(1) Measuring the minimum perceptible odour
(2) Identification tests
(3) Adaptation tests

Objective tests

(1) Using physiological measurements
(2) Evoked responses

Haematogenous tests

Subjective tests

(1) The minimum perceptible odour
Measuring the minimum perceptible level of any sense is the basis of all perceptual investigation. In the case of smell it is still virtually the only one giving relevant values. This can be done in various ways.

(i) Dilution in air   Although this is feasible, the techniques are difficult to maintain as they require a known quantity of odorant in a known volume of air. This can be done quite easily by using larger and larger bottles of air for a smaller and smaller quantity of odorant in solid or liquid form. The results are then given as mg/ml of air. The problem lies in the variable quantity of odorant vaporized from the measured substance.

(ii) Dilution in liquids   It is essential in the first place that the liquid used to dilute the odorant substance should not itself have a smell. Many clinicians have used similar techniques for the past 100 years, the most important contribution being that of Proetz (1924).

Proetz's olfactometer consisted of a rack containing 100 bottles arranged in ten rows to form a square. Each row represented an odour and the bottles in each row a different intensity. He used liquid petrolatum as a diluent because it was odourless and non-volatile and would not react with the substances dissolved in it. The odours he chose represented a general class of compound and could be recognized again. They had to be soluble in petrolatum and not liable to irritate the nasal mucosa. They were—Iodoform, Methylsalicylate, Amylalcohol, Xylol, Nitrobenzol, Phenol, Guaia-col, Cinnamon oil, Eugenol, Coumarin.

Proetz introduced a quantitative element. The minimum perceptible odour (MPO) for a substance recordable by many people he called an 'olfact'. This was expressed in g/l. Each row of bottles contained solutions of $\frac{1}{4}$, $\frac{1}{2}$, 1, 2, 3, 5, 10, 25, 50 and 100 olfacts.

(iii) Controlled-stimulus technique   Many workers became interested in developing a controlled-stimulus technique and Elsberg and Levy a simple blast-injection technique (*Figure 12.1*).

The author (Douek, 1967) aimed at combining Elsberg and Levy's quantitative approach with a qualitative element. The problem here lay in choosing a suitable range of substances. A decision was made to use the seven 'primary' odours of Amoore (Volume 1) not so much because there was incontrovertible evidence that primary odours existed and that if they did these were the ones, but because these were, as a group, the commonest recorded odours. They were—Ethereal, Camphoraceous, Musky, Floral, Minty, Pungent, Putrid.

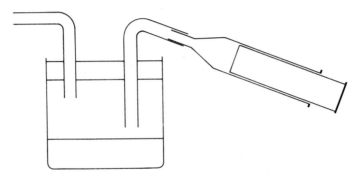

Figure 12.1 Blast olfactometer

The results were recorded in the form of block graphs (*Figure 12.2*) according to the amount of air blown into the nose and expressed in millilitres. It was made clear that these figures could not represent absolute values and that the importance of this method lay principally in that it was able to demonstrate that it was possible to lose the sense of smell for one substance more than for another.

(2) Identification tests

In 1962 Sumner reported an investigation designed to show the ease with which test substances could be identified. Using 200 subjects with a normal sense of smell he found that only two were able to identify all the substances. The majority could identify only half the substances.

If recognition is required, however, it is possible to use the same techniques recording the minimum identifiable odour (MIO) instead of the MPO.

(3) Adaptation tests

The adaptation phenomenon is well-known and very marked in taste and smell. Adaptation time for smell can be measured by running a stream of air carrying an odorant into the nose of the subject and measuring the time it takes for him to cease to be able to smell the substance. If the stream is stopped and the subject is then tested again every half minute until he can smell it again, recovery time can also be measured.

Objective tests

(1) Physiological measurements

Various changes can be recorded in physiological function in response to all types of stimuli. Smell is no exception but, of course, these changes are not specific and have to be considered with great caution. The following have each received attention: (i) The olfacto–pupillary reflex; (ii) Rise in blood pressure—response to unpleasant smells; (iii) Changes in pulse-rate; (iv) Plethysmographic changes; (v) Changes in respiratory rate; (vi) Psychogalvanic reflex; (vii) Electroencephalography—changes in alpha rhythm similar to those seen in response to visual stimuli.

Polygraphic methods have also been used but it is rarely possible to extract more from the use of multiple tests than from a single one when they all rely on the same premise.

(2) Evoked responses

By analogy with visual and auditory electrical evoked responses interest has been raised in a similar approach to testing smell. This has been very difficult for two main reasons. The first is the difficulty of disentangling a response to the olfactory stimulus from that to the trigeminal receptors. The second is the difficulty of producing a stimulus sharp enough to engender a recordable response.

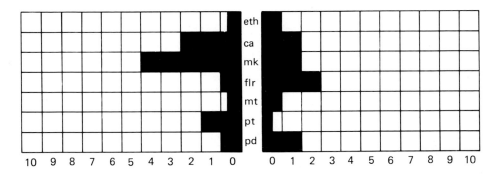

Figure 12.2 Olfactory spectrogram

Finkenzeller (1966) was the first to look at such a possibility and subsequent reports were published by Allison and Goff (1967) as well as Smith *et al.* (1971), Giessen (1970), Alber *et al.* (1972) and Gerull, Giessen and Mrowinski (1975). Herberhold (1972) described a twin potential suggesting an olfactory sensory component and mechano/chemosensory component.

In view of this progress it is likely that olfactory evoked responses will find their place in clinical diagnosis in the not too distant future.

Haematogenous tests

These have not come to fruition in a clinical sense but are ingenious in that they are based on the intravenous injection of a non-toxic odorous substance which, on reaching the olfactory area, produces a sensation of smell.

Lesions causing abnormalities of smell

Lesions of the nose

Simple anatomical abnormalities such as a deviated nasal septum are unlikely to cause any abnormality of smell and a submucous resection is never indicated for the specific purpose of curing hyposmia.

Allergic rhinitis very commonly causes abnormalities of smell. Only rarely is this total, as in most instances careful testing will show that there is more smell present than the patient realizes. A particularly interesting phenomenon occurs when there is loss of smell for only one or two smells as shown by the olfactory spectrogram (*Figure 12.3*). This often results in the complaint that smell has been 'altered' in some way.

This condition responds to anti-allergic therapy and the most valuable agents are topical steroids. Occasionally systemic steroids are required but the side effects of these drugs are such that their use by this route is hardly ever justified.

Nasal polyps are usually superadded to nasal allergy and in these patients true anosmia may occur. Excision will clearly give access to the olfactory area but the underlying allergic rhinitis must be vigorously treated with antihistamines and topical steroids. No promise can be given to the patient that polypectomy will restore the sense of smell.

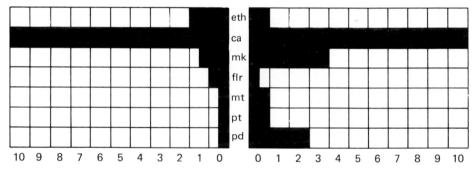

Figure 12.3 Olfactory spectrogram with anosmic zone

Infective rhinitis may damage considerable areas of the olfactory mucosa if it becomes chronic and the areas destroyed will not regenerate.

Tumours of the nose need not be considered here as loss of smell is not an important symptom.

Lesions of the olfactory nerves

There is no doubt that viral infections such as influenza can cause great damage to the olfactory nerve fibres, replacing all the neuronal tissue with fibrous tissue.

A bizarre olfactory experience that many of these patients describe is a single, very weak smell, whatever the substance may be. The author has given the name of Single Non-Discriminating (SND) response to this and the prognosis is invariably bad.

Injury to the olfactory nerves may occur through a direct blow but quite often results from an occipital blow causing a shearing of the nerve fibres.

Usually the loss of smell is total and immediate. Occasionally some recovery occurs but, for legal purposes, if the patient is anosmic after six months it can be taken that there will be no recovery. Sometimes the patient complains of a distortion of smell so gross that it can be very distressing. Again, here the prognosis is also very poor.

Intracranial lesions

There are two ways in which intracranial tumours can affect the sense of smell.

(1) By pressure on the olfactory nerve fibres or the olfactory bulb.
(2) By interference with the intracerebral pathways.

Osteomas or meningomas of the anterior fossa tend to diminish the sense of smell and at first this is unilateral. Large frontal lobe tumours may do the same.

When the tumour lies in the brain substance it may interfere with normal fatigue or adaptation but the patient does not complain of this as a symptom.

Temporal lobe epilepsy may present with an olfactory aura or the fit itself may consist of an olfactory sensation, often a smell of burning accompanied by a taste sensation as well.

Psychogenic disorders

Many psychiatric diseases such as schizophrenia or depression can be accompanied by hallucination of smell. Almost invariably this is a bad smell. Occasionally we see patients complaining mainly of the unpleasant smell and to these Pryse Phillips (1970) has given the name Olfactory Reference Syndrome.

When surveying the field of olfaction and its disorders, and comparing it with other aspects of disease it is impossible not to experience a sense of dissatisfaction. This is due to our great lack of knowledge regarding the nature of this sense. It is possible, however, that with advances in electrophysiology information of a more original quality may become available during the next few years.

References

Alber, K., Mrowinski, D., Giessen, M and Schwab, W. (1972). *Archiv für Ohren-, Nasen und Kehlkopfheilkunde*, **199**, 687

Allison, T. and Goff, W. R. (1967). *Electroencephalography and Clinical Neurophysiology*, **23**, 538

Douek, E. (1967). *Journal of Laryngology*, **81**, 431

Douek, E. (1974). *The Sense of Smell and Its Abnormalities*. Edinburgh & London; Churchill Livingston

Finkenzeller, P. (1966). *Archiv für die gesamte Physiologie des Menschen und der Tiere*, 292

Gerull, G., Giessen, M. and Mrowinski, D. (1975). *EEG-EMG*, **6**, 37

Giessen, M. (1970). *Archiv fur Ohren-, Nasen-, und, Kehlkheilkunde*, **196**, 632

Herberhold, C. (1972). *Archiv fur Ohren-, Nasen-, und Kehlkheilkunde*, 202

Proetz, A. (1924). *Annals of Otology (St. Louis)*, **33**, 746

Pryse Phillips, M. (1970). Personal communication

Smith, D. B., Allison, T., Goff, W. R. and Principato, J. J. (1971). *Electroencephalography and Clinical Neurophysiology*, **30**, 313

Sumner, (1962). *Lancet*, **2**, 895

13 Acute sinusitis
David Wright

Introduction

Inflammation of the paranasal sinuses rarely threatens life, but it causes considerable morbidity. The true incidence is shown by the statistics from the Department of Health and Social Security (1971) estimating that half a million working days are lost in Britain each year on this account. The initial acute infection of the sinuses may well be viral, and anatomical anomalies may predispose towards a chronic infection from which a diversity of micro-organisms may be cultured. Most of the bacteria isolated are normal inhabitants of the upper respiratory tract and proliferate as secondary invaders in a diseased sinus.

Acute sinusitis is a condition usually requiring medical treatment whereas chronic sinusitis often demands surgery. There are certain features in both acute and chronic sinusitis which are common to all the paranasal sinuses and others that differ with each particular sinus and have to be considered separately. These differences usually depend on the anatomy of the individual drainage mechanisms for each sinus. Complications from infection of particular sinuses will be influenced by adjacent structures, for example the ethmoidal sinuses which are barely separated from the orbit.

There may also be variations in size and shape and they may contain bony divisions or septa which may influence the spread of infection.

In this chapter the features which are to a large extent common to acute and chronic sinusitis will be discussed, together with the special aspects of acute sinusitis. These include bacteriological and aetiological considerations as well as conditions which predispose to sinus infection, whether acute or chronic. This will be followed by a discussion of certain specific and rare types of sinus infection, while Chapter 14 concentrates on the special pathology of chronic infection and surgical techniques.

Development of the sinuses

The sinuses develop from small diverticula from the nasal cavity which invade the surrounding bones of the skull. At birth the maxillary, sphenoid and ethmoid sinuses are already present and after draining of amniotic fluid they become aerated during the first few weeks of life. Only the frontal sinus diverticulum is not present at birth but during the first year it invades the frontal bone, so that by the third year it has assumed an inverted pear-like shape. The frontal sinus is fully developed by the age of 15 years and all the other sinuses are usually completely developed by puberty.

The ethmoid sinuses are already fully pneumatized at birth and are the most developed of all the sinuses at this time. They form cavity systems occupying the upper two-thirds of the lateral wall of the nasal cavity.

The maxillary antra are formed from oblong cavities 1 cm long antero-posteriorly and about 0.5cm high. As the floor of the antrum does not descend below the level of the corresponding nasal cavity until the eruption of the second dentition, at about the age of eight, it occupies less than a third of the lateral wall of the nose. The antrum grows in size by 2–3 mm every year, and by the age of nine years the downward growth has been such that its height is now equal to that of the ethmoid.

The relative sizes of these sinuses have some clinical importance for after the age of three or four years the antrum is the sinus most vulnerable to acute infection, but infants are just as liable to suffer from acute ethmoiditis.

The sphenoid sinus is less than 0.5cm long at birth and only 2–3 mm high. It is fully pneumatized by the age of eight years.

Aetiology of acute sinusitis

Sinusitis is most common in the maxillary sinus. This is followed by the ethmoid, the frontal and the sphenoid in that order, but very often there is simultaneous involvement of more than one sinus. There are a number of possible sources which may infect the sinuses and a number of predisposing or contributory features.

Acute rhinitis

By far the most common factor in the production of acute sinusitis is an acute rhinitis spreading to the sinuses and this acute rhinitis is in turn often associated with the common cold

In health, the anterior third of the nose of the adult and that of children over 8–12 months may contain common organisms which appear to have no immediate pathogenicity, and even in those exceptional people who seldom or never have acute nasal infection, these organisms are present. They are present also in the noses of the people of the Arctic region who, in their normal environment, never have colds. In acute infection, whether precipitated by a virus or an extraneous organism, the normal inhabitants increase rapidly in numbers and are found in abnormal situations, namely the eustachian tube and middle ear, the larynx and the sinuses. Thus, infection usually spreads to the sinuses by way of their natural ostia from the nasal cavities.

An acute sinusitis, if not very severe, may develop in this way and remain untreated until chronic changes take place, the patient believing he has a persistent cold. The resulting chronic sinusitis, discharging pus into the nose, then gives rise to chronic rhinitis with its attendant symptoms, and no improvement can be expected until this vicious circle is broken by therapeutic measures. Care should be taken therefore to treat sinusitis early, before irreversible changes have taken place, and to make sure that it has completely resolved before discharging the patient from observation.

Foreign bodies in the nose, particularly in children, set up an infective rhinitis which may easily be followed by sinusitis.

Pharyngeal infection

Although not as commonly responsible for sinus infection as nasal conditions, pharyngeal infections can also spread to the nose and sinuses. Chronic adenoiditis may be an important cause of sinusitis in children and tonsillitis can also act as a focus of infection. Conversely chronic sinusitis may be responsible for chronic tonsillitis. It is not always possible to separate nasal and sinus infection from that of the pharynx and nasopharynx and this fact should be remembered when considering the management of patients with upper respiratory tract infection.

Dental infection

The proximity of teeth to the maxillary antrum makes it the most commonly infected sinus from dental causes. Estimates of the proportion of odontogenic infection in maxillary sinusitis have been put at 10 per cent (Formby, 1960), though there must be wide topographical variations. The condition of the teeth and gums must therefore never be overlooked in a patient with sinus disease.

In 1651, Nathaniel Highmore, who described the anatomy of the maxillary sinus, wrote that 'the bone which encloses and which separates it from the sockets of the teeth does not much exceed a piece of wrapping paper in thickness'. The sinus may continue to expand throughout life, and in some individuals the floor extends to the apices of the teeth and dips downwards into the inter-radicular spaces or into any adjacent edentulous area. Although the thickness of the bone is variable there is often nothing interposed between the apices of the teeth and the sinus cavity other than the mucosal lining itself.

Although the association between dental and sinus infection is not in doubt, the exact manner in which the antrum is affected is not certain.

Two possible ways are:

(1) Chronic dental infection can cause localized areas of granulations in the sinus mucosa where it lines the alveolar recesses of the antrum. The function of this area of the sinus is altered, its ciliary activity is impaired and its mucus-secreting activity affected. This situation predisposes to infection of nasal origin or to blood-borne infection if there is a bacteraemia from some other source. So long as part of the mucous membrane remains in an inflamed condition attempts at treatment are unlikely to be successful.
(2) Bacteria may spread directly from an apical granuloma or a periodontal pocket, or be carried to the antrum by the lymphatics.

Just as the teeth may affect the sinus, an antritis may affect the teeth. The resulting pain and sensitivity to bite affect all the teeth associated with the infected antrum and dental x-rays may suggest oedema of the supporting membranes. The vitality of the teeth is preserved, however, and recovery should take place if the sinusitis is treated.

The dental conditions which can give rise to sinus infection are the following:

Acute peri-apical abscess

Infection which reaches the apex of the dental root has passed through the pulp and out through the apical foramen. The commonest teeth to be involved are the upper first and second molars. An acute peri-apical abscess may occur, but if the infection is of a lower grade a chronic granuloma is formed. In time, the granuloma may suppurate and a chronic peri-apical abscess results. As this infection usually arises from pulpitis the diseased tooth is devitalized.

Dentigerous cyst

An infected dentigerous cyst may develop in relation to an unerupted tooth (*Figure 13.1*). The upper wisdom teeth are the most likely to give rise to a dentigerous cyst. The standard occipito–mental radiographs will not always demonstrate foreign bodies in the sinus and these are better shown on an orthopantogram.

Periodontal abscess

Periodontitis is an inflammation of the membrane which surrounds the root of the tooth. It may be acute or chronic and if it is confined to one tooth it is referred to as 'local periodontitis'; if to many teeth as 'general periodontitis'.

Infection may reach this membrane from the pulp through the apical foramen as has been described above under 'Peri-apical abscess'. More commonly it enters by the

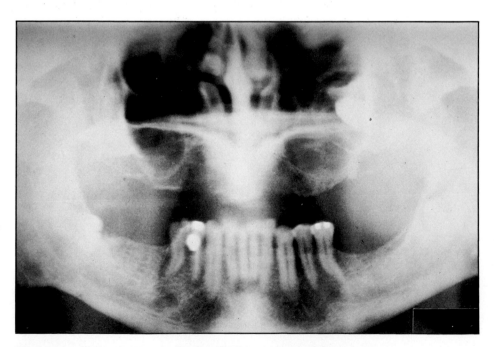

Figure 13.1   Ortho-pantogram showing dentigerous cyst in left antrum

margin of the gum and its lymphatics. Very rarely it may be carried by the bloodstream.

Chronic periodontitis, though rarely causing sinusitis, is a slowly progressive disease whose main feature is loss of alveolar bone through resorption which may lead to gross mobility and eventual exfoliation of the affected teeth. Advanced resorption may create a periodontic pocket so large that it communicates with and infects the sinus. This direct spread is uncommon and in the large majority of cases a low grade infection of the sinus occurs from bloodstream and lymphatic spread (Powell, 1965).

Acute periodontitis spreads in the form of a lateral periodontal abscess which will hasten the progress of the disease. The pus may then reach the exterior by taking a number of different directions. It may break through the outer plate of bone above or below the insertion of the buccinator; it may travel inwards through the inner plate to cause a palatal abscess; it may come out through a tooth cavity or through the gingival sulcus or more rarely through the floor of the nose. Finally, it may break out into the maxillary sinus causing a severe infection of this cavity. It should again be stressed that, however dramatic, this is not the most common manner in which dental infection gives rise to maxillary antritis.

When it does occur it is the second premolar or the first or second molar which is usually responsible

X-rays taken in patients with periodontitis demonstrate sclerotic changes in the floor of the sinus but only rarely show evidence of a communication between the periodontal lesion and the sinus cavity. When this is present it is probably the result of an acute lateral periodontal abscess breaking through into the antrum.

Tooth extraction
During extraction a tooth may be fractured and the root forced into the maxillary antrum by the injudicious use of elevators in the confined space of a socket. The danger of perforation is increased where there is peri-apical rarefaction and the bony floor is already eroded.

Displacement of the root into the maxillary sinus may tempt a dentist to operate in an area which may be outside his field of competence, so that prompt referral is desirable. Unless removal is performed by an experienced operator within a reasonable time, there is a strong likelihood that antritis will develop as well as a persistent oro–antral fistula due to bacterial invasion from the mouth. During extraction of a tooth associated with an apical abscess, infection may be forced into the antrum. The socket may heal but the sinus may become infected if a small amount of pus has been forced into the antrum by the extraction.

The removal of upper wisdom teeth may give rise to sinusitis. Usually there is no evidence of fistula initially but three days later the patient may develop signs of acute sinusitis. It is to be suspected in these cases that the mucoperiosteum of the sinus is directly related to the periodontal membrane of the wisdom tooth.

It has been found that the first molar roots are forced into the antrum more frequently than the roots of other teeth. Although the second molars are more closely related to the antral floor, the roots of the first molar diverge more widely bucco–lingually, increasing the difficulty of forceps extraction and the chance of root fracture. The roots of teeth adjacent to edentulous spaces are most likely to be involved and males are affected more often, probably because the more robust maxillary architecture makes the extraction more difficult. The left antrum has been found to be more vulnerable than the right and this is probably associated with the technique of exodontia.

It is important to decide whether the root is in the sinus, lodged beneath the buccal mucoperiosteum or between the bony floor of the sinus and an intact lining mucous membrane. Extra-oral x-ray films such as those designed to demonstrate an antral infection have only a limited value in locating these roots. Peri-apical and occlusal films usually show a root near the site of perforation, but a small root which may have lodged in a crevice between the bony ridges which cover the apices of adjacent teeth may only be visible on parallax intra-oral views, but if a root cannot be demonstrated radiographically, it does not exclude its presence in the sinus.

Foreign bodies in the sinus
Apart from the roots of teeth, dental prosthetic materials used for root filling have caused antral infection by being inadvertently pushed into the sinus.

The special instance of infection associated with the canine tooth should be mentioned. As the apex of that root is usually above the level of insertion of the circumoral muscles, the signs of a peri-apical abscess may easily be mistaken for a sinus infection. The considerable oedema which results is restricted from the region of the mouth by the muscle attachments; and instead of producing swollen eyelids, give an impression of ethmoiditis due to an infra-orbital cellulitis. The soft-tissue swelling may even suggest an opaque antrum when it is superimposed upon the antrum in the occipitomental radiograph.

A detailed effort should be made in every case of maxillary sinusitis to assess the dental state, as treatment will always fail if an infected tooth or a displaced root is overlooked. In order to recognize these conditions, some knowledge of their pathology is necessary.

Swimming and diving

Water may penetrate into the sinuses, especially in diving, ducking or jumping in feet first. As the natural ostia are not closed due to preliminary swelling as in acute rhinitis, infected water introduced into the nose may easily enter the sinuses, producing an acute inflammation. In rare cases of osteomyelitis of the frontal bone, there is often a history of recent swimming.

Most public swimming pools are maintained at a pH of 7.6 with 1.5 parts/million of chlorine. Levels of pH of 7.2 have been recorded in public baths where there are 4 parts/million of chlorine. The lowered pH is reasonably well tolerated by cilia but the chlorine may be in sufficient concentration to produce a chemical inflammation, as improved facilities encourage children to stay in the pool for longer periods. Anyone who swims or dives during the prodromal stage of a coryza is at a much greater risk with regard to developing acute sinusitis or any of its complications.

Trauma

Trauma to a sinus may lead to infection. It may be brought about in various ways.

Compound fracture of one of the sinuses

The sinuses involved are the maxillary, the frontal and the ethmoid. These fractures are discussed in Chapter 3 and are all liable to become infected. The fracture may open the sinus to the outside or into the nose so that the damaged mucosa and resultant blood clot can easily become infected.

Contusion of the sinuses

A severe blow on the cheek or forehead even without a fracture may produce a contusion of the mucous membrane with extravasation of blood into the underlying sinus cavity. Infecting organisms in the nose or bloodstream may set up, though rarely, a maxillary or frontal sinusitis. Trauma affecting the frontonasal duct can give rise to secondary frontal sinusitis.

Foreign bodies

Foreign bodies other than roots of teeth and dental materials may also cause sinus infection. Penetrating wounds, for example by gunshot, may introduce infecting organisms from the outside.

A foreign body, particularly if a rhinolith has been formed, may erode into the antrum. The erosion is caused by pressure atrophy on the lateral wall of the nose and the associated infection will produce a sinusitis.

Barotrauma

Barotrauma may be produced by rapid changes in barometric pressure during flight or scuba diving. The manner in which this is produced and its pathological changes will be discussed later in this chapter, but if the sinus is invaded by bacteria the resulting acute sinusitis will be little different from any other type.

General health

Poor general health frequently precipitates sinusitis. Among those diseases responsible are influenza, measles, whooping cough and other specific diseases of children.

Contributory and predisposing factors

There are a number of factors which contribute directly to sinusitis or which are believed to predispose to infection. In the latter group it is not always possible to know the exact mechanism which brings about an infection and it is rather that an association between the two conditions has been observed.

Poor general environment

Nasal infection and chronic sinusitis are more common in children with lowered resistance who live in poor housing conditions where there is a greater risk of exposure to epidemic viral infections. Deprived families do not always seek advice early enough. The incidence of upper respiratory tract infection in many children increases with their attendance at play school during their fourth year.

Prolonged exposure

Exposure to large numbers of people during school, travel or at work will increase the frequency of infection. Such conditions exist in crowded cities and affect particularly children in their early years at school when they also have a somewhat lowered resistance.

Exposure to cold is said to reduce the activity of the cilia of the mucosa lining the nose and sinuses and therefore to invite infection. This may happen during a skiing vacation but does not seem to be an important factor under normal conditions. It is the dry atmosphere created by excessive central heating which is much more likely to cause mucosal changes predisposing to sinus infection.

Obstruction

Anatomical obstruction

There can be deformity of the septum or turbinates, excessive enlargement of the bulla ethmoidalis or hypertrophy of the adenoids. All these abnormalities prevent adequate drainage of the nasal cavity and sinuses.

In the case of a simple deviation of the nasal septum where there is compensatory hypertrophy of the middle turbinate on the wider side and atrophy of the turbinate on the narrower side, it is found that the fronto–nasal duct of the maxillary or ethmoidal sinuses are obstructed on both sides (*Figure 13.2*). This is caused by pressure of the septum on the narrower side and by the turbinal hypertrophy on the wider side. This hypertrophy is not only on the medial aspect of the turbinate but also laterally towards the middle meatus, in the region of the ostia opening from the sinuses into the hiatus semilunaris.

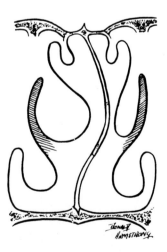

Figure 13.2   Diagram of deviated septum showing how obstruction to the middle meatus may occur on both the wide and narrow sides of the nose

Infective obstruction

Infection of the nasal fossae, post-nasal space or pharynx produces congestion and obstruction by swelling of the mucosa as well as providing a 'focus'.

Allergic obstruction

Allergic states in the nose and sinuses are characterized by mucosal swelling. This may result not only in a narrowing of the passage through the nasal cavity and of the ostia of the sinuses but also of the small intercommunicating openings that exist between the ethmoidal cells. The condition will be further aggravated if there are multiple ethmoidal polypi present.

It should be noted that many of the symptoms caused by allergic rhinitis are often thought to be 'sinusitis' by the patient and referred to as such. Radiographs in these cases usually show considerable mucosal thickening and these changes may be associated with either allergy or a true infective sinusitis.

Tumours

Benign tumours of the nose and sinuses are uncommon but may present as an acute sinusitis; however infection in the sinuses is more likely to be an associated symptom in malignant disease, particularly if the ostium is involved.

Association with chest conditions

It has long been recognized that there is an association between sinus and chest infection. The various chest conditions which have been associated one way or another with sinus disease are as follows.

Chronic bronchitis

A cough is a common symptom in chronic sinusitis but this does not imply that bronchitis is present. Usually adequate treatment of the sinus infection is sufficient to reduce the cough. The aetiology of chronic bronchitis remains closely related to the patient's smoking habits. Routine radiographs of the sinuses taken of patients with bronchitis rarely show a sinus involvement. Chronic bronchitis is less common than it used to be due to the earlier effective treatment with antibiotics and possibly a greater awareness of atmospheric pollution.

Asthma

Many patients are referred from the asthma clinic to the rhinologist because of nasal obstruction and excessive nasal secretion. It is often suspected that sinusitis may be present and causing exacerbation of the chest symptoms. Often an accompanying radiograph shows hazy antra.

It is important to screen carefully the sinuses of these patients, especially those in the later age group who present with intrinsic asthma without signs of atopy, to make sure that there is no evidence of sinus infection.

Examination in most cases shows the typical appearance of allergic rhinitis with a bluish oedematous mucosa. Antral washout usually produces only a mucoid return with no pus cells, but sometimes eosinophils. Although an infected antrum may be present in allergic patients, and indeed the altered mucosa and excessive stagnant secretion may predispose to infection, it would be wrong to imply a direct association.

Bronchiectasis
Bronchiectasis is a condition in which the bronchi are chronically dilated. Patients with bronchiectasis can be broadly divided into two groups.

Congenital
This may be due to a failure of the alveoli and peripheral bronchi to develop normally. It also occurs as a complication of cystic fibrosis where the disease is one of mucus secreting and non-mucus secreting exocrine glands giving an increased viscosity of mucus and high sodium chloride in sweat.

The altered nature of the mucoid secretions may give bronchial blockage resulting in bronchiectasis and for the same reason may lead also to sinusitis. The resulting sinusitis is often accompanied by nasal polyps of an unusual texture and the presence of polyps in children associated with sinusitis and chest infection should make this disease suspect.

Obstruction and infection
These are patients in whom bronchiectasis has followed chest infection caused by measles or whooping cough.

Wax keratosis
Munro Black (1964) observed that there was an association between wax keratosis of the external auditory meatus and chronic sinusitis with cough in children between the ages of five and ten years. He suggested that the wax keratosis may be a reflex oversecretion of exocrine glands related to sinus infection.

Bacteriology

The methods of taking specimens for bacterial culture are as follows:

(1) *From the nasal vestibule*   A routine swab can be used and in about 20–30 per cent of the population a staphylococcus will be cultured.

   The incidence will rise to 60–80 per cent in hospital staff. The staphylococcus may or may not be related to the organism responsible for sinusitis.

(2) *From the posterior nares*   A special per-nasal swab should be used and it may be helpful to compare the organisms grown from this swab with the one used in the anterior nares to build up an overall picture of the organisms present.

(3) *From the sinus*   A true specimen can be obtained by puncture of the affected sinus and aspirating a sample of the sinus content into a syringe. However, the results of cultures from these specimens are often unrewarding as the organisms are sensitive to handling and do not always survive in water or saline. It is necessary to culture for both aerobic and anaerobic organisms. Most patients have had a prolonged course of antibiotic treatment before having a sinus washout and this may also be a factor in producing a negative culture result.

Virus infection

Over 50 per cent of the time lost from work in Britain because of illness is due to upper respiratory tract infection.

In the past few years it has become clear that the vast majority of these infections are viral in origin (Tyrrell, 1965).

Although these respiratory viruses lack disease specificity, they can be grouped into well-defined clinical syndromes. The type of response depends to some extent on the host; thus a respiratory syncytial virus will cause bronchiolitis or pneumonia in the child but only a cold in the adult. This may be due to the presence of antibody in the more or less immune adult.

The patient may be infected by multiple agents and different groups of virus may cause the same clinical syndrome. There is nevertheless some clinical correlation and the coryzal syndrome which leads to acute sinusitis may be caused by any of the following viruses:

Rhinovirus

Para-influenza I and II

Echo 28

Coxsackie A21

Respiratory syncytial virus

Social security surveys based on claims for sickness benefits are only valuable in influenza and more serious illnesses. Records of school attendance show a waxing and waning which indicates a certain periodicity. In Britain, there is an increase of these infections with the start of each school term.

It is very likely that most cases of acute sinusitis are viral in origin. Only subsequently do the sinuses become secondarily infected by bacteria.

Advances made in virus research have so far only been of epidemiological interest and of no help in clinical treatment.

Bacterial infection

It is quite likely that the majority of bacterial infections of the sinuses, other than those of dental origin, are secondary to virus infections.

The organisms which have been found in sinusitis are pneumococci, streptococci, staphylococci, *Haemophilus influenzae*, *Escherichia coli*, *Micrococcus catarrhalis*, *Bacillus pfeiffer* and *B. friedlander*. No rule can be given as to the type of inflammatory reaction they produce; some strains of streptococci and particularly the haemolytic streptococcus, for example, are prone to produce a necrosis of the mucous membrane and an acute suppurative lesion, whereas pneumococci are often found in hypertrophic states.

There is a tendency to grow pure cultures from cases of acute sinusitis and to obtain mixed growths from chronic sinusitis.

The *Haemophilus influenzae* strain which is most commonly associated with sinusitis is the capsular type A (Holdaway and Turk, 1967) and possibly the rare type C. The organism tends to remain dormant in the tissues of the sinuses and give a negative swab and this may be the reason for recurrence. According to Bujuggren and his colleagues (1953), if *Haemophilus influenzae* is present in the sinus then a high level of antibody formation occurs. It is possible that this is responsible for the feature of haemophilus infections which produces a high incidence in winter and spring followed by a decline in the number of cases.

Investigations based on anterior nasal swabs are usually valueless because of contaminants and should be disregarded. Bjorkwall (1950) found the pneumococcus to be the most common organism followed by the streptococcus; Mounier–Khun (1953) observed similar proportions; Dishoek and Franssen (1957) found three times as many cases infected by streptococcus as by pneumococcus and haemophilus, and this finding was later repeated by Palva, Grönroos and Palva (1962). Kinman, Chang and Seung (1967) demonstrated a high (48 per cent) incidence of *Haemophilus influenzae* compared with 29 per cent pneumococcus and only 6.6 per cent streptococcus.

These wide variations may well be related to the geographic distribution. Kinman's patients, for instance, were in Korea. Although there is little practical value in studying reports of this kind when a clinical decision has to be made, it is important in a general sense to be aware of the pattern of behaviour of infection in sinus disease.

Specific infections and fungal infections

Infections due to fungi, syphilis, tuberculosis and leprosy will be discussed in separate sections at the end of this chapter.

Pathology of acute sinusitis

The changes in the mucous membrane in acute sinusitis are those of acute inflammation in any tissue: increased blood supply with outpouring of serum and polymorphonuclear leucocytes associated with local swelling, redness and oedema. The oedema is caused by obstruction to the return of body fluids through the veins and lymphatics, and to the passage of fluid through the walls of the dilated capillaries into the tissues.

The sinus mucosa is able to return to normal after developing extensive swelling, providing the oedema has not been present for too long. It does so by the draining away of fluid by gravity, aided by arterial pulsation and resorption of intercellular fluid into the capillaries and lymphatics.

If the obstruction and oedema persist cell degeneration occurs with cloudy swelling, and necrotic changes will take place if interference with the circulation becomes prolonged.

Clinically in the early stages of infection the response is of hyperaemia and excess of secretion of mucus, but with few leucocytes and little or no destruction of the mucous membrane. If the inflammatory reaction is more severe there will be more extensive extrusion of leucocytes which together with the mucus form the discharge of mucopus. With increasing involvement of the mucous membrane or with severe infections the discharge becomes increasingly purulent and less mucoid until, with a necrotic membrane, frank pus alone will be found.

The acute inflammatory changes can produce very quickly a suppurative sinusitis, particularly with a dental infection involving the maxillary sinus.

Alternatively, an acute inflammation may be accompanied by marked swelling and oedema of the mucous membrane. The mucous glands became hypertrophied and secrete an unusually thick and tenacious mucus and the membrane may become so thickened as to appear to fill completely the sinus cavity.

Polypoid mucous membrane or polypi are often already present. In these cases there may be an allergic background and it is difficult to say which comes first, the allergy or the infection.

This question is fully dealt with in Chapter 10 but the allergic patient is more prone to serious involvement than a normal individual as there is more swelling and the obstruction may be more difficult to relieve.

A low grade suppuration may continue for years without any corresponding hyperplasia and finally degenerate into an atrophic condition.

It would seem that the virulence and type of organism, together with the state of resistance of the patient, determine whether in the early stages the changes are mainly hypertrophic or mainly suppurative.

It is important to decide which type of disease is present as the treatment will be influenced by this decision.

Physiopathology

Interesting studies on the physiopathology of sinusitis have been carried out by Drettner and Lindholm (1967). Most of their investigations were done using a wash-bottle connected to a needle which had been introduced into the maxillary sinus. They noted various forms of obstruction of the ostium; partial obstruction; obstruction transformed into a permanent opening after blowing the nose; valve-type obstruction; and complete obstruction resistant to pressure.

This last situation was present during all punctures for chronic sinusitis but only half of those for acute sinusitis.

When they investigated the permeability and resistance of the ostium in 44 sinuses of 23 patients who had had acute rhinitis for 1–10 days they found that only eight had a patent ostium, 16 had an obstruction which could be overcome by blowing or sniffing and the rest remained obstructed. The ostial obstruction also showed a positive correlation to the radiographic appearance of the sinus.

This work suggests that acute sinusitis probably starts with ostial obstruction.

Clinical features of acute sinusitis

Symptoms

The symptoms of acute sinusitis can be divided into two broad groups.

(1) General symptoms
The symptoms of sinusitis may be slight and not sufficient to prevent ordinary work, or severe and necessitating treatment at home or in bed.

Many people have radiological changes in the sinuses after a cold, although this does not necessarily produce the clinical picture of sinusitis. The general symptoms associated with sinusitis are malaise, headache and fever in the more acute cases, and are indicative of general toxaemia that accompanies acute infection in the sinuses. The fever is not usually high and, when it is, suggests a closed infection or a complication. It is usually remitting but may be intermittent if the sinus is blocked and contains pus. The malaise is a most frequent feature, particularly in the early stages and before the formation and discharge of the mucoid or mucopurulent secretion that usually appears in 48 h. With onset of free discharge the malaise may rapidly improve.

(2) Local symptoms

The local symptoms in the early stages may consist only of a feeling of discomfort in the post-nasal space and clearness of the nasal passages, but this quickly gives place to obstruction on the side of the sinusitis, with loss of vocal resonance. This is particularly noticeable with ethmoiditis, producing the typical 'flat voice'. The sense of smell may be lost or there may be cacosmia.

A diagnostic symptom is the nasal or post-nasal discharge, usually nasal in the early stage or after an exacerbation, gradually becoming post-nasal as the amount of discharge lessens and the cilia deal with the discharge by conveying it into the post-nasal space.

The patient may complain of an unpleasant taste associated with post-nasal drip.

It is unusual for epistaxis to be severe or repeated but such a symptom should suggest an acute infection in one of the sinuses, often the antrum. This may be overlooked and the epistaxis treated by cauterization, packing or even transfusion when an antral washout will quickly prevent a recurrence.

Pain over the sinus concerned may be localized or referred along branches of the nerves involved in the inflammation.

Antral pain   This is characteristically described by drawing the finger from the inner canthus of the eye downwards across the cheek under the eye. It radiates along the upper alveolus and is referred to the teeth or gums on the affected side and may be worse on coughing or bending. Patients with maxillary sinusitis may report to a dental surgeon before consulting a doctor.

Pain referred in the distribution of the supra-orbital nerve is a common symptom and is therefore frequently and mistakenly interpreted as evidence of frontal sinusitis. It may also be referred to the ear but careful examination will show a normal tympanic membrane.

Ethmoidal pain   Ethmoidal pain is localized over the bridge of the nose and inner canthus behind the eye. This is aggravated by moving the eye. Pain may be referred to the parietal eminence and is often localized to a small area.

Frontal pain   The pain of frontal sinusitis is mainly localized to the forehead and is always associated with generalized headache. Infection in the frontal sinus gives rise to the characteristic periodicity of pain more than in any other sinus. It often persists for an hour or two after getting up in the morning and clears during the afternoon.

The symptoms mentioned above vary largely in respect of the acute or chronic nature of the infection and the degree of obstruction at the nasal opening of the sinus involved. If the ostium is patent then, as the natural defences come into action with an outpouring of mucus and leucocytes, there will be a free discharge of mucopus and the symptoms are usually relieved.

In the closed infections, however, in which the natural drainage is obstructed, the outpouring of serum, mucus and leucocytes produces pressure in the inflamed sinus and the symptoms are all increased and prolonged. Pain then becomes a marked feature either locally or referred and may be very severe.

Sphenoid pain   Acute sphenoiditis is usually associated with a pan-sinusitis and in particular with infection of the posterior ethmoidal cells. It may give rise to occipital or vertical headache and sometimes referred to the mastoid process.

Signs

The signs of sinusitis are frequently masked by those of the accompanying acute rhinitis and as an aid to their elucidation it is usual to divide the sinuses into

(1) an anterior group consisting of maxillary, anterior ethmoid and frontal sinuses; and
(2) a posterior group which includes the posterior ethmoid and sphenoid sinuses.

The anterior group drains into the middle meatus and the posterior group drains into the superior meatus and spheno–ethmoidal recess.

External signs   In the case of maxillary, frontal or ethmoidal sinusitis external signs may be present. There may be slight flushing of the cheek with swelling which may spread to the lower lid in the case of the antrum; in frontal sinusitis the upper lid may be affected.

Ethmoiditis rarely gives rise to any external appearances except when complicated by abscess formation. There may then be swelling just above and internal to the inner canthus. This applies particularly to children with ethmoiditis and abscess formation. The lids may also be swollen.

Tenderness over the frontal sinus must be carefully distinguished from tenderness over the supra-orbital nerve, which is more common with maxillary than with frontal sinusitis.

In frontal sinusitis tenderness on pressure over the floor of the sinus just above the inner canthus is diagnostic, although tapping over the inner end of the supra-orbital ridge may cause exquisite pain.

In maxillary sinusitis there may be tenderness over the cheek in closed infections or on palpation of a tooth if the sinusitis is of dental origin.

Anterior rhinoscopy   The general increased redness and mucosal swelling of an accompanying rhinitis may obscure the local signs of an acute sinusitis but when these can be seen they will consist of a localized area of red, shiny and swollen mucous membrane in the neighbourhood of the ostium of one of the sinuses. In acute cases after shrinkage by the application of cocaine and adrenaline it is easier to see the local signs of sinusitis.

If the lateral wall of the nose is easy to examine it may be possible to see a localized area of swelling high up under the anterior end of the middle turbinate and a trickle of pus may be seen coming down from the same area; this would be suggestive of a frontal sinusitis.

The presence of pus farther back in the middle meatus would strongly suggest an antral infection. Ethmoiditis usually gives a more general swelling of the middle turbinate.

From the posterior sinuses pus will trickle from the superior meatus between the middle turbinate and the septum. This is not always easy to demonstrate

Examination of the nasopharynx and pharynx   Pus may be seen on the upper surface of the palate or trickling down the lateral pharyngeal gutter. When there is a free discharge of pus from one of the sinuses it may appear as a curtain across the posterior wall of the pharynx.

Investigations

Bacteriology

An attempt must be made to culture the organism responsible and assess its sensitivities at the same time as treatment is started, but in practice it will be found that most patients will have been already treated by their practitioner with an antibiotic before a culture swab was taken.

This makes it even more important that a suitable antibiotic is selected in the first instance. A culture swab is more likely to be taken if the sinusitis fails to respond to initial antibiotic treatment, though this is not a correct practice.

X-ray examination

Hodgson (1933) developed the usefulness of radiographs of the sinuses. He recommended the upright position and devised a sinus stand with a head clamp for this purpose.

Sometimes the prone or supine position will give more information particularly in demonstrating fluid in a posterior sinus. A horizontal x-ray beam must always be used for demonstrating fluid levels.

The various standard views, their variations, the use of stereoscopic views, tomography and examination with radio-opaque substances are all discussed in Volume I. The diagnostic use of computerized tomography is still in its infancy and may prove helpful in the differentiation between benign polypoidal lesions and malignant tumours. Routine practice is to take the standard occipitomental view to demonstrate the maxillary sinuses and the occipito–frontal view to demonstrate both the ethmoid and frontal sinuses. A lateral or submento–vertical view may also be necessary.

Soft tissue structures such as polypoidal changes in the sinuses are sometimes best demonstrated on a blue medichrome film viewed through a coloured filter.

The x-ray appearances in acute or chronic sinusitis are as follows.

Thickened mucosal lining

The mucosal lining may become grossly thickened but if there is an air space present the appearance of the soft tissue swellings within the cavity will be typical (*Figure 13.3*). Sometimes these swellings are reported as 'polypi'. Mucous cysts give a similar

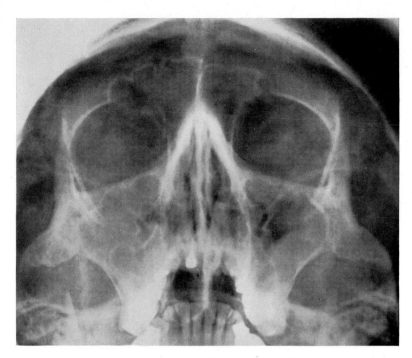

Figure 13.3   Radiograph showing uniform opacity of right antrum and a lining membrane mainly on the outer wall of the left antrum. No fluid level can be seen on either side

appearance although they are more discrete and rounded. If there is no air space present and the soft tissue swelling is gross, then the appearance may be of an opaque sinus.

Opaque sinuses

An opacity of a sinus must be investigated to determine whether the sinus is full of pus or has gross mucosal thickening. An opaque maxillary antrum can be best seen in the occipitomental (45 degree tilt) position (*Figure 13.4*).

Fluid level

This is most commonly visible in the maxillary antrum (*Figure 13.5a*) but may be present also in the frontal sinuses. In the erect position fluid gravitates to the floor of the antrum, often showing a dense area in the lower part with a horizontal upper margin. If the fluid is very viscous the surface may not be quite level and appear with a meniscus. A fluid level may be demonstrated by tilting the head to one side while maintaining the 45-degree extension. Sufficient time must be given for a viscous fluid to take up a new position but the change in position can often be demonstrated, so confirming the presence of fluid (*Figure 13.5b*).

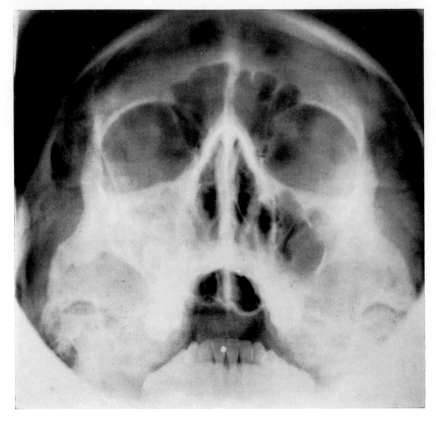

Figure 13.4   Opaque right antrum. Right antral washout yielded offensive pus. The tooth causing the 'dental' infection can be seen in the cavity

A fluid level in the sphenoidal sinus can sometimes be seen on a lateral view taken in the prone or supine position (*Figure 13.6*). Fluid level in the posterior ethmoidal cells can be seen in a view taken in the standard submento–vertical position (*Figure 13.7*).

Differential diagnosis

There are many conditions which may confuse the diagnosis of acute sinusitis. Most of these conditions present with facial pain as the predominant symptom so these are discussed first.

Pain as the symptom of sinusitis is discussed on p. 256. In the differential diagnosis the most common cause of confusion is pain of dental origin.

Dental neuralgia

Caries with or without gross infection may simulate sinusitis and particularly maxillary sinus infection. A carious tooth will in time develop infection of the pulp

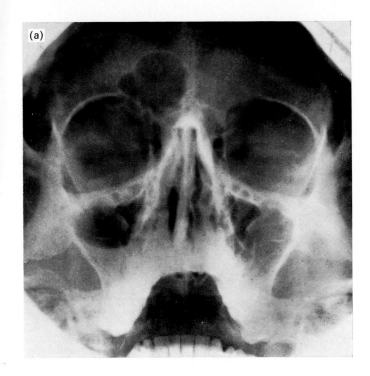

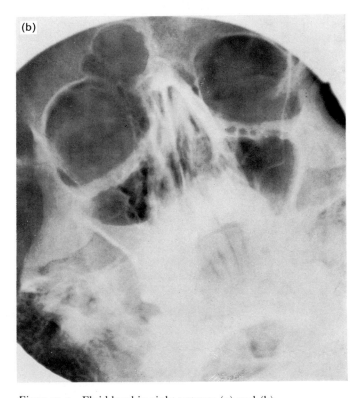

Figure 13.5   Fluid level in right antrum (a) and (b)

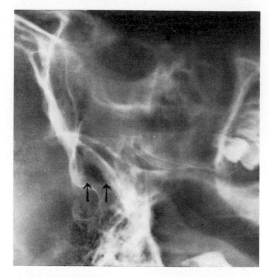

Figure 13.6   Showing fluid level in sphenoid with patient prone

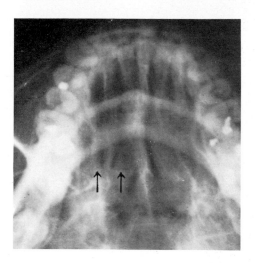

Figure 13.7   Showing fluid level in posterior ethmoid cell

space causing a pulpitis. This is characterized by a poorly localized pain. The affected tooth is sensitive to thermal change but not to percussion until the periodontal membrane is involved by apical extension of the infection. In contrast with pulpitis, the pain of a periodontal infection is constant and may well be localized to the region of the tooth. At this time the affected tooth is sensitive to percussion. Apical infection or apical abscess nearly always gives some swelling of the cheek which is more marked than is found with maxillary sinusitis. An x-ray examination may show thickening of the lining membrane due to the proximity of the infected tooth. It may require a proof puncture of the antrum to prove it is not infected.

Recurring and intense pain often lasting for weeks or months in the region of an extracted tooth will frequently call for an examination to exclude antral infection. It is believed that damage to one of the branches of a dental nerve gives rise to this pain which is similar to causalgia from damage to other peripheral nerves.

Temporo-mandibular neuralgia

Temporo-mandibular neuralgia (Costen's syndrome) is due to alteration in the bite producing stresses and strains in the temporo–mandibular joint. The pain may be dull or severe and usually present when the patient is chewing. The joint itself is often tender to palpation. The pain may radiate forward into the face or upward into the temporalis muscle. The condition can be relieved by prosthetic devices that prevent overclosure of the bite.

Trigeminal neuralgia

The pain of trigeminal neuralgia (tic douloureux) is characterized by its distribution in the area of supply of the fifth nerve only. The main sites have been defined in (1) the mouth–ear zone where the pain spreads from the region of the lower canine tooth back to a position felt deep in the ear and (2) the nose–orbit zone where the pain shoots up from the nostril to the orbit. The pain is characteristic as it starts as a feeling like 'electricity' or 'red-hot needles' and builds up into an excruciating pain that is felt deep in the face. It lasts only a few seconds but is then replaced by a very unpleasant ache or burning sensation. Attacks may vary from one every few minutes to one or two a day. They are usually 'triggered' by chewing, smiling, yawning or hot or cold fluids touching a lower canine tooth.

Atypical facial pain

Atypical facial pain is usually misdiagnosed as being due to dental or sinus disease because the pain is invariably in one or other maxillary region. The pain is described as deep, burning and continuous. In spite of the patient's insistence on the severity of the pain, the response is often inappropriate and the facial appearance is unlike that of a patient with tic. Psychotic facial pain may be an extension of this condition but in these cases the pain is confined to a single area such as the tongue.

Migraine

In migraine the pain is usually unilateral and fronto–temporal, although sometimes it starts in the occipital area and radiates forward to the 'classic' frontal region. A variant often ascribed to sinusitis is where the pain is confined to a position deep in behind the eye (Patten, 1977). Classic migraine has dramatic prodromas such as 'fortification' spectra (seeing zig-zag lines which look like fortifications of a castle), nausea and vomiting. Most commonly they will consist of photophobia with some slight visual blurring. The diagnosis is made from the history for there are no abnormal neurological signs.

Temporal arteritis

Temporal arteritis typically occurs in elderly patients (invariably over 60 years of age) who develop pain and tenderness over an obviously swollen temporal artery on one or both sides.

The other superficial arteries of the head may be involved. The ESR will be raised and biopsy will confirm the diagnosis. A high risk of blindness exists if steroids are not given.

Trigeminal nerve lesions

These lesions involve the trigeminal nerve such as tumours of the cerebello–pontine angle and Paget's disease may alter the anatomy of the apex of the petrous bone and irritate the trigeminal nerve.

Nasopharyngeal tumours

Nasopharyngeal tumours are of the greatest interest to the rhinologist as they may be symptomless for months and facial pain may be the first symptom. If this is associated with conductive deafness and later with immobility of the soft palate or a metastatic node in the neck the diagnosis becomes almost certain (*see* Volume 4).

Brain-stem lesions

Lesions in the brain stem including primary and secondary tumours of the pons and medulla, multiple sclerosis, thrombotic lesions and syringobulbia may also set up facial pain.

Herpetic or post-herpetic neuralgia may simulate the pain of sinusitis but is only likely to be confusing in the early stages before the vesicles appear, or in the later stages without a complete history.

Specific fevers

In acute specific fevers the headache associated with rhinitis, in *measles* for example, may suggest a sinus infection but development of the rash will usually make the diagnosis plain. *Nasal diphtheria* is associated with a purulent nasal discharge and the diagnosis is established by finding the Klebs–Loeffler bacillus on bacteriological examination. It is a rare condition but may easily be overlooked in children. *Typhoid fever* may be mistaken for a sinusitis, usually ethmoiditis, before the diagnosis is confirmed by the Widal reaction. The headache is general but there is often pain behind the eyes aggravated by the jarring of the cough which is a symptom of typhoid fever. *Cerebrospinal meningitis* might be confused in the early stages and meningitis of whatever origin may cast suspicion on the sinuses. *Erysipelas* may cause confusion and the slight swelling and redness over the frontal sinus or the cheek, with swollen lids and headache, malaise and fever, produce a picture that may be misleading. The raised edge to the swelling and the stippling of the surface develop quickly and clarify the diagnosis.

Children may push into the nose *foreign bodies* such as beads, pieces of plastic, etc.

A unilateral and usually profuse purulent malodorous discharge will be present and may suggest a sinusitis.

Angioneurotic oedema

Angioneurotic oedema can cause confusion but only until a rhinological examination is made.

Insect bite

Insect bite of the face may suggest a sinusitis by producing local redness and swelling.

Neoplasms of the sinuses

Tumours of the ethmoid, by obstructing the middle meatus and perhaps causing a secondary chronic rhinitis, may simulate chronic ethmoiditis and a transitional cell papilloma may be confused with a polypus until examined histologically. Carcinoma of the antrum may produce nasal obstruction, swelling of the cheek and dental symptoms. Radiographs should be taken to demonstrate bone destruction.

Treatment of acute sinusitis

The treatment of acute sinusitis is medical, for major surgical procedures should be avoided and even minor ones delayed until antibiotics have begun to have their effect. Active measures should begin immediately after the onset of the infection. Acute sinusitis is hardly ever dangerous if uncomplicated, but the development of a serious complication can be fatal. If it is not adequately treated by conservative measures a chronic condition is easily established which may require major surgery later, or it may persist for 1–3 months by which time permanent damage is done to the mucous membrane and recurrence becomes more likely.

The treatment can be discussed under three headings.

Prophylactic treatment

Prevention of colds by general treatment

Any factor, whether it be environmental or a medical illness which directly affects the health of a patient, has to be considered. If the general resistance is lowered by chronic illness or by physical or mental fatigue, then these factors may influence the preservation or breakdown of the first line of defence in the nose, namely the protecting mucous blanket and the ciliary action. Once these defences are lost and the submucosa is damaged, both general and local treatment are less effective.

Environmental changes of climate and those produced by air conditioning or central heating may markedly affect the state and activity of the nasal mucous membrane. Flying, and swimming with a cold should always be avoided.

Medical treatment

This consists primarily of antibiotics associated with local decongestants and with analgesics as the pain may require. Many patients remain ambulatory but in general it is best to put the patient at rest in a warm, well-humidified room. This is particularly the case in a patient with acute frontal sinus symptoms. The diet should be light and tobacco and alcohol should be avoided as they cause congestion of the nasal mucosa.

Antibiotics

It has been customary to use penicillin for the treatment of acute sinusitis but with the development of antibiotics with a wider spectrum which are effective not only against the pneumococci, streptococci, *Staphylococcus aureus*, but also the *Haemophilus influenzae*, the choice of antibiotics has changed in recent years.

The antibiotics of choice to commence therapy are amoxicillin (Amoxil) or co-trimoxazole (Septrin). Co-trimoxazole is to be preferred if a staphylococcus is suspected as the main organism.

Doxycycline (Vibramycin) is an equally effective antibiotic but being a tetracycline derivative is not suitable for children in view of its adverse effect on developing teeth. Erythromycin may be used in children who are allergic to penicillin derivatives.

Agbin (1974) has shown that doxycycline penetrates the sinus well, for he found effective concentrations of the antibiotic in the secretions of acute sinusitis. Studies by Carenfelt and his co-workers (1975) have shown that values determined in the laboratory do not always give a true description of the sensitivity of bacteria to antibiotics *in vivo* and that the most important factor achieving a maximal effect was to obtain the highest antibiotic concentrations at the site of infection. It is therefore important that antibiotic treatment for sinusitis should be continued for an adequate time and not be stopped as soon as the patient starts to feel well as there is a strong likelihood of recurrence.

Local decongestants

The ideal decongestant is one which will not interfere with the action of the cilia. Ephedrine or xylometazoline hydrochloride (Otrivine) are probably the least harmful drugs to cilia and are best administered in a spray. A spray should be used to clear the nose and then, 20 min later, a steam inhalation with menthol, Friar's balsam or pine oil administered to encourage drainage and give symptomatic relief. It is important that the patient is adequately instructed in the preparation of a steam inhalation.

Douching and forceful nose blowing should be avoided in the acute stage owing to the risk of spreading infection.

Analgesics

Aspirin and codeine preparations are usually sufficient to control the pain and only rarely are opiates necessary.

Heat applied locally by an electric pad or hot water bottle may bring symptomatic relief but if the ostium is blocked sudden heating may aggravate the pain.

Surgical treatment

Surgery is rarely necessary. In the case of maxillary sinusitis antral lavage can be carried out (the technique is described in Chapter 14).

It is perhaps better avoided during the first few days until antibiotic therapy has commenced. In the early stages there may be no return as the lining is so acutely swollen but it may be most valuable in the later stages when the sinus ostium is blocked by thick secretions.

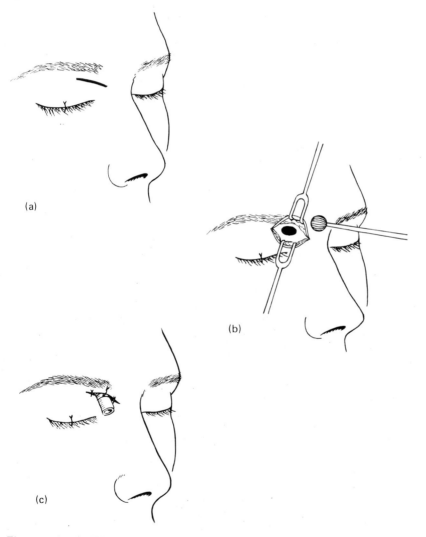

(a)

(b)

(c)

Figure 13.8   (a) The incision for trephination of the frontal sinus. (b) The bony opening can be made with a burr or osteotome. (c) Silicone tubing is inserted into the sinus cavity

Frontal sinusitis is almost invariably accompanied by maxillary infection and antral lavage is usually required as part of the treatment.

Rarely, frontal sinus symptoms continue for more than 2–3 weeks and it may be necessary to carry out a submucous resection of the septum, or to excise part of the middle turbinate so as to clear the fronto-ethmoidal region and permit drainage.

It is recommended that the frontal sinus should be opened and a drain inserted when acute frontal sinusitis does not respond to medical treatment. If the pain is worsening after 72 h, with increasing swelling threatening an orbital cellulitis, or if there is no abatement of pyrexia, a decision must be taken whether the frontal sinus should be drained (*Figure 13.8*). No other operative procedure is necessary at this stage and even this operation is rarely necessary today.

Acute sinusitis in children

As the frontal sinuses are not fully developed in small children it is to be expected that the maxillary antra and ethmoids are those most commonly affected.

Even newborn babies are occasionally infected by their mothers, but it is usually after six months that the condition appears. There is often an increase in incidence at the age of three and a significant rise between five and six years. This corresponds with attendance at play-group and later at school, with exposure to numerous viruses and bacterial organisms, and at the same time to infection and enlargement of the tonsils and adenoids.

It usually starts as an acute rhinitis with, perhaps, more marked constitutional symptoms than in the adult. An ethmoiditis may present with rapid swelling of the eyelids to such a degree that the eye is closed. There may be purulent discharge from the nostril but occasionally it remains dry as no drainage is taking place.

Acute sinusitis in babies has to be differentiated from acute osteomyelitis of the maxilla. This is a staphylococcal infection of an unerupted deciduous tooth and the surrounding bone. The swelling in this condition is usually considerably more extensive than in sinusitis and involves the cheek and hard palate as well as the eyelids. The alveolus is swollen and sometimes a fistula is present.

The treatment of acute sinusitis is the same as for adults; with antibiotics, decongestants and analgesics. If the symptoms and signs do not quickly abate antral lavage is usually necessary. This is carried out under general anaesthesia and a polythene tube can be inserted through a large Lichtwitz cannula and secured in place so that washouts can be repeated on subsequent days.

Agamma-globulinaemia

In cases of congenital or acquired gamma-globulin deficiency predisposition to recurrent sinus infection can be expected, but a search for reduced serum globulin levels in patients with this condition is seldom rewarding. It should be kept in mind, however, when dealing with particularly refractory cases which show recurrent infections of other regions as well.

Sinus barotrauma

Sinus barotrauma was established as a clinical entity in 1942 by Campbell although it had previously been known to be one of the hazards of flight. He had defined barotrauma as 'an acute or chronic inflammation of one or more of the nasal accessory sinuses produced by barometric pressure differences between the air or gas inside the sinus and that of the surrounding atmosphere'.

Rapid descent in an aircraft or rapid ascent during scuba diving can result in sinus barotrauma.

Boyle's law states that at any given temperature the volume of a gas varies in inverse proportion to the pressure exerted on it. Calculations have shown that one volume of air at sea level becomes two volumes at 18 000 ft and four volumes at 33 000 ft (United States Department of the Air Force, 1962). As the air expands during ascent it easily passes through the natural ostia of the sinuses to equilibrate with the ambient air pressure. During descent air must return through the ostia to equalize with the rapidly increasing atmospheric pressure. When the sinus ostia and nasal mucosa are normal the air exchange occurs efficiently and without subjective sensation.

By pressurizing an aircraft cabin to an altitude of less than 8000 ft, as is done in commercial aircraft, minimum stress is placed on this exchange mechanism. Military aircraft, however, can ascend faster than 1 mile/min and descend faster than 10 000 ft/min, subjecting the paranasal sinuses to rapid and high-magnitude barometric stress.

Upon descent, a relative negative pressure occurs in the sinus and a plug of mucus or swollen and redundant mucous membrane may act as a cork, occluding the sinus orifice. Negative pressure in this sealed sinus is resolved by the cavity becoming filled with fluid or blood. With rapid or extreme pressure changes, the mucosa can be ripped from the sinus wall resulting in a haematoma of the sinus.

The frontal sinus is most vulnerable to severe barotrauma because of its long, narrow, bony fronto–nasal duct and a lack of accessory ostia (Weissman and Green, 1972).

Prompt medical treatment is required with the addition of a vigorous course of vasoconstrictors placed in the middle meatus under direct vision.

Fungal infection of the sinuses

In recent years there has been an increasing number of cases of fungal infection of the sinuses reported in the literature.

The circumstances in which fungal infection is known to occur are: (1) trauma of the face, particularly after compound fractures; (2) poorly controlled diabetes; (3) severely debilitated patients such as those with carcinomatosis; and (4) patients who have been treated with immunosuppressive drugs, antibiotics and steroids.

Primary aspergillosis of the sinuses is the type of mycotic infection most frequently reported. It is usually confined to one sinus, primarily the maxillary sinus. It may extend to the orbit, causing pain, proptosis and decreasing vision. Zinneman (1972) reviewed the world literature and revealed only 37 cases; however 17 of these cases were reported by one group of authors (Milosed *et al.*, 1969). It becomes apparent that aspergillosis of the paranasal sinuses is probably much more common than reported.

The chief symptom is usually nasal obstruction associated with nasal and post-nasal blood-stained discharge. In the nose a mass of necrotic fungus can be seen and sent for investigation.

Treatment should be complete excision of the necrotic and diseased tissue if possible by whichever surgical approach is the most appropriate. Antral washings have not proved successful in treatment due to the thick, gelatinous consistency of the fungal mass. Systemic antifungal therapy with amphotericin B combined with tetracycline and nystatin have been used; systematic anti-fungal therapy alone, however, has been unsuccessful and should not be employed since the prognosis is usually excellent with simple surgical intervention (Warder, Chikes and Hudson, 1975).

Tuberculosis of the sinuses

Myerson (1944) collected only 48 cases in the literature and nearly 80 per cent of the 27 cases involving the maxillary sinus were fatal. All the cases in which the other sinuses were affected were fatal, the meninges nearly always becoming involved. The infection was always by the bloodstream from a pulmonary or extrapulmonary focus.

The few cases reported in the last 20 years have been more conservatively treated.

Leprosy

The nasal mucous membrane is involved only by direct spread from the face in the localized or tuberculoid type of leprosy, whereas in the lepromatous type the nasal mucous membrane is always involved and the *Mycobacterium leprae* can always be found in a smear. Secondary purulent sinusitis is very common. Specific leprosy of the sinuses is probably never seen clinically or by pathological examination.

Syphilis

In spite of the rise of early syphilis after the Second World War, the expected rise in tertiary cases has not occurred. Lee (1968) reviewed the literature and described but a single case. The diagnosis is made by biopsy and serology. It must be distinguished from malignancy.

References

Agbin, O. G. (1974). *Clinical Medical Research Opinion*, **2**, 291

Bjorkwall, T. (1950). *Acta otolaryngologica Stockholm*, Suppl. 83

Black, J. Munro, (1964). *Journal of Laryngology*, **78**, 785

Bujuggren, G., Kraepelien, S., Lind, J. and Tunevall, G. (1953). *Svenska Läkartidningen*, **50**, 953

Cambell, P. A. (1942). *Archives of Otolaryngology*, **35**, 107

Carenfelt, C., Enroth, C., Lundberg, C. and Wretlind, B. (1975). *Scandinavian Journal of Infectious Diseases*, **7**, 259

Department of Health and Social Security. (1971). *Digest of Statistics*

Dishoek, H. A. E. van and Franssen, M. G. C. (1957). *Practical Otorhinolaryngology*, **19**, 502

Drettner, B. and Lindholm, C. E. (1967). *Acta Otolaryngologica, Stockholm*, **64**, 508

Formby, M. L. (1960). *Proceedings of the Royal Society of Medicine*, **53**, 163

Hodgson, H. K. G. (1933). *British Medical Journal*, **1**, 5

Holdaway, M. D. and Turk, D. C. (1967). *Lancet*, **1**, 358

Hora, J. F. (1965). *Laryngoscope*, **75**, 768

Kinman, J. Chang, W. L. and Seung, H. P. (1967). *Acta otolaryngologica, Stockholm*, Suppl., **11**, 1

Lee N. Y. (1968). *Ohio Medical Journal*, **64**, 1264

Milosed, B., Mahgoub, E. S., Abdel Aal, O. and el

Hassan, A. M. (1969). *British Journal of Surgery*, **56**, 132

Mounier-Kuhn, P. (1953). *Journal français otolaryngologie*, **11**, 1

Myerson, M. C. (1944). *Tuberculosis of the Ear, Nose and Throat*, Springfield, Illinois; Thomas

Palva, T. A., Grönroos, J. A. and Palva, A. (1962). *Acta otolaryngologica, Stockholm*, **54**, 159

Patten, J. (1977). *Neurological Differential Diagnosis*, London; Starke

Powell, R. N. (1965). *Oral Surgery*, **19**, 24

Tyrell, D. A. J. (1965). *Common colds and Related diseases*, London; Edward Arnold

United States Dept. of the Airforce, (1962). *Flight Surgeons Manual*, **4**, 1

Warder, F. R., Chikes, D. G. and Hudson, W. R. (1975). *Scandinavian Journal of Infectious Diseases*, **7**, 259

Weissman, B. and Green, R. S. (1972). *Laryngoscope*, **82**, 2160

Zinneman, H. H. (1972). *Minnesota Medicine*, **55**, 661

14 Chronic sinusitis
David Wright

Introduction

Chronic sinusitis during the last two decades has become a less common disease. Whereas it was a debilitating disease affecting a significant proportion of any population, it now presents only occasionally but when it does the disease, particularly frontal sinus disease, still carries the same risk of morbidity from the development of serious complications. In many cases it follows an incompletely resolved acute sinusitis, but it may appear insidiously following a cold or dental infection. The maxillary sinus is the commonest to be affected but often other sinuses are involved, at the same time. Chronic ethmoiditis is often associated with nasal polyposis.

In the pre-antibiotic days the need for major surgery was much more common than today for the danger from complications could be very serious. Many operations were designed; almost every approach to every sinus seems to have been explored and the degree of skill attained by some surgeons, particularly in the field of intranasal clearance, was great indeed. To read of the technical achievements of Halle (1907, 1914) and Mosher (1929) in the early part of the century cannot but impress the present-day surgeon.

On the other hand many inadequately treated cases are reported; Negus (1947) recalls a patient who came to him after 17 operations for frontal sinusitis.

The operations used in present-day practice are described in detail in this chapter. Some of them will be required only on rare occasions but the operator should have knowledge of their application and be in a position to perform them when indicated.

Aetiology and bacteriology

The causes of chronic sinusitis, the bacteriology and the factors which predispose to chronic sinus infection are so closely associated with those of acute sinusitis that they have been discussed together in Chapter 13.

Pathology

The pathological changes encountered in chronic sinusitis have been recognized over the years and classified according to the histological changes (Eggston and Wolff, 1947; Rewell; 1963).

Histological changes

(1) Hypertrophic or polypoid sinusitis
(2) Atrophic sinusitis
(3) Papillary hypertrophic sinusitis

Hypertrophic or polypoid sinusitis
In hypertrophic sinusitis the inflammatory changes mainly affect the efferent vessels (*Figure 14.1*) and the lymphatics and the soft tissues are secondarily affected. The inflammation starts as a periphlebitis or a perilymphangitis. If an acute attack subsides completely little damage will be done but repeated attacks will ultimately produce fibrous changes which are permanent and will make subsequent attacks of acute inflammation more likely to become chronic. In chronic inflammation the venous and lymphatic changes produce oedema and a polypoid mucous membrane, polypi, oedematous periosteum and rarefaction of bone.

Atrophic sinusitis
In atrophic sinusitis the condition is associated with much less increase in tissue and such increase is due to an increase in submucous fibrous tissue rather than oedema of the stroma.

Microscopically the main changes can be shown to occur in the afferent vessels, in the early stages there is a cellular reaction around the arterioles and arteries, and the latter vessel walls become thickened and the lumen narrowed; often endarteritis and thrombosis are present (*Figure 14.2*).

These microscopic changes certainly accord with the gross pathological conditions found and with the clinical conditions in so-called hypertrophic sinusitis on the one hand and atrophic sinusitis on the other. Both types may occur side by side in the same sinus producing atrophy or necrosis in one place and polypoid hypertrophy in another.

Papillary hypertrophic sinusitis
This is an uncommon variety of sinusitis which may be mistaken for a neoplasm at operation; but microscopically it will be seen that there is a metaplasia from a ciliated columnar epithelium to a stratified squamous epithelium or to an intermediate form, and throughout the papillary hyperplastic epithelial cells or stroma may be seen numerous inflammatory cells. Eggston and Wolff (1947) believe that this condition follows a virus infection, certain tissue changes being, in their opinion, characteristic of such infection.

Rewell (1963) considers that the distinction between chronic papillary sinusitis and transitional cell tumours may be difficult to make. Fundamentally the inflammatory element is greater and the tumour pattern is less in sinusitis. The final decision may have to depend on whether or not the mass recurs. Neither he nor Eggston and Wolff (1947) consider metaplasia as diagnostic of malignancy.

Eosinophilia

In an attempt to differentiate between allergy and sinusitis Van Dishoeck and Franseen (1957) examined the secretions of patients in which allergy was thought to be an important factor in the cause of their sinusitis and found an eosinophilia in ten out of 100 cases. Blood eosinophilia of 5 per cent or more occurred in only ten out of 62 patients (Kinman, 1967) and only two had over 8 per cent. On the whole, a search for the presence of an eosinophilia in secretions, tissues and particularly blood has not been rewarding as a guide to clinical diagnosis and management (Douek, 1971).

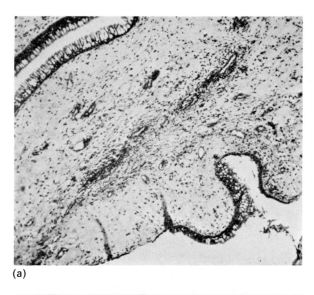

(a)

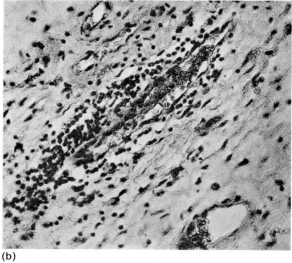

(b)

Figure 14.1 Hypertrophic sinusitis: (a) sloughing epithelium and periphlebitis; (b) high power magnification of the periphlebitis. (Reproduced by courtesy of Williams and Wilkins)

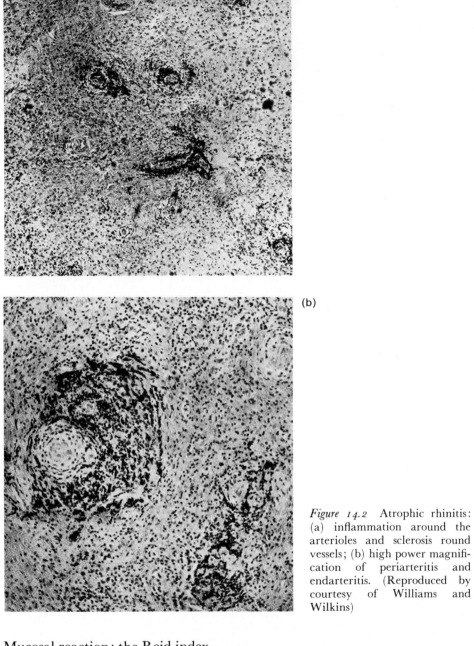

Figure 14.2 Atrophic rhinitis: (a) inflammation around the arterioles and sclerosis round vessels; (b) high power magnification of periarteritis and endarteritis. (Reproduced by courtesy of Williams and Wilkins)

Mucosal reaction; the Reid index

The nose is lined by a respiratory type of pseudostratified, ciliated, columnar epithelium richly supplied with goblet cells; the lamina propria containing numerous racemose seromucinous glands. This is essentially similar to the lining of the bronchi though there appears to be a higher proportion of serous cells in the nasal glands. In the sinuses the mucosa is much thinner, with fewer goblet cells. Racemose glands are scarce and found mostly round the ostia of the maxillary antra. The mucosal reaction which is brought about by longstanding inflammation, including mucous-gland hypertrophy and goblet-cell hyperplasia, is very similar to that found in the bronchial mucosa and this led Cawthorne and Edwards (1966) to postulate that the response of the lining membrane to inspired air will be the same whether it lines the nasal cavities or the lower bronchi.

Goblet-cell hyperplasia was described by Reid (1954) as an early change in chronic bronchitis, and pathological criteria for the diagnosis of chronic bronchitis have now been established and are widely accepted. The major criteria are hypertrophy of mucous glands and an increased proportion of goblet cells in the epithelium.

Reid (1960) described a method of quantitating mucous-gland hypertrophy by expressing the gland size as a ratio of the mucous gland thickness to the total width of the bronchial mucosa. This is generally known as the Reid index but it may be more strongly correlated to smoking than to the inflammation of chronic bronchitis.

Burton and Dixon (1969) used this index to compare the state of the mucosa of the nose, sinuses and bronchi. They came to the conclusion that atmospheric pollution affects the upper and lower respiratory tracts equally but smoking has a particularly adverse effect on the bronchi. This seems to be because smoke is inhaled directly from the mouth. They found no evidence to confirm the belief that simple chronic bronchitis, with no other pulmonary disease such as bronchiectasis, forms part of the so-called 'sinobronchial syndrome'.

Changes in the secretions and cilia

The cilia (*Figure 14.3*) which normally beat at the rate of 1000/min produce a flow

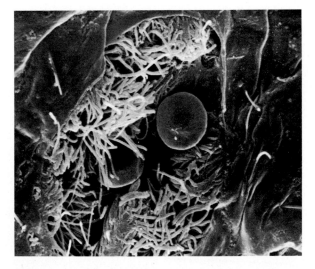

Figure 14.3   Scanning electron micrograph showing mucosal blanket overlying nasal cilia. × 5000, reduced by half on reproduction. (By courtesy of Professor N. Dilly and Mr R. F. Gray)

rate of about 4.2 mm/min at a relative humidity of 43.6 per cent (Ewert, 1965). In smokers the mean flow rate drops to 3.6 mm/min.

In chronic sinusitis it is almost impossible for the cilia to transport the viscous, profuse secretions. The chronic inflammatory reaction has destroyed large tracts of cilia-bearing cells interrupting still further the streaming of mucus towards the ostia, creating a situation where stagnation easily gives rise to re-infection.

The secretions produced by these glands are probably altered in quality as well as in quantity and in particular there is a change in the relationship between protein and mucopolysaccharide. This has stimulated an interest in mucolytic agents and led to study of the shape of the protein–mucopolysaccharide filaments and their depolymer-ization (Bürgi, 1965). These changes have an obvious bearing on pathological states for they produce considerable changes in viscosity. Mélon (1967) noted altered concentrations of protein and inorganic ions in patients with allergic rhinitis. There is no doubt that the chemical constitution and pH of the solution that bathes them affects the function of the cilia (Negus, 1958).

Blood changes

Changes in the systemic blood picture are few for the leucocyte count is usually below 8000/mm³, but occasionally it is slightly raised and the type of infection may reflect changes in the differential pattern. The erythrocyte sedimentation rate is always low, or at least returns to normal soon after treatment has started. This test should always give a normal response in simple chronic sinusitis so if the sedimentation rate is consistently high, the diagnosis must be suspect.

Serum proteins are usually within normal limits but electrophoresis may show a relative decrease in the albumin fraction with a raised gammaglobulin level.

Physiopathology

Drettner's (1967) work as described in Chapter 13 has shown that the resistance of the maxillary ostium is more pronounced in cases of chronic sinusitis than in the normal or acutely inflamed antrum.

Clinical features

Symptoms of chronic sinusitis
The symptoms of chronic sinusitis are very variable. They may be severe enough to prevent the patient from going to work or they may be so mild that the source of his chronic ill-health may never become obvious. Although the symptoms usually suggest inflammation of the nose or sinuses, they are sometimes quite unrelated to this region and the correct diagnosis may be missed.

To aid description they will be considered here under separate headings, but it should be understood that they are often vague, overlapping and changeable.

Symptoms relating to the nose, throat and ear

These symptoms form the most common manner of presentation. A patient may be referred complaining of disturbances in one or more of these regions often slight in intensity but irritating in their persistence.

Nasal and nasopharyngeal symptoms
The main complaints are nasal obstruction, nasal discharge and post-nasal drip, but quite often there may be associated epistaxis, vestibulitis and olfactory abnormalities.

Nasal obstruction
This may have been present prior to the sinusitis for a deflected nasal septum or allergic rhinitis may be one of the predisposing factors. The fact that a patient has decided only later to seek advice may indicate that a new feature has arisen and that the development of chronic sinusitis should be excluded. Polyps of mixed allergic-infective origin may be present and these often cause complete obstruction. Even in a structurally normal nose a sinus infection may set up a chronic rhinitis with nasal obstruction resulting from hypertrophy of the nasal mucosa and turbinates.

The nasal discharge
This may be of varied character. In a primarily allergic case the only change may be an increase in the quantity of clear mucus produced. Excess of nasal secretions is also produced by the accompanying rhinitis and usually frank mucopus is discharged. Blood staining is not uncommon, but a neoplasm should always be suspected in a patient with unilateral symptoms of this nature.

Post-nasal drip
This is a very common complaint and is often the only symptom. The cilia of the nose normally convey the mucopurulent secretions backwards so that a chronic nasopharyngitis develops. It is only if the secretions are excessive that they appear in the form of an anterior nasal discharge. A post-nasal drip is a particularly irritating symptom for it often causes a sensation of dryness and burning at the back of the nose together with an unpleasant taste in the mouth.

Epistaxis
Occasionally it results from the inflammatory vasodilatation in the nose. The possibility of an underlying chronic sinusitis should always be considered in patients with persistent nose-bleeds.

Abnormalities of smell
They are common in sinusitis though often overshadowed by other symptoms. They may take the form of cacosmia in which there is objective unpleasant odour, that is a smell noticeable to other people as well as to the patient; various degrees of hyposmia; and a distortion of smell perception, parosmia, usually present in patients with underlying allergic rhinitis. If the chronic sinusitis can be successfully treated the prognosis regarding the olfactory symptoms is generally very good (Douek, 1970).

Excoriation of the skin around the nostrils is more common in children but may occasionally be seen in adults with excess antronasal secretion, causing a *chronic vestibulitis.*

Pharyngeal symptoms
Pharyngitis may be the main symptom with the patient complaining only of dryness of the throat. The tonsils may become infected and the case may present as one of tonsillitis. Chronic sinusitis should always be excluded when an adult begins to suffer from tonsillitis after having been free from throat infection. When there is pharyngeal or tonsillar inflammation enlarged cervical lymph nodes are common.

Symptoms related to the ears
Nasopharyngitis often includes inflammation and swelling of the eustachian orifice so that symptoms of eustachian obstruction may occur. Occasionally this may turn into an acute otitis media or chronic secretory otitis. Chronic sinusitis may be a cause of persistent otorrhoea in the established chronic ear which does not respond to treatment, or which relapses despite intensive therapy.

Headache

Pain in the head and face are very common complaints in sinusitis. This fact is so well known that patients whose headaches are totally unrelated to the sinuses are often sent to the rhinologist. It is common to find, however, that only a small proportion of all the headaches seen are due to sinusitis. Other causes such as refractive errors, migraine, trigeminal neuralgia, tooth pain and cervical spondylosis have to be excluded. There is often a certain periodicity about a sinus headache, for it gradually becomes apparent during the morning and then wears off during the rest of the day. This has been said to be due to secretions accumulating in the sinuses during the night and then draining away as the patient takes up an erect posture. The cause of sinus headaches is not entirely clear. A theory which has remained popular since the time of Sluder (1918) is that if a drainage opening such as the fronto–nasal duct or maxillary ostium is blocked, a partial vacuum is produced, even in the uninfected sinus, and causes pain. There is little evidence to support this view and Drettner (1967) has produced a measured partial vacuum in the maxillary sinus without any resulting pain. Although the exact cause of this type of headache remains unexplained, it is likely to be associated in some way with inflammation and swelling of the lining mucosa.

The various sinuses present with slightly different pain areas so that these can have a certain localizing value. They have been described in Chapter 13, but may also be present in chronic sinusitis in a milder form.

Eyes

Ocular symptoms are not common and are usually the result of obstruction or infection of the lacrimal passages leading to conjunctivitis.

Respiratory tract symptoms

The continuous descent of infected pus may cause a chronic laryngitis which does not respond to local treatment. All such cases should have a sinus x-ray as part of their investigation.

A post-nasal drip often causes a constant cough which can be mistaken for chronic bronchitis, but a direct association between these two conditions is doubtful.

Digestive tract symptoms

The swallowing of infected secretions often sets up a low-grade gastritis with nausea and digestive disturbances.

General symptoms

General symptoms are surprisingly mild, even in widespread chronic sinusitis. A gradual increase in general ill-health and tiredness may not be always apparent to the patient. In some cases there may be a low-grade pyrexia or attacks of intermittent fever which may point to the wrong diagnosis.

From the point of view of historical interest a word should be said about chronic sinusitis and mental illness. In 1935, Pickworth published a series of 676 autopsies in mental patients and reported some signs of sinus inflammation in the sphenoidal sinuses of 30 per cent of these cases. He described the direct absorption by the brain of toxins resulting from vascular or perivascular transmission from sinus to cerebral capillaries. The suggestion seemed so important in its repercussions at the time that much work was done on this study. It is now generally accepted that there is little evidence in support of this theory. Chronic sinusitis is no more frequent in mental patients than in any section of the population that tends to have a lowered resistance, and a 'toxic' theory for mental illness has found little support.

Signs of chronic sinusitis

There are usually no external signs of chronic sinusitis. Ransome (1964) described six cases of non-malignant expansion of the maxillary antrum, four of which were due to chronic sinusitis with considerable hypertrophy of the mucosa. This rare possibility should be noted, but expansion of the antrum should always arouse suspicion of a neoplasm.

Anterior rhinoscopy
Anterior rhinoscopy usually shows the reddened, swollen mucosa of an accompanying rhinitis. In maxillary sinusitis pus may be seen in the region of the middle meatus. This is often made more obvious after spraying with cocaine. Placing the head down between the knees with the infected sinus upwards and then raising the head again may make the pus appear at the ostium.

Chronic ethmoiditis is very commonly associated with a polypoid hypertrophy of the sinus lining membrane and of the adjacent nasal mucosa. This often becomes a collection of polyps arising from the lateral wall of the nose above the inferior turbinate.

The nasal discharge is not profuse and tends to be inspissated tenacious mucopus. There is usually considerable crusting. Occasionally an ethmoidal infection may take the form of an encysted empyema with swelling of the affected cell. The middle turbinate may be grossly dilated on appearance.

In chronic sphenoidal sinusitis pus may be seen in the olfactory cleft. This is seen better with the help of Killian's nasal speculum.

In frontal sinusitis pus is usually seen in the middle meatus and as this is often associated with infection of the maxillary sinus or ethmoid sinus, it is not possible to distinguish by rhinoscopy the origin of the pus.

Posterior rhinoscopy
A pool of pus on the upper surface of the palate may arise from any sinus but is more commonly associated with infection in the anterior group. If the pus or mucopus is seen trickling over the posterior end of the inferior turbinate from the middle meatus, the sign is consistent with an infection in the anterior group of sinuses.

Local congestion in the region of the spheno–ethmoidal recess may be seen with a post-nasal mirror or nasopharyngoscope and pus may be seen trickling from the area of the sphenoidal ostium, the superior meatus, or from a posterior ethmoidal cell.

Examination of the pharynx
Pus may be seen trickling down the lateral pharyngeal gutter and usually comes from the anterior sinuses; even when no discharge is to be seen, swelling of the lateral lymphoid tissue suggests an anterior sinusitis on the same side. Whenever there is a free discharge of pus from any of the sinuses it may present as a curtain on the posterior pharyngeal wall.

Investigations

X-ray examination

Radiographic findings in chronic sinusitis are very similar to those of acute sinusitis. A radiograph is even more valuable in chronic illness as it is often the only positive finding in a vague complex of symptoms and signs. The appearances have already been described in Chapter 13 and the various views and techniques which demonstrate the sinuses are discussed in detail in Volume 1.

Transillumination

Transillumination can be used as a method to examine the maxillary and frontal sinuses if x-rays are not available.

A small source of light is used with a glass cover that can be easily removed and disinfected. The light is controlled by a rheostat so that the intensity can be varied while the patient is examined in a darkened room or under a cloth.

Transillumination of the antra is carried out by the patient closing his lips over the light source which is place centrally in the mouth. Any dental plate must be removed as it will obscure the test. The antra, if equal in size and normal, will transilluminate equally. This will result in an infra-orbital crescent of light and a brightly-lit eye with glowing pupil (*Figure 14.4*). The interpretation is not always easy, particularly if a similar pathological situation exists in both antra. If either or both do not light up normally it is because the antrum contains pus, mucopus, a thickened lining membrane or new growth; because it is smaller or denser from development or trauma, or because the soft tissues are thickened over the antrum.

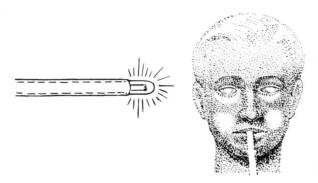

Figure 14.4   Transillumination of the sinuses

McNeill (1963) confirmed by lavage that 68 per cent of cases thought to be infected by transillumination were in fact so. This is 15 per cent less accurate than by x-ray examination. Both are therefore useful subsidiary methods of examination and when considered together and with the clinical picture will usually give an accurate diagnosis.

A striking difference is found if a large cyst is present in the maxillary sinus. A radiograph will show an opaque antrum, but transillumination is brilliantly clear.

It must be pointed out that both methods may be deceptive and in McNeill's series where three cases out of 25 showed the antra to be entirely normal radiologically, pus or mucopus was found on lavage; Ballantyne and Rowe (1949) in a review of 100 cases thought that transillumination was often misleading in the diagnosis.

The value of transillumination of the maxillary sinuses probably depends on the frequency with which it is employed and the experience of the individual surgeon.

Transillumination of the frontal sinus is of even more doubtful value. In this case the source of light is applied to the floor of the sinus above the inner canthus; these sinuses are so frequently unequal in size and shape that translucency merely suggests a well-developed and normal sinus, whereas opacity may only mean an undeveloped one.

Sinus sounding or puncturing

Direct evidence of sinusitis can be obtained by expelling pus or sucking it out of the relevant cavity. This can then be cultured and the sensitivity of the bacteria determined. Although pus obtained from the nose can also be cultured, it is much more likely to be contaminated by staphylococci and other nasal organisms than secretions collected directly from the sinuses.

The maxillary sinus is easily investigated in this manner but the other sinuses are more difficult.

Maxillary sinus

This is normally carried out by puncturing the bone of the inferior meatus. Apart from its value in establishing the diagnosis ('proof puncture') it plays an important part in the treatment of maxillary sinusitis and will be discussed in detail under that section.

Ethmoidal sinus

Puncture and aspiration of the ethmoid cells with an exploring needle and syringe through the bulla or a posterior ethmoidal cell is rarely necessary. If it is required in order to give information as to the bacteriology of an infection it can be done under local anaesthesia. The middle turbinate is made to shrink in size with cocaine and adrenaline and the needle inserted obliquely into the ethmoidal bulla passing it backwards into the posterior cells so as to avoid perforating the orbital plate. Sterile normal saline solution is injected and then withdrawn.

Frontal sinus

It is seldom possible to catheterize the frontal sinus without excising the anterior end of the middle turbinate. It cannot therefore be recommended as a diagnostic procedure, but it will be discussed as part of the treatment of frontal sinusitis.

Sphenoid sinus

The anterior sphenoidal wall is situated 7 cm from the anterior nasal spine, and in the adult is subject to very little variation. The opening of the ostium is in most cases within 10 mm of the roof of the nasal cavity. The anterior wall of the sphenoid sinus slopes downward and backward and consists of a thin nasal part close to the septum in which the ostium is always situated and a lateral ethmoid part.

There are two methods of irrigating the sphenoid sinus, (1) through the natural ostium, and (2) by making an opening in the anterior wall. The method of puncturing the thin anterior wall has certain advantages over the approach through the natural ostium.

For example, a cannula inserted through a natural ostium which is small and occluded with oedematous membrane, makes it impossible to apply suction. A technique of irrigation of the sphenoid sinus has been described by Tremble (1970) who used an indicator probe to identify the natural ostium and then a specially designed trocar and cannula which is either inserted through the natural ostium or is used to puncture the anterior wall close to the ostium. The calibre of the lumen is sufficient to allow aspiration of thick pus, if present.

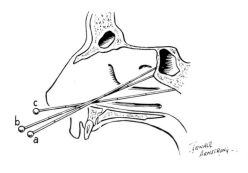

Figure 14.5   Diagram to illustrate the points in identifying the anterior sphenoid wall before puncture of the sphenoid sinus. (a) Sound crossing midpoint of middle turbinate and striking sphenoid wall at 7 cm from anterior nasal spine. (b) Sound identifying angle between anterior sphenoid wall and floor. (c) Sound has passed back along the floor of the sphenoid sinus

The anterior wall of the sphenoid sinus is located by passing the graduated probe through the nose, diagonally across the midpoint of the lower edge of the middle turbinate, so striking the sphenoid wall at 7 cm from the anterior nasal spine (*Figure 14.5*). There is now a margin of safety of 2.5 cm above this point where the thin nasal part of the anterior wall of the sinus may be punctured with the trocar, followed by irrigation of the sinus with normal saline through the cannula. The procedure can be satisfactorily carried out under local anaesthesia; a general anaesthetic is preferable and may be necessary if there are deformities in the septum, preventing access to the anterior sphenoid wall. The position of the probe or cannula can always be confirmed by means of a lateral radiograph.

Bacteriology

It is an essential part of the diagnosis and management of chronic sinusitis to attempt to culture the organisms from sinus washings or nasal swabs, though in practice the results from the laboratory are often disappointing. Chemotherapy can then be started immediately in the knowledge that sensitivities will be available shortly if the treatment proves ineffective.

Diagnosis and assessment

The combination of signs and symptoms aided by radiography and 'proof-puncture' rarely leave the diagnosis of chronic sinusitis in doubt but some further points need to be elucidated:

(1) A conscious attempt should be made to clarify whether a single sinus is involved or whether there is a multisinusitis or a pansinusitis so that the full extent of the disease is determined.
(2) The role of allergy should be assessed in each particular case. This is generally done with the help of the history, the appearance of the nasal lining and its secretions, and the response to anti-allergic treatment. Some like to add a search for eosinophils in the secretions.
(3) The presence of such predisposing factors as infected teeth, a deflected nasal septum and nasal polypi of whatever origin should be noted.
(4) The severity of the symptoms, the length of time they have persisted and the amount and type of previous treatment received already by the patient are all features that must be carefully noted as they will influence future management.

If pain and headache are prominent symptoms, the same questions are posed as in the differential diagnosis for acute sinusitis.

Cysts of dental origin in the maxillary sinus must be recognized (Volume 4). Exclusion of malignant neoplasms in the nose and sinuses can be difficult in the early stages.

Unilateral nasal obstruction, discharge and epistaxis together with persistent pain should arouse suspicion, and the possibility of malignancy must always be kept in mind when considering chronic sinusitis. These conditions are discussed in Chapter 17.

Treatment

The management of acute sinusitis is based on the assumption that complete recovery of the lining membrane of the sinuses is the likely outcome. This assumption cannot be made in chronic sinusitis. Indeed, the management of this condition depends principally on whether the lining mucosa has been irreversibly damaged or not. If recovery is possible, the treatment should be conservative and consists of obtaining adequate drainage of the sinuses by medical and minor surgical procedures such as antrum washouts.

If recovery is unlikely by conservative means then radical surgery has to be considered. Most operations are designed to allow removal of all the diseased mucous membrane in the affected sinus and to create a good drainage system. In the rare cases where the radical operations are not successful, obliterative operations can be carried out, so that the infected sinus ceases to exist as a cavity.

The main flaw in what would appear to be a clear distinction is that it is difficult to define, let alone diagnose, irreversible changes in the sinuses. Surgeons have used many personal criteria as a guide to the condition of the mucous membrane. These include radiographic changes, the nature of the pus obtained from antral washouts etc., but it is clear that judgment of this type can be neither standardized nor compared. Probably the most logical approach is to say that an irreversible state has occurred when conservative treatment has failed. Even this attitude, however, is not without fault when comparing results, as again it is a matter of individual judgment when treatment is considered to have failed or when it is felt to be worth persisting with.

It is in this area of difficult decision that the operation of intranasal antrostomy finds a place, and it is because of this difficulty that it has remained controversial and its role is often not made clear. In this chapter it will be discussed among the minor surgical procedures associated with conservative treatment.

In addition to the treatment of the sinuses, abnormalities which may have contributed to the chronic infection may also have to be dealt with surgically. These operations include nasal polypectomy, submucous resection of the septum and extraction of infected teeth. This aspect of treatment must not be treated as an aside because the operations are not described in this chapter. In many cases removal of polyps may initiate the cure of a troublesome ethmoiditis and resection of a high septal deviation or excision of an enlarged and obstructing middle turbinate may sometimes relieve the most persistent frontal sinusitis.

It should be recognized that a well-established chronic frontal sinusitis is the most disabling of sinus infections and is the most difficult one to treat. In spite of modern advances no operation on the frontal sinus can be guaranteed to give a successful result; it is therefore important to treat early cases thoroughly by conservative measures designed to free the fronto–nasal opening from obstruction and so avoid radical treatment later. Again in this type of case, Negus (1947) insisted that in the external frontal sinus operation only very diseased mucosa need be removed and if adequate drainage were obtained the remaining mucosa would often recover.

Negus' conclusions were based on operations performed on over a 100 patients, so that in this context the term 'radical operations' will not necessarily mean the complete excision of all the lining of a sinus.

The forms of medical and surgical treatment available will be described in detail as well as the manner in which a choice can be made. *Table 14.1* summarizes the therapeutic options to be considered in the management of chronic sinusitis.

Table 14.1   Treatment of chronic sinusitis

Conservative
  Medical
    Antibiotics, antihistamines, decongestants etc.
  Surgical
    Antral puncture and washout
    Intranasal antrostomy, and, if necessary, polypectomy, submucous
      resection, dental treatment.
Radical (if conservative therapy fails)

DRAINAGE OPERATIONS

'Single' sinusitis		*Multisinusitis*
Maxillary	Caldwell–Luc operation and modifications	External fronto–ethmosphenoidectomy,
Ethmoid	Intranasal ethmoidectomy	Patterson's operation
	External ethmoidectomy	Transantral ethmoidectomy
Frontal	Intranasal drainage	
	External drainage	
Sphenoid	Intranasal drainage	

OBLITERATIVE OPERATIONS

Maxillary	McNeill's operation
Frontal	Excision of anterior wall
	Osteoplastic flap; unilateral
	bilateral

Conservative treatment

Medical

Inhalations and nasal decongestants
These are unlikely to effect a cure in chronic sinusitis, but can give considerable relief of symptoms and so may be used as a supportive treatment while other methods are dealing with the infection.

They must therefore be given with this end in view for a limited period and their role should be explained to the patient. The symptomatic relief that may be given by decongestants may encourage continued use, without clearing up the infection, and eventually producing a chemical rhinitis which may be difficult to cure or even distinguish from the chronic infection.

Anti-allergic drugs

There is no doubt that allergy plays an important part in the development of some cases of chronic sinusitis and it is often difficult to decide which changes of the lining mucosa are due to allergy and which to chronic infection. If the appearance of the nose is that of allergic rhinitis then anti-allergic treatment should be started together with the other forms of medication.

A number of workers have stained the nasal secretions to show eosinophils and in this way have drawn attention to the high proportion of cases with underlying allergy. This knowledge has also helped to classify chronic sinusitis on an aetiological basis, but when, in an attempt at rationalizing treatment, the suggestion is made that such investigations be routinely applied, practical considerations make it rarely possible.

Such a large number of patients have shown eosinophils in their nasal secretions that there is probably a place for a trial of anti-allergic drugs as part of the treatment in most patients with chronic sinusitis, particularly those with pansinusitis.

Antibiotics

Although many of the symptoms of chronic sinusitis are due simply to malfunction of the lining membranes resulting from past infection, whenever there is evidence of existing bacterial infection antibiotics should be tried.

Usually it is possible to wait for the result of bacteriological investigations of pus from the nose or sinus washings, before starting the treatment with the appropriate antibiotic. If there appears to be a subacute exacerbation and the infection warrants treatment without delay, then a broad-spectrum antibiotic such as amoxicillin (Amoxil) or doxycycline (Vibramycin) can be started while the swabs are being plated for sensitivities. The bacterial flora in chronic sinusitis as opposed to that in the acute form are not as likely to respond to antibiotics. It may be necessary to set up anaerobic cultures to identify significant pathogens.

The course should be longer than usually recommended, lasting 10 to 14 days if a favourable response occurs.

At one time there was an interest in the direct instillation of antibiotic solutions into the maxillary sinus through a cannula or polythene tube, but this has been abandoned now that some of the new antibiotics are found in sufficient therapeutic concentrations in the sinus secretions (Carenfelt *et al.*, 1975).

If the pus obtained from a chronically infected sinus appears to be sterile, a broad-spectrum antibiotic should be given nevertheless, as systemic antibiotic therapy in chronic sinusitis is valuable in preventing complications such as meningitis and osteitis. The effect on the sinusitis itself, however, is usually disappointing.

Displacement therapy

Displacement therapy is rarely used now and fuller details of this technique were described in earlier editions of this book. Air is drawn from the sinuses by suction, allowing fluid to flow into the sinuses through the ostia from which air has been withdrawn. This technique was introduced by Proetz (1939) using a special syringe for both diagnosis and treatment.

Enzymes and mucolytic drugs

Reports describing the use of mucolytic enzymes and chemicals of different types have recently appeared in the literature. These can be administered directly into the maxillary sinus by aerosol or taken by mouth. It is difficult to assess their value as their effects are only marginal, and it is doubtful if they alter the course of the disease in any way.

Analgesics

Early institution of drainage is the best form of therapy for headache, but aspirin and codeine are often necessary. These are usually sufficient and more powerful potentially addictive drugs are not indicated.

Shortwave diathermy

This can raise the temperature in the sinuses by 1.7 or 2.2 °C. In a closed sinusitis this sudden heating may prevent rather than encourage drainage and thereby aggravate the pain. It should be avoided in acute sinusitis.

Opinions vary as to the value of this procedure but on the whole it gives disappointing results. It may be tried in cases of subacute or incompletely resolved sinusitis with continual pain which does not appear to be improving.

Changes of environment

This is mentioned because so many papers on the therapeutic results of seaside resorts, spas and other health-restoring stations, appear in the literature of countries which are endowed with such places. There can be no doubt of the beneficial effects of rest and fresh air to city dwellers, but this is not specific to chronic sinusitis, although a change of environment may well improve an allergic nose. Poor social conditions and their effects, however, must not be forgotten, and chronic sinusitis, particularly in children, may justify a recommendation for better housing.

Minor surgical procedures

No procedure in the nose should ever be carried out unless every step can be clearly seen without being obscured by bleeding. There are many ways of improving haemostasis:

(1) The nose may be sprayed with a 10 per cent solution of cocaine.
(2) Pledgets of cotton wool moistened in cocaine solution can be placed directly upon the area to be operated. If these are soaked in a mixture of equal parts of 1 : 1000 adrenaline and cocaine solution, then 10 per cent cocaine should be used as the vasoconstriction prevents absorption.
(3) A paste containing 25 per cent cocaine with desiccated adrenal gland in soft paraffin may be applied with a wool carrier.
(4) Sluder's method—cocaine paste is smeared onto wool-carrying probes. One is passed backwards to rest on the region of the sphenopalatine ganglion. This is between the posterior end of the middle turbinate and the septum. A second probe is used to anaesthetize the branches of the anterior ethmoidal nerve. It is placed directly upwards and anteriorly in the nasal fossa as far as it will go.
(5) Moffet's method—a solution consisting of equal parts of 8 per cent cocaine hydrochloride and 1 per cent sodium bicarbonate is mixed with a quarter part of 1 : 1000 adrenaline. It is instilled into the nostrils and the head is turned into three different positions, to allow the solution to reach all parts of the nasal fossae.

These methods also give adequate anaesthesia for out-patient procedures.

(6) When more extensive procedures under general anaesthesia are to be carried out the nose is carefully painted with cocaine hydrochloride crystals moistened with 1:1000 adrenaline, or 25 per cent cocaine paste by means of a cotton-wool applicator. This is done under careful inspection with a good light and every part of the operative field should be lightly painted. In the case of ethmoidal operations when polypi or polypoid mucous membrane is present the middle meatus must be very carefully and gently explored with the local anaesthetic.

Packing the nose before operation may be equally satisfactory for haemostasis if carried out by the surgeon, but if this packing is done by someone less experienced, haemostasis may not be complete and the risk of post-operative adhesions is considerable if the packing is carelessly or roughly inserted.

Antral irrigation

Irrigation of the maxillary sinus is the simple surgical procedure of choice in cases which fail to respond to medical care. The antrum is usually punctured through the antro–nasal wall in the inferior meatus. The antrum may also be irrigated through the natural ostium, puncturing through the middle meatus.

Puncture through the inferior meatus   The advantage of puncture through the inferior meatus is that it does not interfere with the middle meatus. It can be used as a diagnostic procedure as in 'proof-puncture' in subacute or chronic maxillary sinusitis or as a therapeutic measure. A 'proof-puncture' of the antrum will give not only the most definite evidence in confirmation of the presence of infection, but also information with regard to the type of inflammation and the nature of infecting organisms.

In a hypertrophic sinusitis the washouts will give blobs of mucopus in an otherwise clean return, whereas in a suppurative condition with damage to the mucus-secreting glands, the fluid will be milky and perhaps contain cheesy inspissated debris of pus cells, organisms and sometimes altered blood clot. On puncture, a thin clear yellow fluid may run out of the needle and if collected in a dark receiver the presence of cholesterol crystals can be seen. This is usually associated with a longstanding sterile obstruction of the sinus as may be found with a polypoid mucous membrane.

In the case of a swollen mucous membrane, whether due to an acute exacerbation of a chronic hypertrophic condition or an allergic swelling, the ostium may be so narrowed that fluid cannot escape even with considerable pressure. In the case of obstruction of the ostium by a polypus or polypoid mucous membrane, the flow may be intermittent due to a ball valve-like action.

Repeated antral puncture and lavage once or twice a week is often successful in clearing up a suppurative condition and reducing it to one with little or no secretion.

A thickened lining membrane then resolves spontaneously. Opinions differ as to the number and frequency of punctures that should be carried out. It is often found that after one puncture a frankly purulent washout may on the next occasion be mucopurulent and that, as recovery takes place, the secretion will become more mucoid and less purulent until a clear return is obtained. This procedure may be repeated a number of times if there is continued improvement with each successive washout.

Technique The technique of antral puncture may vary but certain rules render it a safe and useful method of examination and treatment.

In children it should be performed under general anaesthesia and the most suitable way of positioning the head is with a Boyle–Davis gag in the routine adenotonsillectomy position. In this way the fluids may be collected from the post-nasal space with no danger of inhalation of the washings.

The procedure is usually satisfactorily carried out under local anaesthesia in adults. The nose should be sprayed with 10 per cent cocaine solution as this shrinks down the inferior turbinate and opens up the inferior meatus.

It may also open up the middle meatus and ease the passage of washings through the ostium. The inferior meatus is then painted with cocaine ointment or with a paste of cocaine crystals and adrenaline carried on a fine and slightly bent silver wool carrier until satisfactory anaesthesia is achieved. The antrum is then pierced with a Tilley–Lichtwitz trocar and cannula. The tip of the trocar and cannula is passed along the lateral wall of the inferior meatus near the roof. The tip will naturally tend to be arrested at the point where the wall bulges medially. The tip is then withdrawn 3 mm and pointed in the direction of the tragus of the homolateral ear (*Figure 14.6*). The lateral wall of the meatus should be thinnest in this area and it lies behind the opening of the naso–lacrimal duct. The needle will enter the antrum with a greater or lesser 'crack' depending on the thickness of the bone. The needle is withdrawn and the cannula is then pushed in until it reaches the posterior wall and then withdrawn 1.25 cm. A Higginson's syringe is filled with clean tap water or sterile normal saline at 37 °C and connected to the cannula. The patient is asked to lean forward over a large receiver and asked to breathe through his open mouth while the washout proceeds. The fluid usually passes easily through the natural ostium and out of the nares.

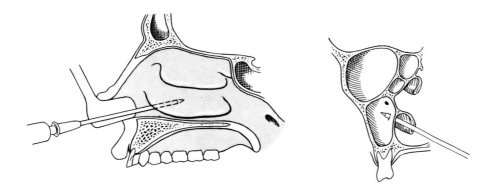

Figure 14.6 Line of introduction of trocar and cannula into maxillary sinus

Any pathological contents in the washings can be sent for bacteriological and cytological examination. Undue pressure should never be used and if the natural ostium is closed by oedema it may be necessary to insert a second cannula into the antrum alongside the first. Washout then proceeds through one cannula and out of the other. Air should never be passed through the cannula as this had been known to cause a fatal air embolus (McNab Jones, 1976). Water should be left in the antrum and the patient warned that this will continue to drain for the next hour or so.

Difficulties and dangers The difficulties of antral puncture must be recognized to be avoided:

(1) There is the possibility of the needle failing to enter the antrum. If too far forwards under the inferior turbinates, it may even be inserted into the soft tissues in front of the pyriform aperture.
(2) The needle may enter the antrum but be pushed on into soft tissues of the cheek or into the orbit.
(3) Pain seldom accompanies the lavage but if it does it must be seriously considered. It is due (a) to the presence of acute inflammation or (b) to a false puncture. The pain will be felt in the cheek or eye. If local swelling occurs there may be a fine crepitus or surgical emphysema if the syringe contains air.
(4) Similar symptoms occur with a congenital fissure or with recent and sometimes long-standing fracture of the maxilla.

If an antral washout is carried out under general anaesthesia it is most important to leave the eyes uncovered by towels. Their position acts as a guide to the needle and if orbital swelling results from irrigation it can be quickly noticed.

Contraindications to antral puncture   The bony antro–nasal wall should not be punctured in the febrile stage of an acute maxillary sinusitis. There is a risk of osteomyelitis of the maxilla commencing from such a puncture.

In cases of trauma there may be an associated haematoma of the antrum. There is no indication for puncture for most cases will drain without infection. If they become infected, puncture and washout, even if carefully performed without undue pressure, may be sufficient to force infected material through a crack in the bone or along the track of a foreign body. If drainage is necessary an intranasal antrostomy is preferable, although such cases may call for surgical investigation of the tract of the injury.

Sounding the natural ostium
The natural ostium is not usually employed for the passage of a cannula for, even with the most careful instrumentation, the mucous membrane of this small aperture is likely to be irritated and the risk of subsequent swelling and obstruction is to be avoided. This method was advocated by Van Alyea (1934) and Lederer (1947), but both authors agreed that between 15 and 20 per cent of natural ostia could not be entered and that the attempts should not be too persistent as the irritation may offset the advantages.

Puncture through the middle meatus
Puncture with a trocar and cannula through the middle meatus has few advantages, although the membranous antro–nasal wall will often be punctured, but the risk of injury to the orbit if the floor happens to be low is sufficient to prevent its general acceptance. Moreover, the reactionary swelling after instrumentation in the middle meatus interferes with the natural drainage from the antrum and later scarring may block the ostium.

Attempts at increasing the drainage of the maxillary sinus through the natural ostium by spraying or packing the nose with vasoconstrictor solutions to cause shrinkage of the turbinates have been used and even fracturing the middle turbinate towards the septum after cocainization of the nose has been done to open up the middle meatus, but it is doubtful whether the trauma produced is compensated for by the increased drainage that may be obtained.

Sinus operations

More radical measures are required if adequate conservative treatment has failed. A variety of operations with modifications have been described and no doubt each surgeon will continue to modify them according to his own approach and to the needs of the individual patient.

It is with this in mind that the standard operations will be described. Operations which have been directed towards treating a single sinus will be described first, and later those used to obtain a clearance of more than one sinus at the same time.

Maxillary sinus operations

(1) Intranasal antrostomy

This operation can be performed as a conservative drainage operation in cases which the operator feels are potentially reversible. It is particularly helpful in a patient who is subject to subacute or recurrent maxillary sinusitis which recovers between attacks. Excessive discharge can therefore drain out during the phase of infection when the mucosal cilia do not function adequately, and washouts are also more easily carried out if required. This operation has been favoured by many operators (Mawson, 1951; Scott-Brown, 1965).

There has been for many years discussion surrounding the advantages and disadvantages of this operation compared with the Caldwell–Luc operation. It is a shorter and simpler procedure and there is less risk of damage to the nerve or blood supply of the teeth. It is only a suitable operation if most of the mucous lining of the antrum is to be conserved where it is hoped that it will recover and form a new satisfactory lining.

The Caldwell–Luc operation allows better inspection of the mucosal lining so that there can be more selective removal of the diseased lining, for any mucosa that is removed will be replaced by fibrous tissue usually covered by cubical, non-ciliated epithelium.

There are many theoretical arguments, some based on the excellent work of Hilding (1941) in which he showed in dogs that any foreign particle placed in the floor of the antrum after intranasal antrostomy was always evacuated via the same but not the shortest route, bypassing the antrostomy to reach the natural ostium. He was unable to demonstrate that any of the foreign particles passed through the intranasal antrostomy. In contrast the work of Grossan (1975) showed that the normal ciliated membrane drains the sinus of mucus in 15 min. The thicker and more tenacious the mucus the more rapidly it can be evacuated, but with greatly increased volumes of mucus, whether associated with infection or allergy, the cilia become overtaxed and drainage then occurs through the antrostomy.

Technique   The operation is done under general anaesthetic with a cuffed endotracheal tube and pharyngeal packing; the nose is then prepared as described on p. 289.

The inferior meatus is exposed by inserting a long-bladed Killian nasal speculum lateral to the inferior turbinate and displacing the turbinate medially by opening the blade of the speculum. The antrum is punctured with an elevator of the Hill's type, as for antral puncture, or by a Myles' gouge, and the outer blade of a Luc's or Henckel's forceps is inserted through the new opening and the antro–nasal wall lowered as close to the floor as possible. This now allows the introduction of Ostrum's forward-cutting forceps to allow enlargement of the hole forwards and downwards.

It is essential that the opening should be: (a) large, so that it remains permanent; (b) situated as close to the floor of the nose as possible.

To ensure its permanence it is important that the opening should be as cleanly punched out as possible, so leaving mucous membrane spreading up to the cut edge of the bone on each side. This ensures quick healing over the cut edge and with less contraction. If, on the other hand, the edges are left rough or, worse still, are rasped then this will ensure heaping up of granulations on the edge of the bone with delayed fibrosis and later contraction of the fibrous ring, causing closure of the antrostomy.

Even though the antrostomy is made near the floor of the nose, this will not be at the same level as the floor of the antrum, as this lies at a lower level (*Figure 14.7*).

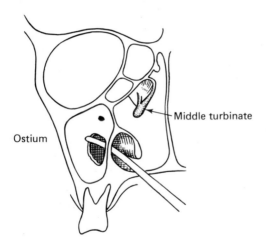

Middle turbinate

Ostium

Figure 14.7   Intra-nasal antrostomy

Usually it is unnecessary to remove any part of the inferior turbinate and the routine excision of part of this structure is to be deprecated. It does not aid drainage in a well-constituted antrostomy and it opens the antrum to cold air and may sometimes be the cause of a post-operative neuralgia. If the turbinate is fractured medially at the beginning of the operation then it must be suitably repositioned at the end.

(2) Caldwell–Luc operation
The earliest use of this type of operation was by Heath of University College Hospital, London, in 1819. He trephined the antrum in the canine fossa but made no antrostomy. In 1892 Robertson of Newcastle upon Tyne removed diseased mucosa through a hole made by a hammer and chisel in the anterior wall of the maxilla, but

he also made no antrostomy. In 1893 Caldwell reported in the *New York Medical Journal* his method of opening the antrum and making an antrostomy. In this article he refers to Heath's method. In 1897 Henri Luc of Paris carried out an operation identical to Caldwell's. Luc's name became attached to the operation in Europe and Caldwell's name became associated with it in the USA, and in some way the names became fused (Goodman, 1976).

The indications for the Caldwell–Luc operation have been given by McNab Jones (1976) as follows:

(1) when there is irreversable disease involving the mucosa of the maxillary sinus;
(2) removal of foreign bodies, usually the root of a molar or premolar tooth from the sinus lumen;
(3) inspection and biopsy of a suspected neoplasm;
(4) surgery for closure of an oro–antral fistula;
(5) surgery for dental cysts involving the antrum;
(6) as part of the approach to the pterygomaxillary fissure and sphenopalatine fossa;
(7) for adequate removal of a recurring antrochoanal polyp;
(8) for elevation of a fractured orbital floor with stabilization by an intra-antral pack.

Technique The operation may be done under local anaesthesia by maxillary nerve block but it is more commonly carried out under general anaesthesia, with a cuffed oral endotracheal tube, and with packing in the pharynx.

An injection of 1 in 200 000 adrenaline is made into the tissues of the canine fossa and into the inferior meatus of the side concerned following prior consultation with the anaesthetist.

An incision is made in the gum margin below the gingivo–labial fold from the posterior edge of the lateral incisor to the first or second molar. This incision is sometimes made with the cutting diathermy to reduce bleeding. The tissues deep to the mucous membrane are divided down to the bone. A large incision such as this requires less stretching and pulling with retractors, and there is therefore less swelling of the cheek afterwards. To diminish the risk of a fistula the incision should be backed by bone and not lie across the antral opening when the operation is completed (*Figure 14.8*).

An alternative incision can be made along the gingival margin elevating the mucosa from the necks of the intervening teeth. The U-shaped incision is completed by an anterior and posterior upward extension to the buccal sulcus. In the edentulous patient the incision is made along the margin with a similar upward and downward extension. The advantages of this incision are that there is less bleeding from the edges of the mucous membrane and less scarring in the gingivo–buccal sulcus.

After making one or other incision, the mucoperiosteal flap is dissected upwards towards the infra-orbital foramen and gently retracted. Any post-operative soft tissue swelling is related to the force used in the retraction of the flap. A window is cut in the anterior wall of the maxilla with a dental burr or a gouge and enlarged by punch forceps. If possible the mucous membrane is kept intact as the bone is removed, as this will assist later in the complete removal of the membrane. Care should be taken not to damage the roots of the teeth or the infra-orbital nerve. Bleeding from the bone edges is controlled by diathermy or with a diamond burr.

If it has been decided to remove the mucous membrane of the maxillary sinus

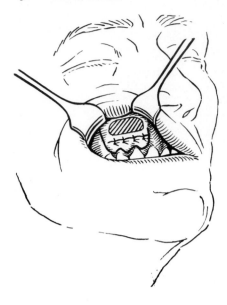

Figure 14.8 Showing the site of the opening into the antrum in the canine fossa above the line of incision or suture

completely then this must be done with meticulous care if the sinus is to develop a fibrous lining and eventually become obliterated. Bleeding during this part of the procedure is often troublesome and suction dissection is useful.

A large intranasal antrostomy is created below the inferior turbinate from within the antrum (*Figure 14.9*). It is not necessary to fashion mucosal flaps from the nose as the opening will persist if it is of satisfactory size.

If a simple linear incision has been used in the mucosa, sutures may not be required but if the U-shaped flap has been used then sutures should encircle the neck of the tooth and be tied on the palatal side of the tooth neck.

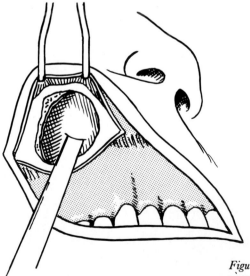

Figure 14.9 Caldwell–Luc: making the intra-nasal antrostomy into the nose

Usually two sutures are sufficient. The anterior upward extension of the incision is closed by one suture, but the posterior limb is left open to allow drainage of the blood from the soft tissues (Goodman, 1976). Post-operative swelling can be reduced with ice packs. The patient should avoid blowing his nose for two weeks after the operation. If the patient has upper dentures they can be worn the following day. The nose will probably require gentle suction on about the third day.

The cavity in the antrum gradually becomes obliterated by granulation tissue and in time by fibrous tissue. The aim of the operation is to leave a small medial air-containing space draining into the nasal cavity through the antrostomy, or possibly through the natural ostium.

Complications are fortunately few. Haemorrhage from branches of the spheno–palatine artery rarely occurs, but when it does the nose and sinus may need packing. Anaesthesia of the region supplied by the infra-orbital nerve can be very troublesome if the nerve has been stretched. It may last for a few weeks or even months. If care has been taken not to damage the roots of the teeth, devitalization is very rarely seen.

Paavolainen, Paavolainen and Tarkkanen (1977) examined the effect of the Caldwell–Luc operation on the permanent teeth of Finnish schoolchildren between the ages of 14 and 16 years. Hyperaesthesia was sometimes present in the first incisors but no teeth died as a result of the operation.

If the sublabial incision has not been carefully made a fistula may remain on rare occasions.

Modifications of the Caldwell–Luc operation

(1) Canfield's operation An intranasal incision is made just behind the vestibule. The periosteum is elevated laterally over the edge of the pyriform aperture and into the canine fossa. This anterior angle of the maxillary sinus is chiselled off to expose the antral contents and then the opening is continued backwards into an intranasal antrostomy.

(2) Denker's operation The incision is made as for a Caldwell–Luc but continued further medially so that when the tissues are elevated from the bone, the nasal cavity is exposed as well as the canine fossa. The antrum can be opened as in the Caldwell–Luc. This approach gives good access to the lower part of the nasal cavity and antrum.

(3) Obliteration of the maxillary sinus McNeil (1966) described an operation for obliteration of the maxillary sinus. He made an inverted-U incision over the anterior wall of the antrum and then perforated the bone so as to open it downwards as a flap hinged inferiorly to the soft tissues. Through this opening the lining mucosa was completely removed and the periosteal layer of the antral wall gently burred. Fat taken from the anterior abdominal wall was placed in the cavity so as to fill it completely. Successful results are claimed for this operation but the indications to perform it are rarely present.

Ethmoid operations

(1) Intranasal ethmoidectomy
The operation can be carried out under local anaesthesia but is usually carried out

under a general anaesthetic. In either case it is essential to provide a bloodless field to improve the already limited visibility. The nasal mucous membrane should be prepared as described on p. 289, with particular attention to the middle turbinate and the region of the spheno–palatine vessels.

In this operation it is important to try to open the ethmoid sufficiently to relieve any obstruction and to allow drainage and ventilation of the air-cells.

It is not necessary to try and clean up every vestige of diseased hyperplastic mucous membrane; in fact, this would be dangerous (Eichel, 1972).

Technique   The middle meatus should be opened out by fracturing the middle turbinate medially exposing the uncinate process and ethmoidal bulla, then removing the bulla with Luc's or Grunwald's forceps and so opening the labyrinth. During the procedure it is essential that the lateral edges of the forceps are used so that the points are directed away from the lateral wall. Sharp instruments run the risk of penetrating the orbital wall or cribriform plate. Their action should be in a downward and medial direction so that they glance away from structures.

Although many variations exist in the arrangement of the cells, the boundaries are fairly constant and must at all times be borne in mind. The lateral wall which separates the ethmoid cells from the orbit is thin, but no damage is done by removing this plate so long as the periosteum that encloses the orbit is not injured.

Posteriorly the anterior sphenoidal wall is easily identified although it may be so thin that the sphenoid is entered through the posterior ethmoidal wall.

Superiorly the roof of the ethmoid is distinguished in much the same way as the tegmen in a mastoid operation. The smooth and white bone warns the operator that the limit of the cells is reached and the cranial fossa will be opened if further bone is removed.

The roof of the ethmoid capsule is always at a higher level than the cribriform plate (*Figure 14.10*). A blunt-ended graduated probe, if inserted between the middle turbinate and the septum, will always penetrate 3–6 mm further when inserted in the same direction lateral to the middle turbinate if all the cells have been opened and the plate of bone covering the anterior fossa has been exposed.

The failure of most intranasal ethmoid operations lies in the difficulty of clearing the anterior cells. It is usually very difficult, if not impossible, to eradicate with safety and certainty the anterior ethmoidal cells and the agger nasi region.

It is rarely necessary to interfere with the middle turbinate as free drainage of the ethmoid will induce shrinkage of turbinate hypertrophy, but if there is any gross turbinal enlargement then careful and minimal removal of the middle turbinate may be undertaken.

Surgery of the ethmoid carries a greater risk of serious complications than operations on any other sinus. This is related to both the limited access and the intimate relationship of the ethmoidal cells to the orbit and anterior cranial fossa (*Figure 14.11*). The principle damage is from injury to the roof of the ethmoidal cells or cribriform plate. Damage to these structures, particularly in the presence of sepsis, invariably leads to meningitis or cerebrospinal rhinorrhoea. There have been many publications reporting orbital complications. This is usually related to direct trauma to the optic nerve or to the production of oedema or a haematoma. If the sphenoid fails to pneumatize, the bone is invaded by posterior ethmoidal cells which may come into

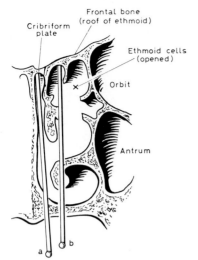

Cribriform plate

Frontal bone (roof of ethmoid)

Ethmoid cells (opened)

Orbit

Antrum

Figure 14.10   Diagram to demonstrate that the roof of the ethmoid is at a higher level than the roof of the nasal cavity

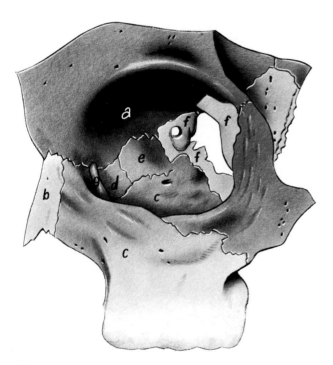

Figure 14.11   Diagram to show bones and suture lines on outer side of ethmoid capsule and floor of frontal sinus. (a) Frontal; (b) nasal; (c) maxilla; (d) lacrimal; (e) ethmoid; (f) sphenoid; (g) naso-lacrimal duct

intimate relationship with the optic nerve so that the intervening bone between the optic nerve and a posterior cell is only of paper-thinness. Proptosis or reduction of vision after operation is an indication for immediate exploration and decompression.

(2) External ethmoidectomy

The external operation is the most effective means of exenterating the ethmoid cells under direct vision with the help of the operating microscope if needed, but it has the disadvantage of requiring an external skin excision.

The original ethmoid operation was described by Ferris Smith in 1933, but there have been many modifications described since. The original operation was designed to control suppuration of the fronto–ethmoid complex which was a serious condition in pre-antiobiotic days, but it is now used for chronic irreversible mucosal changes in the ethmoid sinuses or when there is a recurrence of nasal polypi following intranasal procedures. It has also been incorporated in a method of approach to the pituitary fossa (Bateman, 1963).

Technique   The operation requires a general anaesthetic as the contents of the orbit are likely to be retracted during the operation. A hypotensive anaesthetic is helpful if it is not contraindicated as this will give a drier field. The eyelids should be sutured to prevent accidental trauma to the cornea. A curved incision is made through the naso–facial fold onto the nasal bones through both skin and periosteum. The periosteum is then elevated to reveal the nasal processes of both the maxilla and the frontal bone and the medial wall of the orbit. The lacrimal sac is elevated and displaced from its groove. Periosteum over the lamina papyracea is gently elevated until the ethmoidal vessels are identified as they enter the nasal cavity. A self-retaining retractor designed with a blade to protect the orbital contents is inserted to allow division of the anterior ethmoidal artery (*Figure 14.12*). The thin lamina papyracea of the ethmoid is perforated exposing the ethmoid cells.

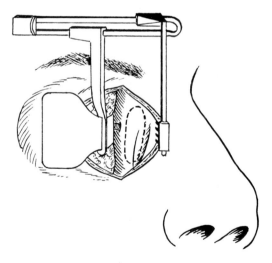

Figure 14.12   External ethmoid operation: site for opening the ethmoid cells

At this stage the operating microscope with a 300-mm objective lens can be used. The cribriform plate is identified superiorly and as the cells are removed the middle and superior turbinates will come into view. Removal of the medial portion of the orbital floor allows entry into the maxillary sinus and the sphenoid can be opened through posterior ethmoid cells and its anterior wall. After exenteration of the anterior ethmoidal cells, the floor of the frontal sinus can be exposed as for a fronto–ethmoidectomy.

Before closure of the skin good aposition càn be assured by drawing together some of the muscle fibres of orbicularis occuli to give an acceptable cosmetic result.

Complications are few, but include temporary epiphora if the lacrimal duct has been disturbed.

(3) External fronto–ethmoidectomy

This valuable operation was popularized in Britain by Howarth (1936), but it was used by Lynch in 1920 and it is by his name that the operation is known in the USA.

The operation consists of an external ethmoidectomy, middle turbinectomy and resection of the entire floor of the frontal sinus.

A plastic or similar tube is placed in the exposed ethmoid labyrinth so as to lie between the frontal sinus and the nasal cavity. This tube remains in place for one to three months. This operation has stood the trial of many years and as a general rule has proved to be a very effective procedure for the control of chronic frontal sinus disease, but it has a failure rate sufficient to stimulate the search for a better operation. If the sinus mucous membrane is not completely removed recovery can be complicated by the development of a mucocoele or pyocoele and if the reconstructed fronto–nasal duct becomes stenosed the frontal sinus condition may recur.

There have been many varieties of this operation, for example by Killian (1903) who opened the frontal sinus through an external incision and removed the anterior and inferior walls but left a bridge of bone along the supra-orbital ridge to avoid a 'repulsive deformity'. To him goes the credit of lining the fronto–nasal duct with a mucoperiosteal flap from the ethmoid and lacrimal bone. Since then many other modifications have been developed, including skin grafting of the fronto–nasal duct.

Linthrop described an operation in 1914 which entailed unilateral or bilateral anterior ethmoidectomy with middle turbinectomy.

The frontal sinus septum was removed making a large opening from the frontal sinus into the nasal cavity by connecting the two fronto–nasal ducts, with resection of a portion of the superior nasal septum. The operation was used for dealing with bilateral frontal sinus disease.

Technique   The incision is made along the inferior margin of the eyebrow extending downwards halfway between the inner canthus and the dorsum of the nose and onto the lateral aspect of the nose (*Figure 14.13*). The ethmoid cells are exposed and removed as described in the operation for external ethmoidectomy.

The frontal sinus is approached by way of the ethmoid sinus. A superiorly based mucosal flap may be fashioned from the upper lateral wall to use later in the reconstruction of a fronto–nasal passage.

The frontal sinus cavity is opened by removing bone from the medial orbital plate to the beginning of the osseus frontal sinus floor and continuing until the entire floor of the frontal sinus is removed. The mucosal lining of the frontal sinus is meticulously removed *in toto*. This may prove difficult if there are superior or lateral extensions of the sinus and this represents one of the shortcomings of this approach.

If the mucous membrane is not completely removed, the procedure may later be complicated by the development of a mucocoele.

An adequate passage is established from the frontal sinus to the nasal fossa by removing the anterior and posterior ethmoid cells and as much of the middle turbinate as is necessary. The position of the cribriform plate can be demonstrated by placing

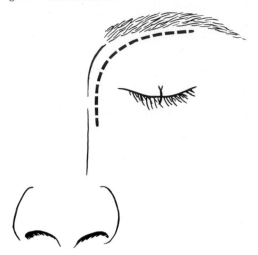

Figure 14.13   The incision for the external fronto–ethmoidectomy operation

a probe through the nasal cavity until it comes into contact with the olfactory slit (*Figure 14.9*). The sphenoid sinus can be opened, if this is indicated, through the anterior wall when the posterior ethmoid cells have been removed.

If a mucous membrane flap has been fashioned from the lateral wall of the nose, it can be turned upwards to line the medial wall of the newly-formed fronto–nasal opening and supported by packing or a plastic tube. If a flap has not been formed, the passage may be established by simply using a plastic tube with the upper end in the floor of the frontal sinus and the lower end lying in the nasal fossa, just above the vestibule (*Figure 14.14*). This should be retained for at least one to three months. The tube may alternatively be covered with a split skin graft. Even when these requirements are met, stenosis of the newly-formed fronto–nasal passage may still occur.

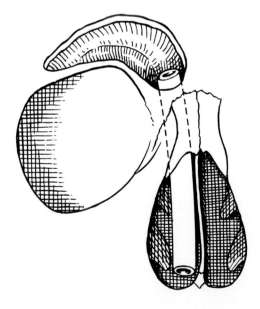

Figure 14.14   Fronto–ethmoid operation: diagram showing position of silicone tube

(4) Sphenoid sinus operations
This sinus can be cleared as part of a fronto–ethmoid operation as previously described, or it can be opened intranasally. Drainage operations for chronic infective sphenoid sinusitis are uncommon and probably the most frequent requirement for exposure of the sphenoid sinus is in an approach for hypophysectomy. This is easily achieved through a trans-septal approach. A partial removal of the cartilage and bony structures of the nasal septum allows inspection of the ostia of the sphenoid sinus after inserting a long Killian nasal speculum between the layers of the septum. The ostia can be enlarged or the anterior wall of the sphenoid sinus can be removed. The mucous membrane of the sinus can then be closely examined with the operating microscope using the 300-mm objective lens.

Surgery for chronic frontal sinus disease

The treatment of chronic frontal sinusitis has always presented a problem for the surgeon. Not only has there been disagreement regarding the value of intranasal and external operations but also differences as to the type of external operation when this route has been decided upon.

It must be realized that in view of such uncertainty there is no royal road to success and the various methods described each give satisfying results in the hands of the particular operator who describes them. In some instances, chronic frontal sinusitis can be cured by correcting intranasal disorders, which either interfere with the proper drainage by way of the fronto–nasal passage or initiate re-infection. Submucous resection of the nasal septum, removal of intranasal polyps or the anterior portion of the middle turbinate, and intranasal ethmoidectomy are all procedures that can be used to establish drainage. A complete external ethmoidectomy may be required if chronic purulent ethmoiditis is present.

If the above conservative intranasal surgery is not successful, then opinions differ as to the most effective form of frontal sinus surgery that is indicated. Intranasal probing, cannulization and enlargement of the fronto–nasal duct and orifice have been practised, particularly in the pre-antibiotic days, but these procedures are condemned by those who favour external surgery, particularly those who support the osteoplastic flap procedure, by reasoning that once the fronto–nasal duct has been violated, inevitable scarring and stenosis will follow.

Intranasal drainage by enlarging the fronto–nasal duct was promoted by Halle (1914) and the technique is well described by Scott-Brown (1965). It may still have its merits as long as mucosal changes are thought to be reversible and simple drainage only is necessary. External operation is then avoided.

External frontal operations

(1) Trephination of the frontal sinus
This is described in the previous chapter on the management of acute frontal sinusitis.

(2) Fronto–ethmoidectomy
This is described on p. 301 of this chapter.

(3) The osteoplastic frontal sinus operation

This operation is based on an inferiorly hinged 'trap door' of bone made from the anterior wall of the frontal sinuses. Although the operation was described in the nineteenth century, it was revived by Macbeth (1954) and further developed by Goodale and Montgomery (1958) and Montgomery (1971).

The operation may be used for unilateral or bilateral frontal sinus disease. The approach affords direct access to the entire contents of the frontal sinus and an excellent view of the fronto–nasal orifice from above. By using this technique, the diseased tissues can be readily removed and either adequate drainage from the frontal sinus through the nasal fossa can be established or the frontal sinus can be obliterated completely by the implantation of fat. This modification was described by Berganara and Itoiz (1955). It is important that the fat, which is usually taken from the abdominal wall, is not traumatized, and as long as both the mucosal and inner cortical linings of the frontal sinuses are completely removed, the fat will revascularize and resist infection. A further advantage of the osteoplastic flap is that there is no resultant facial deformity as the incision is made in the hairline, unlike the *simple obliterative operation* where the anterior wall of the frontal sinus is removed after making an incision below the line of the eyebrows extending from one temple to the other. The periosteum and soft tissues are elevated as far as the upper limit of the frontal sinuses. The sinuses are opened with a gouge or burr and after removal of all the diseased and remaining healthy mucosa, the soft tissues are then allowed to fall into contact with the posterior wall of the sinus. This obliterates the sinus cavity but causes a most ugly deformity. This may be corrected a year or so later by soft tissue grafting (Hughes, 1976).

Technique of the osteoplastic operation   Pre-operative preparation: Radiographs are taken before surgery to determine the extent of the disease. A template of the outline of the sinuses is made by placing an exposed transparent x-ray film over the fronto–occipital view and outlining the sinus with a marking pencil. A template may also be made from lead sheeting as this is easier to sterilize. The pattern should be slightly smaller than the actual dimensions of the sinus so that the cuts made through the bone lie within the sinus boundaries. A culture of the nasal cavity should be taken some days before the operation. The abdomen is shaved and prepared so that subcutaneous fat can be obtained. The hair of the head should be shampooed with hexachlorophene solution.

Incisions: Either an eyebrow or coronal incision can be used for the bilateral osteoplastic flap (*Figure 14.15*). If a coronal incision is used, the hair is shaved 4 cm behind the anterior hairline so that an incision can be made approximately 2.5 cm behind this line. This is the most suitable incision for female patients.

The coronal flap is elevated inferiorly in a plane between the frontalis muscle and the periosteum over the frontal bone. The flap is developed as far as the supraorbital rims and nasal processes of the frontal bones. Haemostasis is obtained with skin clips.

The eyebrow incision if used should be made along the entire length of the upper margin of the eyebrows and extend horizontally over the nasal process of the frontal bone.

The template is then placed over the frontal periosteum and the inferior aspect of the template is cut across horizontally at a level just above the cribriform plate. The periosteum is incised around the outline of the template after it has been accurately located to the supraorbital rims. A horizontal incision is made in the periosteum over

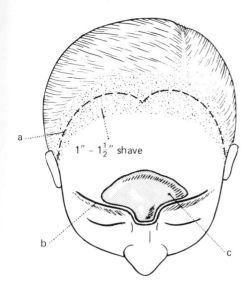

1″ – 1½″ shave

Figure 14.15   Incisions for bilateral osteoplastic flap. (a) Coronal incision, (b) eyebrow incision, (c) x-ray template

the nasal process of the frontal bone. Superiorly the bone incision is made on a bevel to make sure it enters the frontal sinus (*Figure 14.16*). The osteoplastic flap is elevated with a chisel at the superior aspect of the bone until a fracture forms across the floor of the frontal sinus. It may be necessary to divide the interfrontal septum before attempting to elevate the flap. The interior of the sinuses can now be inspected and the diseased tissue removed from the frontal sinus, at the superior margin of the fronto–nasal orifice (*Figure 14.17*).

The inner cortical lining with the remains of the interfrontal septum is removed with a burr to ensure complete removal of mucous membrane so that an adequate blood supply will develop to nourish the fatty implant.

Subcutaneous fat is taken through a horizontal left rectus incision sufficient to fill both frontal sinuses completely and close off both fronto–nasal ducts.

The osteoplastic flap is returned to its normal position and the periosteum sutured. The incision is sutured in one layer of interrupted sutures. A pressure dressing is placed over both eyes and the forehead for 24–48 h. No special post-operative treatment is required other than the administration of antibiotics and later the removal of the skin sutures.

Unilateral osteoplastic operation

This operation is suitable for unilateral disease of the frontal sinus which cannot be controlled adequately by the fronto–ethmoidectomy operation (Montgomery, 1971).

The skin incision is made along the upper margin of the eyebrow and it should extend the entire length of the eyebrow (*Figure 14.18*).

The x-ray template which has previously been prepared from a tracing around the outline of the sinus taken from a fronto–occipital x-ray view is used to outline the incision in the periosteum. The periosteum over the frontal bone is exposed by dissection to the plane deep to the frontalis muscle (*Figure 14.19*). The bone is cut as for the bilateral operation and should be bevelled to facilitate replacement and

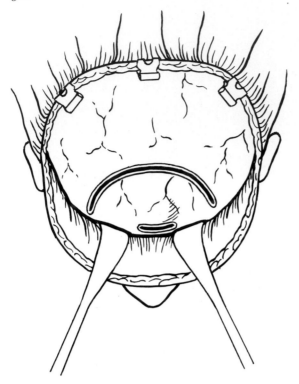

Figure 14.16   The coronal flap has been reflected inferiorly: incisions through the periosteum and bone are shown

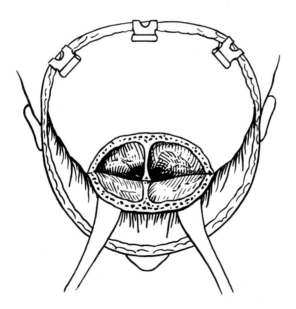

Figure 14.17   The osteoplastic flap has been elevated, exposing the contents of the frontal sinuses

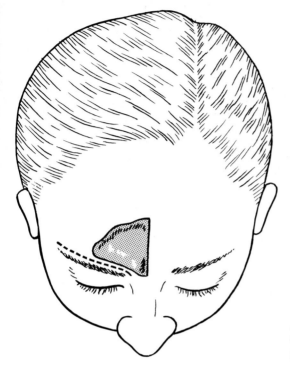

Figure 14.18 Skin incision for unilateral osteoplastic flap. X-ray template in position

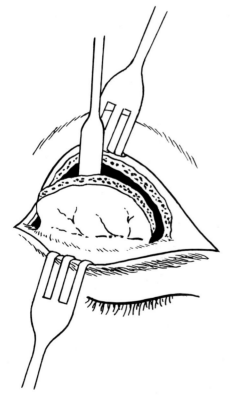

Figure 14.19 Elevation of unilateral osteoplastic flap to expose right frontal sinus

prevent inward displacement. The flap is elevated by prising the upper margin with a chisel to allow the osteoplastic flap to be reflected inferiorly. The interior of the frontal sinus can then be inspected. A culture should be taken and a specimen, if required, obtained for histological examination.

If a benign tumour, such as an osteoma is present, it can be removed and no further surgery is required if the mucous membrane is healthy and the fronto–nasal duct is unaffected. If the mucous membrane of the frontal sinus is irreversibly diseased it should be removed completely as described for the bilateral operation, and the sinus obliterated with abdominal fat.

Other sinus operations

Patterson's operation

Patterson first described this operation in 1939. The incision begins 6 mm below and external to the inner canthus and corresponds to a sulcus which passes onwards and downwards into the cheek (*Figure 14.20*). The orbicularis oculi fibres are separated by blunt dissection and the tissues held apart by a self-retaining retractor. The periosteum is incised and elevated from the maxilla as far upwards as the attachment of the internal tarsal ligament and nearly as far outwards as the infraorbital foramen. It is also raised over the inner part of the floor of the orbit and from the bone which forms the anterior and inner part of the roof of the antrum.

A portion of the roof of the antrum is excised, exposing the naso–lacrimal duct as it passes into the bony canal, and allowing it to be carefully mobilized along its whole length.

The periosteum of the inner wall of the orbit is elevated so that the lamina papyracea and ethmoid cells can be excised (*Figure 14.21*). The mucous membrane of the nose is then incised in front of and medial to the lacrimal duct so that diseased cells may be excised all round it. The sphenoidal sinus may be opened from the posterior ethmoidal cells.

The antrum may also be inspected from this opening and a further permanent opening made into the nose.

The wound is closed by approximating the fibres of orbicularis oculi before closure of the skin.

This operation can be performed to clear the ethmoid sinuses together with the sphenoid and maxillary antrum. The main objections raised against this operation are that access to the ethmoidal cells are not as good as in the external ethmoid operation, while access to the maxillary antrum is not as good as in the Caldwell–Luc operation. Its sole merit seems to be that both areas can be dealt with through one incision, but there is no doubt that it can give excellent results in skilled hands (Hargrove, 1944).

Transantral ethmoidectomy

This operation was originally described by Jansen in 1894 and further recommended by Horgan (1926) for cases which require exploration of the maxillary antrum as well as an ethmoidectomy.

A preliminary Caldwell–Luc operation is carried out and the ethmoid cells opened with a pair of forceps pushed through the postero–medial angle of the roof of the antrum into the ethmoid.

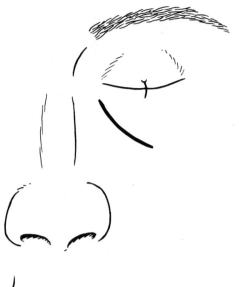

Figure 14.20 Incision for Patterson's operation

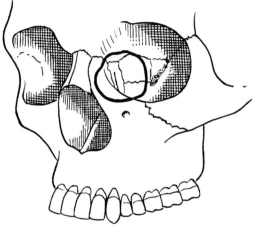

Figure 14.21 Patterson's operation. Area from which bone can be removed

The instrument is directed towards the opposite parietal eminence and this manoeuvre brings it into the posterior ethmoidal cells. The hole is then increased in size with biting forceps and the other ethmoidal cells opened with the sphenoid if this is indicated.

It is almost impossible to excise the anterior ethmoidal cells or the fronto–ethmoidal cells using this technique, but the anterior ones can be opened intranasally. By combining these two approaches a satisfactory clearance of the ethmoidal cells can be obtained.

The choice of treatment

All the methods of treatment described above have a place and deserve to be recorded, either because of their value in specific cases, or because they have produced good results in the hands of those who practise them. They all have their merits and a choice of treatment must therefore be made. This can only be based on the needs of the individual patient and on the familiarity of the surgeon with a particular operation.

There is no doubt that conservative treatment should be tried first. Features such as nasal polyps or a severely deflected septum may require surgical treatment before there is any hope of bringing the associated chronic infection under control.

In the case of chronic ethmoiditis with numerous polyps, it is rarely sufficient to excise a few polyps at a time in the out-patient department and a wider clearance is usually necessary under general anaesthesia. Part of the ethmoidal labyrinth is excised with the polyps and this should be recorded as a 'partial ethmoidectomy' and not as an 'ethmoidectomy', a term which should be reserved for complete exenteration (*see* Chapter 11 for treatment of nasal polypi).

If there are no such features present then treatment should consist of broad-spectrum antibiotics, controlled if possible by bacteriology, supportive decongestant therapy and antrum washouts if the maxillary sinus is involved. Punctures of the ethmoid or sphenoid are not routinely practised, and instrumentation of the fronto–nasal duct is better avoided altogether other than in very exceptional cases.

The question often arises as to how long should antral washouts continue to be repeated before more radical measures are taken. The traditional statement that if after six washouts there is still pus present, then a radical operation should be performed, is not always helpful. If the nature of the washings alters in character from frank pus to mucopus and then becomes progressively more mucoid, the likelihood is that a cure can shortly be obtained.

The ease with which the puncture can be performed may be dependent on the anatomy of the particular nose, and the manner in which the patient will accept this form of treatment can also influence this decision. It is true that a patient often becomes less apprehensive with time and the wish to avoid admission to hospital may make him more receptive to out-patient treatment, but occasionally some people will not tolerate antral puncture even in the first instance and an anaesthetic must be given.

Intranasal antrostomy when accompanied by other forms of medical tratment is often very successful in the milder, shorter-lived but persistent cases. It is useful in bilateral cases where it is preferred to avoid radical treatment on both sides. The antrostomy is not as likely to remain patent as in the Caldwell–Luc operation but in selected cases this may not matter.

If conservative treatment has failed and an ethmoiditis or frontal sinusitis persists despite antibiotics, decongestant treatment of the maxillary sinus rather than radical operations must be considered.

Extensive intranasal operations on the ethmoid or frontal sinuses should not be undertaken other than by surgeons trained in these particular methods of approach. They should not be considered minor simply because no external incision is made.

The external fronto–ethmoid operation has much to recommend it as it permits the same approach for frontal, ethmoid and sphenoid disease. In times when antibiotics have made these operations uncommon the need to acquire familiarity with a standard approach is an important consideration.

In deciding what surgery is necessary a careful assessment of the extent of the infection must be made. In cases of chronic maxillary sinusitis associated with polypoidal ethmoiditis and a clear frontal sinus, Horgan's transantral ethmoidectomy is probably the best approach.

Radical operations on the maxillary, sphenoidal and ethmoidal sinuses are generally successful but this is not always the case in frontal sinus surgery. This has led to the development of obliterative surgery which is suitable for well-established disease of the frontal sinus which has shown no response to simple measures.

The aim should be to cure the symptoms without external disfigurement. Finally, it should be emphasized that no external operation on the the frontal sinus should be undertaken until it is quite certain that any maxillary sinusitis has been adequately treated and that the nasal orifice of the frontal sinus has been freed from obstruction by a deviated septum, an enlarged middle turbinate or polyps.

Chronic sinusitis in children

Sinusitis is unlikely to develop before the age of two to three years and chronic sinusitis in infants and young children is a rare condition. The symptoms are nasal obstruction, persistent mucopurulent discharge and frequent colds. There is often an association with a chronic cough. Examination shows pus in the nose with excoriation of the nostrils and pharyngitis. Infected and enlarged adenoids are nearly always present in the post-nasal space.

There is a high incidence of maxillary sinusitis in children with cleft lips and palates. Jaffrey and Fand de Blanc (1971) found that 62 per cent of children with this type of deformity had maxillary sinusitis.

They related it to the regurgitation and irritation of food and saliva as well as to structural abnormalities of the septum, turbinates and maxillae.

Additional factors predisposing to sinusitis in children may be any other condition causing nasal obstruction, such as nasal allergy, choanal atresia, deviated septum, polyp, foreign bodies or tumour. Debilitating diseases such as leukaemia may be rare contributory factors.

In contrast to adults, infected teeth are rarely responsible for sinusitis in children because of the distance of the deciduous teeth from the floor of the sinus and by the intervening buds of the permanent detention. An abscess from a deciduous tooth invariably drains into the buccal cavity (Bernstein, 1971).

Radiography may show an opaque antrum but this is not always meaningful as a thickened lining membrane due to allergy or a cold may almost completely fill a small antrum in a child even if no pus is present.

There is no place for proof puncture of maxillary sinuses under local anaesthesia in children, and few surgeons would suggest carrying it out under general anesthesia before a trial of medical treatment.

This should consist of a course of decongestant nose drops and antibiotics given with bacteriological control. Often this can be usefully supplemented by an antihistamine syrup. Most children respond to this treatment which should be accompanied by an adenoidectomy if, as is common, the adenoids are enlarged and infected.

Rarely, chronic sinusitis persists in a child and in this case antral washouts should be carried out under general anaesthesia. If pus is found, indwelling polythene tubes can be inserted through the cannulae and attached to the cheek or forehead. Daily washouts can be performed in this way until the return is clear.

Very occasionally a child may need an intranasal antrostomy. A technique of making intranasal antrostomies using the microscope has been described by Dixon (1976). A Caldwell–Luc operation is not a suitable procedure for young children.

Finally, it should be mentioned that one of the most common problems presenting in the paediatric out-patients is the child with a running nose and constant cough.

The vast majority are between the ages of three and seven years; this corresponds more or less with the age incidence of 'glue ears'. The chest x-ray is usually clear and sinus x-rays are often performed in desperation with the mildest opacity being taken as the cause of all the symptoms. Treatment as for chronic sinusitis usually produces some degree of improvement only to recur on cessation of treatment. Antral washouts produce either clear washings or a mucoid return and have no beneficial effect. There is no evidence that these children have bronchitis and the cough may be due to the secretions of nasal allergy. They should certainly not be classified as having a 'sinobronchial syndrome' and it must be remembered that bronchiectasis is now very uncommon in children. The severe chest infections that used to follow measles and cause bronchiectasis are now rarely seen and the measles vaccine is likely to reinforce this, so that virtually the only cases occurring will be the rare Kartagener's syndrome and mucoviscidosis. The parents often need reassurance and are informed that the condition is likely to improve within one or two years; in the meantime the symptoms are allayed with symptomatic treatment.

References

Ballantyne, J. C. and Rowe, A. R. (1949). *Journal of Laryngology*, **63**, 337

Bateman, G. H. (1963). *Proceedings of the Royal Society of Medicine*, **56**, 393

Berganara, A. R. and Itoiz, A. O. (1955). *Archives of Otolaryngology*, **61**, 616

Bernstein, L. (1971). *Otolaryngology Clinics of North America*, **4**, 1, Philadelphia; Saunders

Bürgi, H. (1965). *Schweizerische medizinische Wochenschrift*, **95**, 274

Burton, P. A. and Dixon, M. F. (1969). *Thorax*, **24**, 180

Carenfelt, C. T., Enroth, C. M., Lundberg, C. and Wretlind, B. (1975). *Scandinavian Journal of infectious Diseases*, **7**, 259

Cawthorne, T. and Edwards, W. G. (1966). *Journal of Laryngology*, **80**, 359

Dixon, H. S. (1976). *Laryngoscope*, **86**, 1796

Douek, E. (1970). *Journal of Laryngology*, **84**, 1185

Douek, E. (1971). In *Diseases of the Ear, Nose and Throat* 3rd Ed. London; Butterworth

Drettner, B. (1967). *International Rhinology, Leiden*, **5**, 100

Eggston, A. A. and Wolff, D. (1947). *Histopathology of Ear, Nose and Throat*, Baltimore; Williams and Wilkins

Eichel, B.-S. (1972). *Laryngoscope*, **82**, 1806

Ewert, G. (1965). *Acta Otolaryngologica Stockholm*, Suppl. 200

Goodale, R. L. and Montgomery, W. W. (1958). *Archives of Otolaryngology*, **68**, 271

Goodman, W. S. (1976). *The Maxillary Sinuses, Otolaryngology Clinics of North America*, Philadelphia; Saunders

Grossan, M. (1975). *American Academy of Ophthalmology and Otolaryngology Exhibition*

Halle, J. (1907). *Laryngoscope*, **17**, 115

Halle, J. (1914). *Archives of Laryngology and Rhinology*, **29**, 73

Hargrove, S. W. G. (1944). *Lancet*, **1**, 3

Hilding, A. (1941). *Annals of Otology*, **50**, 379

Horgan, J. B. (1926). *Journal of Laryngology*, **41**, 510

Howarth, W. (1936). *Journal of Laryngology*, **51**, 387

Hughes, R. G. (1976). *Operative Surgery, Nose and Throat*. 3rd ed. Ed. by Rob, C. and Smith, R. London; Butterworth

Jaffrey, B. and Fand de Blanc, C. B. (1971). *Archives of Otolaryngology*, **93**, 479

Killian. (1903). Quoted in St. Clair Thompson and Negus V.E. (1948). *Diseases of the Nose and Throat*. London; Cassell and Co. Ltd.

Kinman, J. (1967). *Acta Otolaryngologica Stockholm*, **64**, 37 .

Lederer, F. L. (1947). In *Diseases of the Ear, Nose and Throat*, 5th ed. Philadelphia; Davis

Macbeth, R. G. (1954). *Journal of Laryngology*, **68**, 465

McNab Jones, R. F. (1976). *Operative Surgery, Nose and Throat.* 3rd ed. London; Butterworth

McNeil, R. A. (1963). *Journal of Laryngology*, **77**, 158

McNeil, R. A. (1966). *Journal of Laryngology*, **80**, 953

Mawson, S. R. (1951). *St. Thomas's Hospital Report*, **7**, 72

Mélon, J. (1967). *Acta Otolaryngologica, Stockholm*, **67**, 158

Montgomery, W. W. (1971). *Otolaryngology Clinics of North America*, Philadelphia; Saunders

Mosher, H. P. (1929). *Annals of Otology, St. Louis*, **138**, 890

Negus, V. E. (1947). *British Medical Journal*, **1**, 135

Negus, V. E. (1958). *Comparative Anatomy and Physiology of the Nose and Sinuses.* Edinburgh and London; Livingston

Paavolainen, M., Paavolainen, R. and Tarkkanen, J. (1977). *Laryngoscope*, **87**, 613

Patterson, N. (1939). *Lancet*, **1**, 558

Pickworth, F. A. (1935). *Chronic Nasal Sinusitis and its Relation to Mental Disorder*, London; Lewis

Proetz, A. W. (1939). *The Displacement Method*, St. Louis; Annals Publishing Co.

Ransome, J. (1964). *Journal of Laryngology*, **75**, 196

Reid, L. (1954). *Lancet*, **1**, 275

Reid, L. (1960). *Thorax*, **15**, 132

Rewell, R. E. (1963). *Pathology of the Upper Respiratory Tract*, London; Livingston

Scott-Brown, W. G. (1965). In *Diseases of the Ear, Nose and Throat* 2nd ed. London; Butterworths

Sluder, G. (1918). *Headaches and Eye Disorders of Nasal Origin*, St. Louis; Mosby

Tremble, G. E. (1970). *Annals of Otology and Laryngology*, **79**, 840

Van Alyea, O. E. (1934). *Archives of Otolaryngology*, **191**, 370

Van Dishoeck, H. E. E. and Franseen, M. C. C. (1957). *Practical Otorhinolaryngology*, **19**, 502

15 Complications of acute and chronic sinusitis
J D K Dawes

Sinusitis which is a mucosal disease becomes complicated through involvement or dissolution of the bony walls whereby infection spreads into the adjacent orbital and intracranial tissues.

Apart from infection in an individual sinus causing infection in neighbouring sinuses, other infective or allergic associated lesions may arise in other parts of the upper and lower respiratory tracts.

Although complications of sinusitis are relatively uncommon due to the widespread use of antibiotics, they usually follow an acute exacerbation of chronic sinusitis.

For convenience, the complications are considered in groups as they clinically present: (a) those of the anterior group of sinuses; (b) those of the posterior group of sinuses; (c) a miscellaneous group; and (d) the secondary lesions of the respiratory tract.

Anterior group of sinuses

Of the anterior group of sinuses, the frontal sinus and the anterior and middle ethmoid cells which form the thin compact bony roof and anterior part of the medial wall of the orbit are also closely related to the anterior cranial fossa and are consequently a common source of orbital and intracranial infections. The maxillary sinus, although it forms the floor of the orbit, is rarely a source of orbital infection unless an acute exacerbation of chronic sinusitis spreads to the neighbouring sinuses of the anterior group and secondarily to the orbital and intracranial tissues. An acute sinusitis is often a multisinusitis involving all of the anterior group and, therefore, it is not surprising to find evidence of an acute or chronic lesion in all of them although only one of the group has produced the complication; usually the frontal sinus in adults and the ethmoid cells in children.

To produce a complication the disease must spread through the bony walls of the sinus by osteitis in the case of compact bone, or by osteomyelitis where diploeic or cancellous bone is present.

For clinical purposes the frontal sinus may be regarded as an anterior ethmoid cell which develops at about the age of 8–10 between the inner and outer plates of the frontal bone in close contact with the diploe. Only a very thin lamina of compact bone, often only 100–130 μm thick, separates the sinus mucous membrane from the very vascular diploe. The anterior wall of the frontal sinus consists largely of cancellous bone; the posterior wall although more compact is still largely diploeic bone whereas the floor separates the sinus from the orbit by a thin plate of compact bone. The veins of the mucosa freely communicate with those of the diploe and dura mater.

An acute infection or an acute exacerbation of a chronic sinusitis in the frontal sinus, particularly if pus collects under pressure, may produce a thrombophlebitis of the mucosal veins which spreads rapidly to the diploe to cause osteomyelitis or more commonly spreads through the thin orbital plate to produce a cellulitis of the orbit (*Figure 15.1*). The orbital spread is at first evidenced by a progressive swelling of the

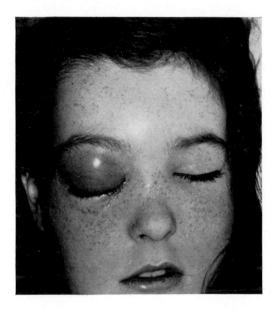

Figure 15.1   Orbital cellulitis and osteitis of the frontal bone complicating frontal sinusitis. Note the slight swelling of the forehead associated with the marked inflammatory lesion of the orbit

upper eyelid attended by all the local signs of inflammation. Within 48 h a subperiosteal abscess forms on the medial side of the orbital roof and the floor of the frontal sinus becomes carious. With development of an increasing subperiosteal abscess the globe becomes displaced downwards and outwards—the degree of displacement is best assessed by studying the pupillary displacement. If untreated the oedema and inflammation spread to the lower eyelid, the lids can no longer be opened voluntarily and chemosis of the conjuctiva appears, the globe becomes more proptosed and displaced and ocular movement is limited. Uncontrolled progression of the lesion disrupts the periosteum and the subsequent suppurative orbital lesion destroys the globe and the orbital contents will slough. Perhaps during the later stages a thrombophlebitis of the superior and inferior orbital veins may develop and lead to a cavernous sinus thrombophlebitis. The earlier stages of the lesion are predominantly an orbital cellulitis with or without a subperiosteal abscess; the later stages which rarely develop are a suppurative destruction of the orbital contents. Simultaneously with the development of the orbital cellulitis, an osteomyelitis of the frontal bone may co-exist and swelling of the forehead with formation of a subperiosteal abscess occurs. Orbital cellulitis is often accompanied by the manifestations of septicaemia, but should a pyaemia be present the cavernous sinus is probably involved.

On occasion, the subperiosteal abscess of the orbital roof or of the forehead points and ruptures through the neighbouring skin to produce a fistula (*see Figures 15.11* and *15.12*) which may relieve the patient's acute symptoms, but the fistula itself will not heal unless the underlying cause is treated. A subperiosteal abscess which lies in the roof or medial wall of the orbit rarely tracks backwards because of the adherence of the periosteum to the suture lines of the frontal and ethmoid bones with the sphenoid.

The direction of spread and rapidity of progression are dependent upon the virulence of the infection, the local anatomy and the patient's resistance, both local and general. A rapid spread of the disease is encouraged by a local dehiscence in bone due to injury, but even without this help the most virulent infections progress at an alarming rate. Antibiotic therapy has modified this pathogenesis and a slower progression of the lesion is more commonly seen.

The most slowly progressive lesion which erodes any one or all of the bony walls of the frontal sinus to cause displacement of the orbit and perhaps expose dura is a mucocoele (*Figure 15.2*). No active signs of inflammation accompany a mucocoele unless it becomes secondarily infected to form a pyocoele and then the structures exposed by the erosion of bone are directly exposed to attack.

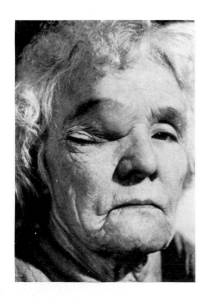

Figure 15.2 Mucocoele of the right frontal sinus. Despite the marked displacement sight was good. (From Dawes (1961), reproduced by courtesy of the Editor of *Journal of Laryngology and Otology*)

The most common method of spread of infection from the frontal sinus is by thrombophlebitis and osteitis. Thrombophlebitis of the vessels in bone causes osteomyelitis or osteitis and therefore local bone caries may predominate in one case, and a diffuse thrombophlebitis in another, and indeed one may see the two modes actively operating in different directions concomitantly. Perivascular lymphatics, although present, contribute more to the development and progress of a thrombophlebitis rather than as an independent potent factor.

Thrombophlebitis and osteomyelitis may affect the posterior wall of the frontal sinus at the time of a developing orbital cellulitis. The insidious and more dangerous symptoms and signs of the killing intracranial suppurations may be overlooked by the observer who directs his whole attention to the orbital lesion.

Ethmoid lesions

In children the frontal sinus is undeveloped and orbital cellulitis not uncommonly follows an ethmoiditis. The appearances are similar to those already described (*Figures 15.3* and *15.4*).

In adults, the ethmoid cells are surrounded by thin compact bone and the problem of osteomyelitis does not arise unless the frontal sinus is coincidentally infected. Loculation of pus under pressure in the ethmoid cells may lead to rupture into the orbit through the lamina papyracea to produce a subperiosteal abscess and progressive signs similar to those of frontal sinus ruptures. Furthermore a rupture can occur into the anterior cranial fossa through the cranial surface of the ethmoid to produce sequential intracranial tissue plane infections.

Mucocoeles may develop in the ethmoid cells but then tend to present in the middle meatus, but quite often they are linked with the frontal sinus to produce a large fronto–ethmoid mucocoele which may destroy the whole of the ethmoid labyrinth.

Management

The clinical history obtained can be extremely helpful in assessing the problem and the stage of orbital cellulitis reached. Symptoms of the preceding illness and any precipitating incident such as injury or swimming are sought. The chronological order of progression and rate of development should be recorded. The only local relevant symptoms are those of local discomfort, diplopia and changes in sight. Any pain should be accurately described if possible, and any change in its character noted. Other symptoms of the illness must be sought, sometimes by direct questioning, for if they are present and not directly a result of orbital cellulitis, they may be the first evidence of intracranial spread (*see below*). The temperature and pulse should be recorded four-hourly. The upper respiratory tract should be examined but radiological examination may occasionally have to be postponed until the acute presenting lesion has been treated.

The most important factors in management are the use of antibiotic therapy, drainage of subperiosteal abscesses and sinuses when necessary, and finally the management of the underlying cause. The organisms responsible are usually one of the pyococci or *Haemophilus influenzae* and they respond satisfactorily to an adequate dose of the appropriate antibiotic given systemically.

Some severe classic presentations will next be described to illustrate the management of orbital cellulitis.

A young child who may have jumped into a polluted river or into a swimming pool while he had an acute upper respiratory tract infection may within a few hours become very ill and develop orbital cellulitis, possibly associated with a swelling of the scalp. Clearly, it is too soon for suppuration to have occurred and the problem is one of acute osteitis or osteomyelitis with a true cellulitis of the orbit. Intensive antibiotic therapy by intramuscular injection is indicated, for this is a very virulent infection. As the organism is unknown, a combination of penicillin, streptomycin and sulphame-zathine will cover all likely organisms and protect the intracranial tissues. The lesion

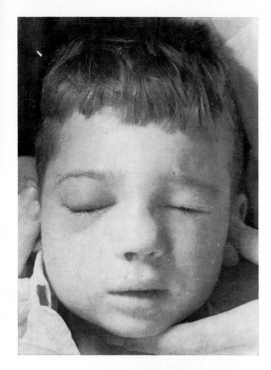

Figure 15.3 Orbital cellulitis complicating maxillary and ethmoidal sinusitis

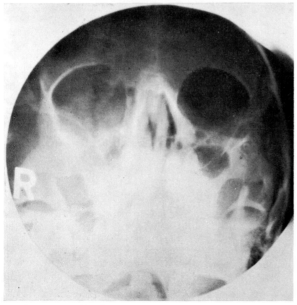

Figure 15.4 Right orbital cellulitis and right maxillary sinusitis

will probably recover by this treatment alone if the organisms are sensitive but a careful watch must be maintained for evidence of deterioration or the development of subperiosteal abscesses.

An adult may have had frontal sinusitis associated with severe local pain indicating pus under pressure for several days prior to the development of orbital cellulitis. This patient has a subperiosteal abscess as well as pus in the frontal sinus so, in addition to adequate antibiotic therapy, it is necessary to open the abscess and drain the frontal sinus through its floor. If the frontal sinusitis complicated a common cold the lesion will settle quickly. The drainage tube may be removed as soon as the fronto–nasal duct is known to function satisfactorily, as shown by the appearance in the nose of fluid injected into the sinus cavity. However, if the initial frontal sinus lesion complicated an acute exacerbation of a chronic maxillary sinusitis, it is preferable to do a Caldwell–Luc operation as soon as the acute lesion has settled and before removing the frontal sinus drain.

In some instances, the patient's history suggests that the orbital cellulitis complicated an infected mucocoele. Relief of the acute lesion by incision and drainage under cover of antibiotics can be obtained, but as the lesion is a true pyocoele then recovery of fronto–nasal duct function cannot be expected. Therefore after the acute lesion has settled the pyocoele should be excised through an external fronto–ethmoidectomy and the fronto–nasal duct reconstructed. If the patient has a chronic maxillary and ethmoid sinusitis these should be treated by transantral ethmoidectomy before embarking on the fronto–ethmoidectomy some days later.

In the child, the acute ethmoiditis which caused the orbital cellulitis usually responds to antibiotics alone but if there is no change for the better within 48 h the subperiosteal abscess should be drained by an incision at the inner canthus.

When antibiotics are given for the management of orbital cellulitis they should be given in high dosage not only to control the acute lesion but also to protect the diploe and intracranial tissues against further spread. In general, the acute lesions settle with antibiotics and drainage and only when these are under control should any underlying chronic pathology be treated. Even then further surgery must be under antibiotic or chemotherapeutic cover.

A striking feature of the early stages of orbital cellulitis is that if this is the sole complication of sinusitis present the patient is not very ill but if the patient is extremely sick other complications such as osteomyelitis or intracranial suppurations are present and these too require treatment (*see below*).

Mucocoele

A mucocoele is a characteristic cystic swelling of the frontal sinus, ethmoid sinus or fronto–ethmoid which contains mucous secretions. The cyst occupies the whole of one sinus or by progressive enlargement and dissolution of the thin intervening bony walls incorporates the other members of the fronto–ethmoid group. Finally the containing bony walls become thin, expanded and at last disrupted so that the cyst may displace the orbital contents, or expose the dura and arachnoid mater.

This mucocoele is lined by cubical epithelium, and contains, as a rule, thick tenacious white or opalescent mucus with cholesterin crystals. Occasionally the contents are straw coloured and serous. The contents, even though occasionally discoloured green or brownish, are always sterile.

The cause is uncertain but the fronto–nasal duct is always sealed either by bone or fibrous tissue and a previous history of injury or surgery of the frontal sinus or chronic sinusitis is frequently obtained. Other patients have had severe nasal allergies or osteomas involving the frontal sinus (Bordley and Bosley, 1973). Perhaps obstruction of the ostium alone leads to retention and accumulation of secretions within the sinus leading to a gradual thinning and expansion of its walls. Some authors believe that a mucocoele arises from a cystic dilatation of a mucous gland.

The patients commonly complain of headache localized to the frontal region and the clinical picture is characterized by the development of a slowly progressive non-inflammatory painless swelling within the orbit over a period of months or years. The swelling causes little inconvenience at first and may only be accidentally noticed. As the orbital contents become further displaced *(Figure 15.5)* the patient may complain of diplopia.

The swelling can be felt within the orbit at the inner canthus or occupying the medial half of the orbital roof deep to the supraorbital ridge; rarely does it extend below the level of the medial palpebral ligament. The swelling is round, smooth, feels rubbery, is tender, cannot be compressed or emptied, and is characterized by the absence of inflammatory signs *(see Figure 15.2)*. Very occasionally, an eggshell crackling may be felt if the bone is thin and just breaking, but if the bone has totally disappeared, fluctuation may be demonstrated. The presence of pulsation indicates that the inner table of the frontal sinus has been eroded and the dura exposed. Dawes

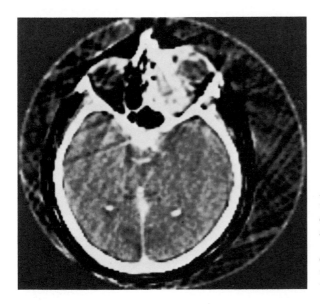

Figure 15.5 Gross proptosis of the right eye with a large mucocoele encroaching on the medial and posterior aspects of the orbit. (By courtesy of the Department of Neuroradiology, Royal Victoria Infirmary, Newcastle upon Tyne)

(1961) found in 14 cases of mucocoele that one had exposed dura and another was in communication with a meningocoele. Two of the 54 cases reported by Bordley and Bosley (1973) had cerebrospinal fluid leaks due to erosion of the posterior table of the frontal sinus.

Radiology

The radiograph *(Figure 15.6)* usually shows the affected frontal or ethmoid sinus to be larger than that of the opposite side; there is decreased density of the involved sinus; the border of the frontal sinus loses its scalloped appearance and the ethmoid cells

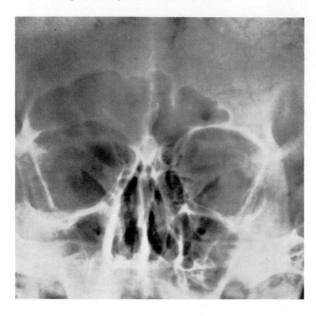

Figure 15.6   Radiograph of mucocoele of right frontal sinus
showing general expansion of the
sinus and 'bulging' of the sinus
septum into the left sinus. The
loss of 'scalloping' is well seen

appear to be replaced by one cystic cavity. Marginal densities become rarefied,
smooth and regular and a deficiency in the bony roof of the orbit apparent. A lateral
view of the frontal bone may show erosion of the inner table.

Intracranial extension of a mucocoele originating in the sinuses can be demonstrated
by computerized tomography (EMI scan) (*Figure 15.7*).

The majority of these cases have been treated by means of a fronto–ethmoidectomy
(Tamari and Bear, 1953; Wilkerson, 1945; Dawes, 1961). By an external approach
the cyst may be totally excised and a wide opening into the middle meatus created
accurately. If the mucosal lining is satisfactory much of it may be left. Goodyear
(1944) advocated simple intranasal drainage (*Figures 15.8* and *15.9*) with preservation
of the mucous walls of the cyst but this method is probably only indicated for the few
where there is a bulge of the mucocoele into the middle meatus or where the lesion is
confined to the bulla. Macbeth (1954), Goodale and Montgomery (1958) and Bordley
and Bosley (1973) recommended an approach through a frontal osteo–plastic flap
with removal of all mucous membrane. Recurrences are common and result from
leaving fragments of mucous membrane and these cases are best treated by the osteo–
plastic frontal flap approach.

Pyocoele

A pyocoele is an indolent purulent collection within the ethmoid or frontal sinuses
with obstruction of the fronto–nasal duct by swollen mucosa, granulation tissue,
polyps or bone produced by chronic sinusitis. In some cases, it may be an infected
mucocoele.

The history may be of a recurrent mild inflammatory swelling appearing and
disappearing at the inner canthus with upper respiratory tract infections or
exacerbations of sinusitis. Each disappearance of the swelling may be associated with

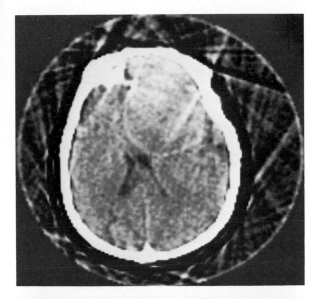

Figure 15.7 The same patient as in *Figure 15.5* showing the massive intracranial extent of a lesion which was a *mucocoele* originating in the *frontal sinus*. (By courtesy of the Department of Neuroradiology, Royal Victoria Infirmary, Newcastle upon Tyne)

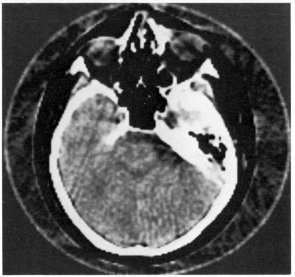

Figure 15.8 The same patient as in *Figures 15.5* and *15.7* after the mucocoele has been drained, the proptosis is considerably diminished. (By courtesy of the Department of Neuroradiology, Royal Victoria Infirmary, Newcastle upon Tyne)

a discharge of pus from the nose. When the swelling appears the local signs of a mild inflammation may be present or absent but local tenderness over the swelling is apparent. The ocular displacement is slight but recognizable as downwards and outwards. If such a case is operated upon during a quiescent period a deficiency of the bony wall is apparent and the sinus is full of inspissated pus. During the acute phase, active inflammation is obvious and, if severe, produces the classic picture of orbital cellulitis (*Figure 15.10*). On examination of the nose the pyocoele may be seen presenting in the middle meatus, but there are usually definite signs of a multisinusitis with pus and polypi present, perhaps also involving the other side. Most cases of pyocoele are truly cases of chronic purulent sinusitis of the ethmoid and frontal sinuses which, by repeated mild exacerbations, has led to disruption of the thin bony walls protecting the orbit and at the same time causes stenosis of the fronto–nasal duct. Some

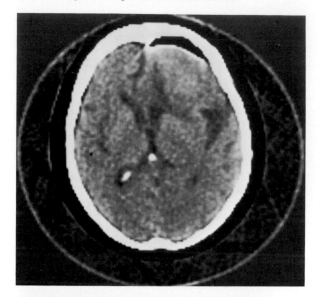

Figure 15.9   The same patient as in *Figures 15.5, 15.7* and *15.8* after surgery. The intracranial extension of mucocoele is very much less. Some post-operative air is present over the right frontal region. (By courtesy of the Department of Neuroradiology, Royal Victoria Infirmary, Newcastle upon Tyne)

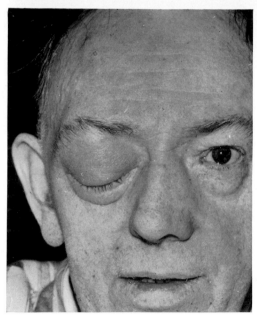

Figure 15.10   Pyocoele of right frontal sinus. This lesion was complicated by an extradural abscess and sequestration of the posterior wall of the frontal sinus. (From Dawes (1961), reproduced by courtesy of the Editor of *Journal of Laryngology and Otology*)

of these pyocoeles rupture through the skin at the inner canthus to produce a fistula; in others the fistula follows incomplete healing after incision and drainage. These pyocoeles can also expose dura or arachnoid and of course an acute exacerbation rapidly produces an intracranial complication. Pyocoeles may occur bilaterally.

The treatment is dependent on the method of presentation. If as an orbital cellulitis, the abscess must be incised and drained first and when the acute exacerbation has settled it may be treated as a quiescent pyocoele. As a chronic multisinusitis is usually present, it is wisest to treat these coincidental lesions first before tackling the fronto–ethmoid pyocoele some days later. Antibiotics should be continued throughout the whole period of surgical treatment for surgical trauma itself may precipitate an oesteomyelitis of the frontal bone. Furthermore it is advisable to continue the antibiotics for some weeks post-operatively to control infection within the nose in the hope of preventing a further stenosis of the fronto–nasal duct by granulation or scar tissue.

Fistulae

Persistent fistulae arising from sinus lesions occur as a rule above the level of the medial palpebral ligament. The commonest site is at the inner canthus but other sites are the upper eyelid, the superior fornix of the conjunctival sac and the forehead (*Figure 15.11*).

These fistulae may develop spontaneously or post-operatively and will not heal until the underlying cause, usually pyocoele or osteomyelitis, is cured.

The presence of a chronic purulent discharge from a fistula above the medial palpebral ligament is diagnostic of its origin. The development of a fistula may have so relieved the patient of his initial discomfort that he delays attendance at hospital. If this delay has been prolonged the fistulous orifice shows marked scarring and contracture may produce an ectropion of the upper lid (*Figure 15.12*).

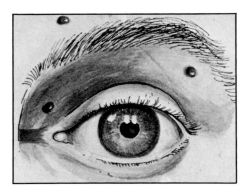

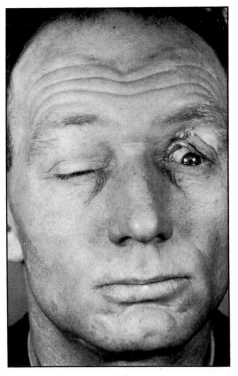

Figure 15.11   Common sites of fistulae. (From Dawes (1961), reproduced by courtesy of the Editor of *Journal of Laryngology and Otology*)

Figure 15.12   Patient with a right-sided pyocoele. The previous left-sided pyocoele had been incised and a persistent fistula had been present for three years. Note the secondary contracture producing the left-sided ectropion. (From Dawes (1961), reproduced by courtesy of the Editor of *Journal of Laryngology and Otology*)

Fistulae are often associated with chronic disease in the whole anterior group of sinuses and if this be the case these lesions should be treated sequentially as for pyocoele. Once the pyocoele or osteomyelitis is cured the fistula heals spontaneously. Often, however, by virtue of its situation the fistulous opening can be included in the incision for an external fronto–ethmoidectomy and then it is worth while excising the fistulous track.

Radiology is useful in determining the state of the other paranasal sinuses, or demonstrating an osteitis or sequestrum, but little help is gained by injecting the track with an opaque dye for the dye often fails to reach a sinus already overfull with pus. Probing of the track prior to surgery is rarely helpful.

Rhinogenic intracranial suppuration

Intracranial complications usually follow infection of the frontal or ethmoid sinuses. The mucosal veins of these sinuses communicate with those of the dura mater and extension from the sinus to the intracranial tissue planes is either by thrombophlebitis or local bone caries involving the posterior wall of the frontal sinus or the cranial surface of the ethmoid labyrinth. A pre-formed pathway may exist through previous fracture or surgery. Mucocoeles and pyocoeles, as we have seen, may expose dura and arachnoid by dissolution of bone.

The lymphatics of the periphery do not communicate directly with the cerebral dural lymphatic system and play no part in dissemination of infection. The special route provided by the perineural spaces of the olfactory nerves is rarely if ever a route used by infection spreading from the paranasal sinuses.

Surgery may indirectly cause intracranial spread by initially producing an osteomyelitis of the frontal bone.

The same methods of dissemination operate for orbital cellulitis, osteomyelitis and intracranial suppurations, and all three may co-exist in the same patient. However, the greatest difficulty arises when the patient has no obvious signs attracting the attention of the observer to the frontal or ethmoid sinuses and the patient merely presents with a pyogenic intracranial suppuration without obvious cause. Of the 33 rhinogenic intracranial complications reported by Dawes (1961) 23 of the patients had either an osteitis of skull or orbital cellulitis. By far the majority had osteitis. The persistent killing diseases, even in this antibiotic era, are cerebral and subdural abscesses, whereas the overwhelming acute suppurative intracranial lesions of the past such as meningitis or longitudinal sinus thrombophlebitis recover (*Table 15.1*).

The intracranial complication may develop during the course of acute frontal sinusitis, or after the sinusitis has apparently recovered. Sometimes it is precipitated by surgical intervention in the frontal sinus, and often accompanies osteomyelitis of the frontal bone.

The medical attendant may only become aware of the development of an intracranial complication during the course of the illness by paying close attention to symptoms. A suspicion of intracranial spread must be the starting point of investigation, for to delay diagnosis and effective therapy may endanger the patient's life. The frontal lobe is a silent area of the brain, and early changes in judgment and character or defects of memory are only recognizable by close relatives and in a sick

Table 15.1   Intracranial complications of frontal sinusitis seen at the Royal Victoria Infirmary, Newcastle upon Tyne 1930–1967

1930–37

8 cases	6 deaths	4 multiple intracranial lesions with brain abscess.
		2 meningitis (1 with sup. long. sinus thrombosis)
	2 recoveries	1 frontal lobe abscess
		1 extradural abscess

1938–44 (Sulphonamides)

8 cases	5 deaths	1 cerebral abscess with subdural abscess
		1 cerebral abscess
		2 meningitis
		1 sup. long. sinus thrombosis
	3 recoveries	2 extradural abscess
		1 brain abscess

1945–67 (Antibiotics)

21 cases	5 deaths		4 brain abscesses
			1 meningitis (moribund on admission)
	3 probably died	—	Brain abscesses
			5 extradural abscess
			1 encephalitis
	13 recoveries		6 meningitis
			1 brain abscess

patient may pass unnoticed. Furthermore these character changes are only evident in the chronic lesion. Therefore the frontal lobe behaves relatively even more silently than usual. The symptoms and signs of raised intracranial pressure may be the only evidence, and as an intracranial abscess must be in existence for at least two weeks before papilloedema is present, headache and vomiting are the only evidence of an early frontal lobe lesion. Headache is common to frontal sinusitis, osteitis and all intracranial lesions and it may be very difficult to assess the exact time of onset of intracranial disease. However, careful questioning of the patient may elucidate a change in the character of headache. Vomiting is also common to all intracranial lesions but does not as a rule occur with frontal sinusitis or osteomyelitis, and therefore its occurrence may be of great significance, and certainly should stimulate interest as to whether an intracranial lesion exists.

A patient who is ill out of proportion to the expectation of local signs should awaken suspicion. Drowsiness is definite evidence of involvement of grey matter and progression to coma with fixed dilated pupils indicates a gross supratentorial hydrocephalus demanding immediate relief by frontal burr hole and aspiration of the brain abscess. Rigors suggest pyaemia and if repeated probably indicate superior longitudinal sinus thrombosis.

An epileptiform fit suggests cortical irritation probably due to thrombophlebitis possibly arising from a subdural empyema. Certainly if Jacksonian epileptic attacks are repeated the diagnosis should be considered to be subdural empyema and urgent treatment by multiple burr holes undertaken.

The meninges of the anterior fossa are far removed from the basal cisterns and neck rigidity which accompanies basal meningitis may be late in appearance. The only symptoms indicative of meningitis in the early stages are headache and vomiting. Neck rigidity may be an accompaniment of subdural empyema as well as meningitis.

Often the most useful physical signs may be seen in the temperature and pulse chart—a marked and dramatic change in either direction may be indicative of intracranial suppuration. A sudden falling pulse and temperature indicates a raised intracranial pressure due to an abscess or a sudden rise of temperature and pulse with rigors a longitudinal sinus thrombosis.

The occurrence of epileptiform fits and focal paralysis with or without neck rigidity are almost certain evidence of subdural empyema. Focal paralysis involving the motor area is rarely due to a frontal lobe abscess for by the time an abscess has extended to this degree it is most likely to have ruptured into the anterior horn of the ventricle producing terminal signs of meningitis, whereas free spread of pus throughout the subdural space may produce diffuse focal signs of rapid onset (*Figure 15.13*). A definite suspicion of intracranial disease is all that can be obtained with absolute certainty on clinical grounds. Unless the physical state of the patient demands urgent burr holes to relieve a subdural empyema or a frontal lobe abscess causing supratentorial hydrocephalus, time may be available to investigate the lesion.

The commonest method of examination is lumbar puncture. However, many patients with headache complicating sinusitis who have been subjected to lumbar puncture have died soon afterwards as a result of a frontal lobe abscess rupturing into the ventricle. A brain abscess is always preceded by a thrombophlebitis and it takes 2–3 days for suppuration to develop. Therefore if the time of onset of the intracranial lesion is known, it is safe to do a lumbar puncture within the first 2–3 days. After this, lumbar puncture should not be done and even if the diagnosis is not really suspected the lumbar puncture should be done circumspectly and only in conditions where it is possible to treat a frontal lobe abscess urgently. An EMI scan (*Figures 15.14* and *15.15*) is the most certain diagnostic investigation for a suspected frontal lobe abscess and should precede lumbar puncture. If this technique is not available a cerebral angiogram is not only safer than lumbar puncture but also a more certain method of detecting a lesion in the frontal lobe (*Figure 15.16*).

Some cases of pyococcal meningitis present without a definite sinus history, but all such cases should have the ears and paranasal sinuses examined to exclude lesions in these sites for an osteitis of the posterior wall of the frontal sinus may produce only headache with meningeal signs and no other overt manifestation of the initial lesion. Fortunately the majority of acute lesions clear up with the treatment given for meningitis.

Extradural abscesses of themselves only cause headache and are usually only diagnosed and demonstrated during surgical exploration of the frontal sinus.

Osteomyelitis

Oesteomyelitis of skull bones only occurs in diploe and therefore apart from those cases in which diploe is exposed to infection by a direct open or penetrating injury, the commonest cause is infection from a paranasal sinus. The frontal sinus is the

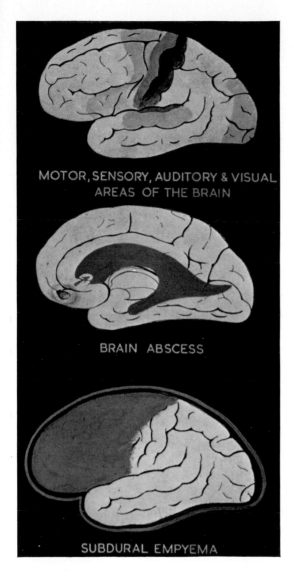

MOTOR, SENSORY, AUDITORY & VISUAL
AREAS OF THE BRAIN

BRAIN ABSCESS

SUBDURAL EMPYEMA

Figure 15.13   Diagram to explain the different symptomatology of subdural and cerebral abscess. A frontal lobe abscess usually ruptures into the ventricle before it is large enough to produce upper motor neurone paralysis, whereas rapid spread of infection throughout the subdural space readily causes cortical thrombophlebitis, epileptiform fits and focal paralysis. (From Dawes (1961), reproduced by courtesy of the Editor of *Journal of Laryngology and Otology*)

commonest source of such infection, and the maxillary sinus is the second most common.

Ostemyelitis of the frontal bone

By virtue of its situation between the inner and outer plates of the skull the frontal sinus is closely in contact with diploeic tissue. Its mucosal veins also freely communicate with those of the diploe and dura and a thrombophlebitis of the veins rapidly sets up osteomyelitis.

Osteomyelitis is usually classified as post-operative or spontaneous. Prior to antibiotic therapy post-operative osteomyelitis was almost invariably virulent and fatal. Therefore, surgical procedures which open diploeic tissue in the presence of

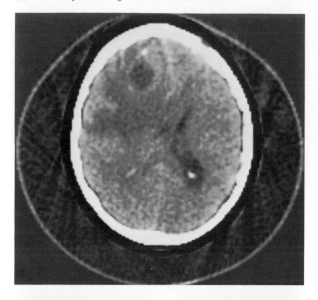

Figure 15.14   EMI scan showing a *frontal lobe abscess* which appears as a round low density area surrounded by oedema. (By courtesy of the Department of Neuroradiology, Royal Victoria Infirmary, Newcastle upon Tyne)

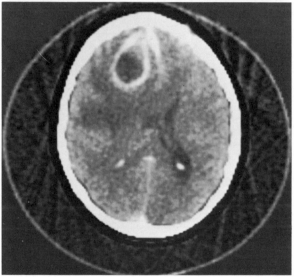

Figure 15.15   Same patient as in *Figure 15.14* after the intravenous injection of contrast medium. The wall of the abscess shows marked enhancement. (By courtesy of the Department of Neuroradiology, Royal Victoria Infirmary, Newcastle upon Tyne)

infection are to be deplored. In the antibiotic era, it may be permissible to open diploic tissue provided the acute lesion has been brought under control and the patient is covered by the appropriate antibiotic during such surgery. During the acute phase of the lesion the frontal sinus should only be drained through the thin orbital plate of compact bone, and bone must not be curetted. Later, when the acute lesion is under control bone curettage should still be avoided but infected mucosa can be carefully stripped out.

Whereas post-operative osteomyelitis is always rapidly spreading due to the opening of virgin diploe to infection, the spontaneous type takes varied forms largely dependent on the balance between the virulence of the infection and the resistance of the patient as modified by the use of antibiotics.

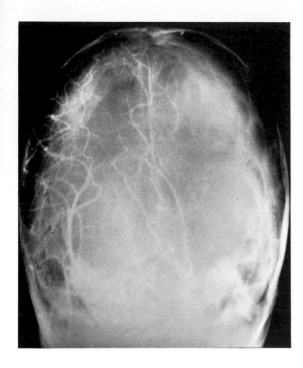

Figure 15.16 Cerebral angiogram showing displacement of the anterior cerebral artery and the absence of filling in the region of the abscess. (From Dawes (1961), reproduced by courtesy of the Editor of *Journal of Laryngology and Otology*)

Accidental trauma, swimming and in particular jumping into a swimming pool without nipping the nose may precipitate an osteomyelitis, particularly in a patient who already has sinusitis.

Although the presence of pus under pressure within the frontal sinus is regarded as the condition most likely to produce osteomyelitis it is not essential, for a patient may within hours of onset of an acute frontal sinusitis develop a fulminating rapidly spreading osteomyelitis of the skull.

Osteomyelitis is due to infection of diploeic bone and osteitis is an infection of compact bone. The thin compact bony floor of the sinus is usually the first and sometimes the only wall to be involved, but one in four of these will later show definite osteomyelitis in the diploeic bone (Dawes, 1961).

Bacteriology
Usually it is the organisms which are responsible for the sinusitis which cause the osteitis but the common organisms of sinusitis are pneumococci and *H. influenzae*, whereas those of osteomyelitis are an anaerobic streptococcus or staphylococcus.

Pathogenesis
The lesion is essentially a thrombophlebitis of diploe. However, within the diploe are large valveless veins known as Breschet's canals and infection of these may lead to rapid dissemination throughout the frontal bone producing the main osteomyelitic lesion well removed from the frontal sinus. More commonly the osteomyelitis is in intimate association with the frontal sinus. Osteomyelitis may be rapidly spreading or localized. Massive tissue death with gross sequestration may occur in one, and in another there is only microscopic necrosis. In others a marked sclerosis of bone is the predominant feature. Despite this variety in pathological pictures the basic lesion is

thrombophlebitic. The chronic cases are really cases of prolonged acute disease, and the pattern may change depending on the degree of control or exacerbation of the lesion.

As with osteitis at other sites, the common manifestation is the development of a subperiosteal abscess, its extent being limited by the suture lines. In the case of the frontal bone the outer surface is covered by periosteum and the cranial surface by adherent dura which provides a large portion of its nutrition. An extradural abscess is therefore a type of subperiosteal abscess. When dura is lifted off the bone by an abscess, necrosis and sequestration will most likely follow. Not surprisingly therefore the first evidence of bone necrosis may be seen on the intracranial surface of the bone. The association of a subperiosteal abscess with an extradural abscess and osteomyelitis of the bone between is a typical 'Pott's puffy tumour'.

Symptoms and signs
The fulminating case.   Soon after surgery or a virulent sinusitis the patient becomes ill, develops a marked pyrexia with possibly a rigor, and has a diffuse headache. An oedematous swelling develops over the forehead and may progress rapidly over the whole scalp in the worst cases. If death does not supervene rapidly from intracranial disease the patient localizes the lesion and develops subperiosteal abscesses at different sites over the skull.

Spreading type.   This is less dramatic; the patient may have a high temperature, looks progressively ill, and develops headache with cellulitis of the orbit and the forehead (*Figure 15.17*). The temperature may persist, the cellulitis becomes a subperiosteal abscess and, despite drainage, the patient develops another subperiosteal abscess over the parietal bones and perhaps later over the occipital bones. In each of these areas sequestration (*Figure 15.18*) may occur and typical multiple Pott's puffy tumours associated with local extradural abscesses develop over the skull. The most rapidly spreading lesions are those of fulminating disease, but the rate of spread is greatly variable. In the maltreated or untreated case, the whole calvarium may become carious.

Localized type.   At the other extreme, the patient may develop a subperiosteal abscess over the frontal bone without suffering any other discomfort (*Figure 15.19*). This is usually a result of a chronic sinus lesion producing a local necrosis of bone and rupturing through a fistulous track on to the outer surface. Sequestration does not occur as a rule. The patient may notice that, if he compresses the abscess of the forehead, pus pours out of his nose. Frequently, on examination of the nose, pus may be seen coming from the fronto–nasal duct and there may be other evidence of a chronic multisinusitis.

Sclerosing osteitis.   In this form of localized disease discomfort also may be slight or non-existent. A long history of a local abscess of the forehead is obtained but radiology demonstrates a marked sclerosis of the frontal bone slowly obliterating the frontal sinus itself (*Figure 15.20*).

The more usual presentation of osteomyelitis is that of a slowly progressive lesion wherein the patient first develops an orbital cellulitis associated with headache, and then a day or two later a subperiosteal abscess of the forehead appears which, if

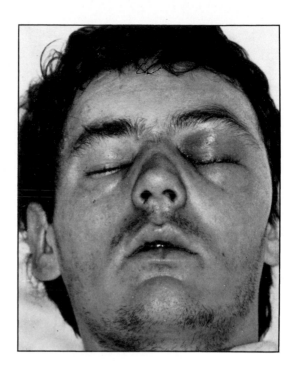

Figure 15.17 Patient who had a spreading osteomyelitis of the skull: 24 h after this photograph the patient had a large fronto-parietal abscess drained

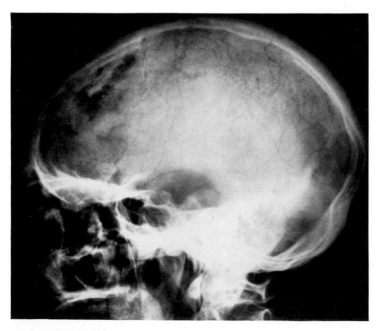

Figure 15.18 Spreading osteomyelitis of the skull with sequestration. (From Dawes (1961), reproduced by courtesy of the Editor of *Journal of Laryngology and Otology*)

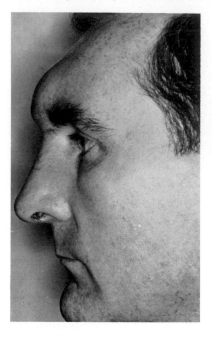 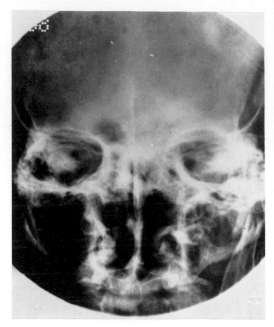

Figure 15.19 Localized type of osteo-myelitis of frontal bone. The abscess had been present for several months and pressure on the abscess produced pus from the anterior nares.

Figure 15.20 Sclerosing osteitis of the frontal bone. (From Dawes (1961), reproduced by courtesy of the Editor of *Journal of Laryngology and Otology*)

untreated, persists and spreads and later leads to a massive sequestration of bone (*Figure 15.21*).

All of these clinical pictures are modified by treatment and many of the classic pictures are only seen when treatment has been ineffective or delayed due to a misdiagnosis.

Recurring attacks of osteomyelitis of the frontal bone frequently follow surgical treatment for removal of sequestra or the anterior wall of the frontal sinus to obliterate a sinus, or to remove osteitic bone. Most of these cases were in fact relapses due to not giving the patient adequate antibiotic therapy for a long enough period to sterilize the bone, for microscopic areas of necrosis within the bone may continue to harbour organisms for a long period of time.

Radiology

Radiological evidence of untreated osteomyelitis does not show for 7–10 days, therefore almost all diagnoses in the early stages must depend on the characteristic clinical picture. However, when the frontal sinus suppuration ruptures through the posterior wall to produce an extradural abscess the clinical picture may be obscure, treatment is consequently delayed and the first definite evidence of osteomyelitis may be radiological. The use of antibiotics modifies the disease so greatly that radiological evidence of osteitis may be delayed for some weeks if the disease is persistent, or if the disease is treated and cured, radiological confirmation of the diagnosis may not be forthcoming.

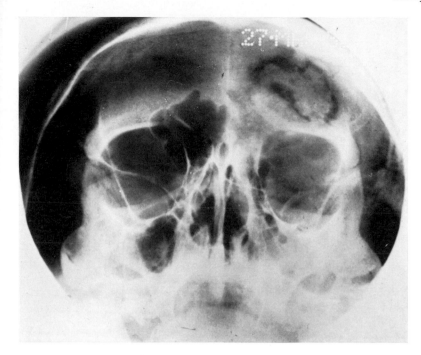

Figure 15.21 Large sequestrum of frontal bone. (From Dawes (1961), reproduced by courtesy of the Editor of *Journal of Laryngology and Otology*)

When radiological changes are demonstrable the first sign may be a moth-eaten appearance of the intracranial surface of the posterior wall of the sinus. Areas of rarefaction may be seen throughout the frontal bone (*Figure 15.22*), bone defects or sequestra may be demonstrable (*see Figures 15.18, 15.21* and *15.23*) and, at other times, marked sclerosis (*Figure 15.20*). Occasionally sclerosis of bone at the superior edge of the frontal sinus may be the only radiological evidence.

Management
Patients do not die from osteomyelitis of the skull, they die from intracranial infections or septicaemia. Therefore, during management it is important to be continually on the look-out for manifestations of these complications (*Table 15.2*).

Since the advent of antibiotics the prognosis has greatly changed—death should be a rare outcome today. Modern treatment is essentially that of giving an intensive dosage of an appropriate antibiotic, most frequently penicillin and sulphonamides. The latter should be incorporated for penicillin does not readily cross the blood–brain barrier and it is essential that the intracranial tissue planes should be protected while treating the osteomyelitis. If subperiosteal abscesses develop these should be opened and at the same time the frontal sinus should be drained through the compact bony floor. Once pus is obtained this should be cultured and the sensitivity of the organisms determined so that the antibiotic may be changed if need should arise. Sequestra should be removed when they develop through a carefully planned non-deforming incision. However, if the sequestrum is very large and its removal leads to a bony deformity of the anterior wall of the frontal sinus this may be repaired 1–2 years later by ilium or

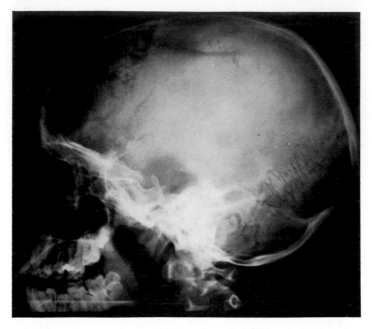

Figure 15.22 Spreading osteomyelitis of the skull showing areas of rarefaction in the frontal bone. (From Dawes (1961), reproduced by courtesy of the Editor of *Journal of Laryngology and Otology*)

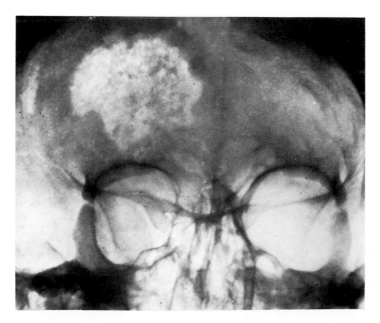

Figure 15.23 Marked destruction of the frontal bone due to osteomyelitis. This patient also had a frontal lobe abscess

Table 15.2   Prognosis of cases of osteomyelitis of skull seen at the Royal Victoria Infirmary, Newcastle upon Tyne, 1930–1967

1930–37		
10 cases	6 deaths	1 anaesthetic 5 intracranial lesions
1938–44 (Sulphonamides)		
12 cases	4 deaths 8 recoveries	—All intracranial complications
1945–59		
22 cases	2 deaths	—Both intracranial complications
1959–67		
13 cases	All recovered	

a tantalum plate. In every case of osteomyelitis antibiotics should be continued in reduced dosage for three months to prevent relapse. In chronic cases the antibiotics should be continued for perhaps as long as six months. In the extremely rare event of the patient's osteomyelitis continuing to spread because of an infection due to organisms insensitive to any known antibiotics then the whole of the diseased bone should be removed. This is usually done through an incision made from ear to ear behind the hairline. Burr holes are made and joined by a Gigli saw at least 2 cm clear of the diseased bone.

Osteomyelitis of the maxilla

Of the skull bones only the frontal bone is a more common site of osteitis than the maxilla. The alveolar portion of the maxilla is not only tooth-bearing, but is composed of cancellous bone between two thin plates of compact bone, whereas the remaining walls are largely composed of compact bone. As the air sinus increases with age the relatively largest volume of cancellous bone exists in the suckling and younger age groups. Therefore, it is not surprising to find that acute osteomyelitis occurs most commonly in these age groups, whereas chronic osteitis is seen more often in the adult.

Maxillary sinusitis of itself rarely causes osteitis unless the infection is virulent or the disease is neglected. Surgical or accidental trauma by exposing cancellous bone to infection, possibly already present within the sinus, may lead to osteomyelitis. Surgical trauma usually occurs during intranasal antrostomy when the lower margin of the antrostomy is enlarged, particularly so if done by rasping. Curettage of the sinus walls close to areas of cancellous bone during a Caldwell–Luc operation may be dangerous. Radiotherapy given for an antral carcinoma in the absence of adequate drainage for infection, may occasionally cause osteitis.

By far the commonest cause is dental infection. In the majority of these cases the osteitis is localized but occasionally it may become extensive. In sucklings the developing tooth buds, which are embedded in the relatively large mass of spongy bone, may become infected from an infected nipple of the mother's breast (Macbeth, 1952) and then be followed by a rapid and extensive spread throughout the maxilla. Asherson (1939) after studying the cases in the literature concluded that the origin was haematogenous, and others have thought it to arise from the lacrimal apparatus.

The causative organisms are usually a staphylococcus or a streptococcus, aerobic or anaerobic.

Osteomyelitis tends to be localized but a fulminating lesion may follow once the infection has produced a thrombophlebitis within the cancellous bone. Once established, osteomyelitis causes subperiosteal abscesses over the anterior wall of the maxilla, along the palatal surface, within the pterygoid fossa or the orbit. The orbital abscess produces proptosis and ophthalmoplegia, possibly blindness, and through thrombophlebitis of the ophthalmic veins may cause a cavernous sinus thrombophlebitis. If the osteomyelitis is of the spreading or fulminating type the lesion may cross suture lines to reach the frontal bone or zygoma.

As the blood supply of the maxilla is derived almost entirely from branches of the maxillary artery which are freely joined by arterial arcades, sequestration tends to affect only small portions of the bone but on the occasion when the major trunk becomes thrombosed a massive sequestration of the maxilla may follow. Recovery from an extensive osteitis produces bone sclerosis and if the initial lesion occurs in the young, maldevelopment of the teeth and maxilla follows. This marked bone sclerosis can obstruct the lower end of the naso–lacrimal duct. As the maxilla has a poor subperiosteal network of vessels loss of bone is followed by fibrous healing rather than new bone formation.

The more chronic forms of osteitis produce bone sclerosis rather than necrosis and the two features of sclerosis and halisteresis of bone may co-exist in different sites and stages of the lesion.

Symptoms and signs
Adults The more localized forms of osteitis following dental infection cause pain, tenderness and swelling over the affected tooth. Commonly the subperiosteal abscess or 'gumboil' is found over the canine fossa or over the palatal surface. Spontaneous rupture of such an abscess may occasionally produce a persistent discharging fistula. The 'dry socket', which is a localized osteitis following a dental extraction, causes localized persistent discomfort and may be accompanied by a minor sequestration of bone.

The spreading type of osteitis which is usually post-operative causes a dull boring pain over the maxilla accompanied by a brawny progressively extending swelling over the anterior wall of the maxilla or its palatal surface. The nose becomes totally obstructed due to a massive mucosal oedema and this is accompanied either by an increase in the purulent nasal discharge or a continuous serous drip. Such a lesion is accompanied by pyrexia and intense pain, trismus and epiphora, and the patient is extremely ill. An orbital cellulitis with proptosis and blindness may occur. Such severe infections may be accompanied by septicaemia and pyaemia, or may terminate with intracranial suppuration. Spread to other skull bones can be seen in the progression of the inflammatory signs and sequestration.

Less severe and more slowly spreading lesions may produce subperiosteal abscesses which rupture on to the buccal and palatal surfaces, or point over the nasal process or within the orbit. These abscesses may be followed by sequestration. Each of these abscesses produces local signs of disease and if they rupture on to a surface produce a persistent discharge from the wound. A purulent nasal discharge accompanies the disease. Occasionally the palatal process may necrose to produce a large oro–antral fistula. Chronic sclerosing osteitis in the adult produces the symptoms of a chronic maxillary sinusitis and the diagnosis is dependent on the radiological appearance (*Figure 15.24*).

Children   Osteomyelitis of the maxilla in a suckling of a few days to a few months old produces a characteristic clinical picture (*Figure 15.25*). A rapidly increasing brawny swelling develops in the cheek, producing oedema of the lower eyelid in a pyrexial and ill child. This is soon followed by a unilateral purulent nasal discharge and swelling of the palate of the affected side. After 48 h an abscess frequently presents

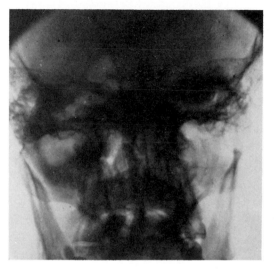

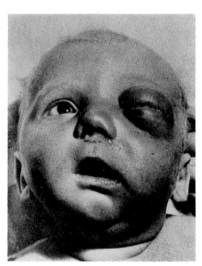

Figure 15.24   Chronic osteitis of maxilla. Note the immense thickening of the bone walls

Figure 15.25   Osteomyelitis of maxilla. Note the considerable swelling of left side of face and eyelids and homolateral nasal discharge. (From Macbeth (1952), reproduced by courtesy of the Editor of *Journal of Laryngology and Otology*)

over the nasal process or the alveolus. Sequestration may occur, tooth buds may be rejected and often destroyed. In the suckling osteomyelitis is usually due to a staphylococcus.

Radiological appearances

Apart from the local findings in relation to the dental roots, the radiographic appearances of acute osteitis of the maxilla are not characteristic. Loss of translucency of infected sinuses may be the only finding. Later when sequestration has occurred the bone loss may be demonstrable, and later still the bone sclerosis of a healed lesion can be recognized.

In the suckling radiographs are singularly unhelpful and unnecessary.

In the case of chronic osteitis which accompanies chronic maxillary sinusitis the only finding is a marked sclerosis and thickening of the bony walls of the antrum (*see Figure 15.24*).

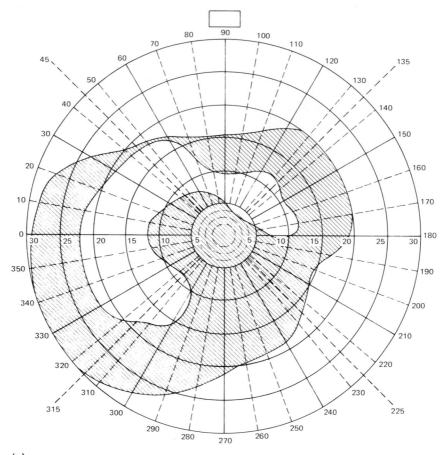

(a)

Sequelae
Osteitis in the young may have destroyed tooth buds of the primary and permanent dentitions and consequently teeth of either dentition may not appear. A more severe osteitis with or without bone loss may lead to maldevelopment of the affected maxilla. Bone sclerosis obstructing the nasal orifice of the naso–lacrimal duct will cause epiphora. An oro–antral fistula may be produced, and in the more severe cases blindness follows infections of the orbital apex or cavernous sinus.

Prognosis
With the advent of antibiotics sequelae are now rare, for the disease may be recognized early on clinical grounds alone. The rapid exhibition of systemic antibiotics not only cures the lesion but reduces the morbidity and sequelae.

Treatment
At all ages intensive dosage of the appropriate antibiotic will not only cure the lesion but also may prevent abscess formation if instituted early. Abscesses should be drained and sequestra removed when they have formed. Antibiotic therapy should be continued in reduced dosage for several weeks after apparent resolution of the lesion to prevent recurrence.

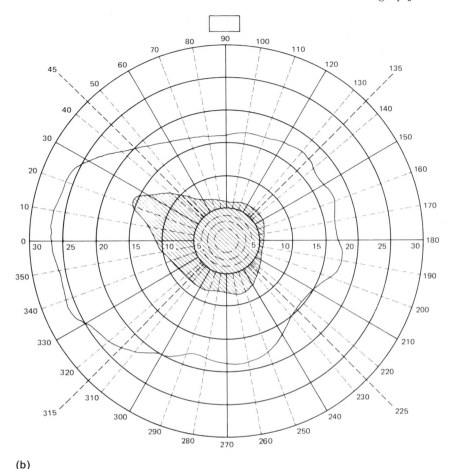

(b)

Figure 15.26 (a) Vision pre-operatively. (b) Vision two months post-operatively. (Both measured using the Hamblin Scotoma Chart)

Posterior group of sinuses

The posterior group of sinuses, comprising the posterior ethmoid cells and the sphenoid sinus, are closely related to the orbital apex. At the orbital apex three openings are present: (1) the optic foramen for the optic nerve; (2) superior orbital fissure transmitting the ophthalmic veins, the first division of the trigeminal nerve and the third, fourth and sixth cranial nerves; and (3) inferior orbital fissure for the second division of the trigeminal and the infraorbital artery.

The orbital apex syndrome is rare and due to involvement of the vessels and nerves passing through the superior orbital fissure and optic foramen. The full clinical picture is that of ptosis, ophthalmoplegia, impaired vision and pain over the distribution of the ophthalmic division of the trigeminal nerve. If vision is normal the symptom complex is called the superior orbital fissure syndrome.

Suppuration, mucocoeles or pyocoeles of the posterior ethmoid and sphenoid sinuses occasionally cause these syndromes. Pus tracking from a frontal sinus, subperiostally along the orbital roof towards the apex, may affect the vessels and nerves of the superior orbital fissure and optic foramen. More commonly the syndromes are caused by syphilis, neoplasia of the nasopharynx, posterior group of sinuses and pituitary, idiopathic granulomas and aneurysms.

Isolated optic neuritis is very rarely due to infection of the posterior group of sinuses (*Figure 15.26a* and *b*). If so, surgical drainage produces improvement in vision. More frequently these isolated cases are manifestations of multiple sclerosis.

Radiographs of the sinuses and the EMI scanner can help to differentiate lesions at the orbital apex.

Intracranial complications rarely follow lesions of the posterior sinuses, and the surmise so frequently made that in the past cavernous sinus thrombosis was due to sphenoiditis is not substantiated in clinical practice. The gangrene of the sphenoid mucosa so often seen in fatal cases of cavernous sinus thrombophlebitis probably was due to retrograde thrombophlebitis spreading from the cavernous sinus to the sphenoid sinus rather than in the reverse direction.

Cavernous sinus thrombophlebitis

Despite the fact that cavernous sinus thrombophlebitis is rarely due to paranasal sinus disease, the description of this disease is always linked with the complications of paranasal lesions. This is presumably for two reasons: (a) the difficulty which may be encountered in distinguishing between orbital cellulitis and sinus thrombophlebitis; and (b) the common autopsy finding of a gangrenous mucosa in the paranasal sinuses.

Orbital cellulitis presents all the conditions for the development of cavernous sinus thrombophlebitis but rarely does so. In 55 cases reviewed at the Royal Victoria Infirmary in Newcastle upon Tyne almost all the cases arose from furuncles or skin sepsis of the face, nose and forehead; several others followed lateral sinus thrombophlebitis due to ear disease and three cases followed a quinsy. The only one that was suspected to have cavernous sinus thrombophlebitis due to orbital cellulitis recovered in the pre-antibiotic era—an unlikely event.

The usual precipitating factor in the case of skin infections is squeezing of a boil or continued interference with the lesion. Soon after this the patient develops a high temperature, headache, rigors, becomes extremely ill and the ipsilateral eye becomes swollen, both eyelids are affected, proptosis develops, then chemosis of the conjunctiva. Finally ocular movements become restricted, venous engorgement of the retina is seen and finally blindness (*Figure 15.27*). The discoloration of the eye is bluish due to venous engorgement. During the development of proptosis etc. in the ipsilateral eye it is usually noticed that the other eye also is becoming involved. Thrombophlebitis of the veins can be seen on the forehead and along the course of the facial vein. If the case is far advanced, a surface suppuration of the skin venules may occur and in one case these extended over the whole scalp to the occiput. In the untreated case death follows inevitably and is associated with meningitis, cerebral thrombophlebitis, possibly other intracranial suppuration and pyaemic abscesses throughout the body.

As a complication of ear disease, the lesion is preceded by a thrombophlebitis of the lateral sinus or the inferior petrosal sinus and the first evidence of its development is oedema of the upper and lower eyelids.

In the case of quinsy the sinus thrombophlebitis is often accompanied by a 'pipe stem' neck in which a marked thrombophlebitis of the internal juglar vein is evident. The direction of spread can be either by the internal jugular vein or the pterygoid venous plexus.

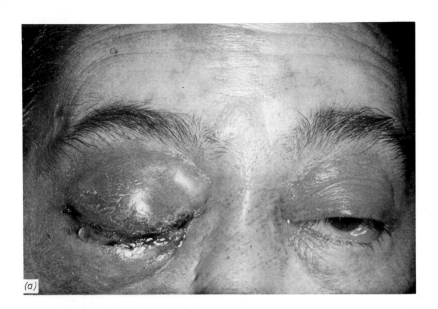

(a)

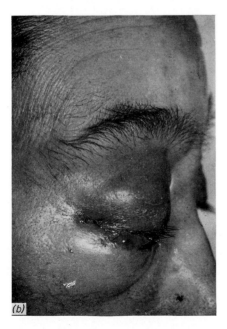

(b)

Figure 15.27 Cavernous sinus thrombosis: (a) frontal view. The patient's right eye was blind. Note the left peri-orbital swelling and the thrombophlebitis of the forehead; (b) lateral view of right eye. (From Dawes (1961), reproduced by courtesy of the Editor of *Journal of Laryngology and Otology*)

All the manifestations of septicaemia and pyaemia are seen, including a marked polymorphonuclear leucocytosis, and blood cultures may be positive. The organisms causing the disease are usually staphylococci or streptococci

Differential diagnosis

This is from orbital cellulitis. The initial lesion, the chronological order of events, the affliction of both eyes, the presence of thrombophlebitis in skin vessels, the skin discoloration, the retinal engorgement, the direction of ocular displacement (directly forwards in sinus thrombophlebitis and downwards and outwards in orbital cellulitis) all help to make the distinction.

Treatment

Intensive treatment by intramuscular penicillin together with streptomycin and sulphamezathine have altered the prognosis and most patients now recover, whereas in pre-chemotherapeutic days they all died. Early recognition of a spreading thrombophlebitic lesion permits early institution of treatment and prevention of cavernous sinus thrombophlebitis. Anticoagulants have been used but have little part to play in management.

Oro-antral fistula

The oro-antral fistulae most frequently calling for surgical treatment are those which result from dental extraction. The most common teeth involved are the second premolar and first molar but extraction of any tooth from the canine to the third molar may produce an alveolar fistula, for the roots of these teeth may be separated by only a thin lamina of bone from the antral mucosa in a well-developed air sinus. Osteitis around a tooth root may have destroyed this lamina so that on extraction a fistula is produced. Sometimes, a tooth root is displaced into the antrum and occasionally the alveolus is fractured and comes away with an ankylosed tooth during extraction. In removing a dental cyst a communication with the antrum may be created which could lead to fistula formation.

Many fistulae are unrecognized at the time of extraction and the track which seals with blood clot heals by primary intention. If the dentist does recognize the presence of a fistula immediately after extraction, he should not syringe, pack or probe the track for these acts break the seal, and delay healing. However, it is probably wisest to suture the gum, trimming the bony margins when necessary, so that the suture line is not under tension (Reading, 1955; Bosley, 1963), and the patient should be given systemic antibiotics in case the antrum has been contaminated. If an oro–antral fistula has been produced by extraction, the dentist should be forewarned that other tooth roots on the ipsilateral side may be close to the antral mucosa, or that similar conditions are likely to exist on the contralateral side. Oro–antral fistula produced by removal of a dental cyst should also be treated by primary wound suture. Even some of the larger traumatic fistulae resulting from removal of ankylosed teeth may heal by primary intention if carefully sutured immediately; in these instances a dental plate should be worn for support.

When a tooth root is lost in a sterile antrum, this should be confirmed radiologically, then the root should be removed by a Caldwell–Luc approach, an antrostomy made beneath the inferior turbinate and the bony edges of the fistulous track trimmed and the gum sutured. Careful planning of the incision for the Caldwell–Luc approach can usually include the gum edge of the fistula so leaving only a single suture line.

In the unrecognized case the patient may return in a few days complaining that fluids and food particles pass into his nose or that he can blow air from his nose into his mouth. The patient may also develop signs of acute maxillary sinusitis with pain or tenderness over the antrum and a mucopurulent or purulent nasal discharge which may rapidly become offensive. Similarly acute sinusitis may complicate those cases which had a primary repair. Treatment should be primarily by systemic antibiotic therapy and antral lavage via the inferior meatus when necessary; the majority of cases recover satisfactorily. However, a small proportion do not respond to these methods of treatment and if a fistula is present for 14 days it usually will not heal spontaneously and can be regarded as a chronic fistula. Some of these have a purulent discharge from the fistula and oedematous antral mucosa may prolapse into the oral cavity. One of the reasons for failure to heal by primary intention is that the patient at the time of fistula creation may have had a chronic maxillary sinusitis, possibly due to apical infection of the tooth which required extraction. The fistulous track may therefore be continually bathed in pus preventing spontaneous closure. These patients frequently develop an acute exacerbation of their chronic sinus lesion after extraction and although the acute exacerbation is controlled by antibiotics the fistula remains patent. In these chronic fistulae the antral infection is important and a potent factor in their persistence. Reading (1955) recommended closure of the fistula and an intranasal antrostomy unless teeth or pieces of bone are present in the antrum or an offensive discharge is present. He quotes the temporary anaesthesia or devitalization of teeth as a reason for avoiding the sublabial approach to the antrum. He reports only three failures out of 29 cases of intranasal drainage and plastic closure of the fistula. The majority of surgeons, however, feel the need to explore the antrum through a Caldwell–Luc approach, to remove any foreign bodies and assess the state of the antral mucosa, removing it if necessary, and creating an antrostomy beneath the inferior turbinate before immediately proceeding to a plastic closure of the fistula.

For very large fistulae or those fistulae which have failed to heal after simple suture, a plastic closure is obtained by using either a palatal or buccal flap or a combination of the two. Before closure by these flaps the lining of the bony track should be removed and the outer bony edge trimmed so that the soft tissues may fall into and obliterate it. In general, closure by a palatal flap is more reliable than a buccal flap but each individual case must be assessed as to which flap will provide the best closure with the least tension on the suture line. In some cases, if by no means all, it may be preferable to have a dental plate prepared to protect the suture line.

The palatal flap

The palatal flap is made from the mucosa of the hard palate and must be large enough to swing right across the fistulous opening to join the buccal flap. It is essential that the sutures between the flaps should not be immediately over the fistula but well lateral to it and flap approximations should be meticulous (*Figures 15.28* and *15.29*). The flap must also be long enough to ensure that there is no tension and not too much twisting at its base. The denuded area of the palate heals quickly and requires no dressing but great care must be taken in obtaining haemostasis for post-operatively a haematoma may form beneath the palatal flap so endangering the repair.

The buccal flap

The buccal flap claims the advantage of a more mobile flap with no denuded area, but the constant tension and movements of the lip and cheek prejudice the result.

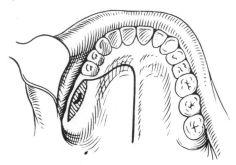 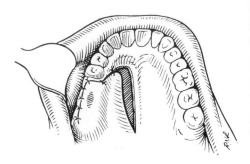

Figure 15.28 Incision to excise the fistula and to outline the plastic flap

Figure 15.29 The 'flap' swung into position over the fistulous track through the alveolus

If the buccal flap is used, the best results are probably obtained by an incision along the gum margin of two teeth on each side of the alveolar fistula. A muco–periosteal flap is raised up to the canine fossa where the periosteum is incised to free the flap. This procedure gives a very mobile flap which can be carried medially over the fistulous opening after it has been prepared. A short palatal flap is elevated along the palatal gum margin and the two flaps are carefully sewn without tension.

The sublabial fistula

The sublabial fistula follows a failure of healing of the Caldwell–Luc incision. This is a rare occurrence even if the incision is not sutured, and less frequent if the wound is carefully sutured. These fistulae are usually closed by an incision around the fistula, sewing the edges of the fistulous opening together after undercutting and inverting the edges. This line of sutures is then buried by undercutting the outer flaps and bringing them together with a second line of sutures (*Figure 15.30*). It is possible by cutting

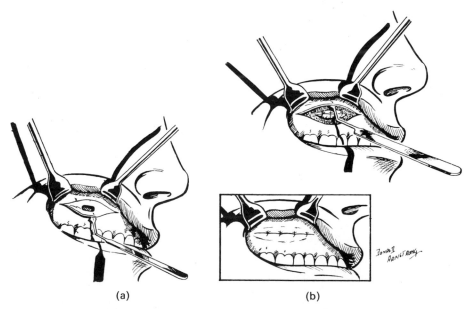

(a)   (b)

Figure 15.30 (a) Shows incision around oro-antral fistula; (b) shows undercutting of edges which are brought together over the closed fistula

unequal flaps to arrange that the two suture lines do not lie directly over one another. In old or decrepit patients an oro–antral fistula may be satisfactorily occluded by an obturator or a dental plate.

Miscellaneous fistulae

Oro–antral fistulae may be produced by penetrating injuries, osteitis of the maxilla, carcinoma of the antrum or palate, malignant granuloma or syphilis. The management of these conditions, is discussed elsewhere but large surgical fistulae deliberately created for observation of an antral carcinoma are best filled by a dental obturator. Where a benign antral neoplasm has been excised and the patient is left with a large opening into the antrum some plastic surgeons advocate repair of the opening by pedicled skin. However, skin covering the defect in the hard palate does not withstand wear and tear satisfactorily and the majority of these patients are better managed by the use of a dental obturator.

Secondary effects

Apart from the rare development of a transitional cell carcinoma from chronic hypertrophic papillary sinusitis the majority of the complications of sinusitis are minor and occur in other parts of the upper and lower respiratory tracts. Most of these are associated with acute sinusitis or an acute exacerbation of chronic sinusitis. Often the other lesions of the respiratory tract begin at the same time or shortly after the onset of the acute lesion, for example, acute otitis media, particularly in children, acute pharyngitis and acute tracheobronchitis.

However, in chronic sinusitis pus may be continually swept over the eustachian tube cushion causing acute otitis media, serous, catarrhal or purulent. Persistent non-smelly discharge from an antero–central perforation is frequently found to result from chronic sinusitis.

Lateral wall pharyngitis, in which a hypertrophied injected lymphoid band is seen behind the posterior pillar of the fauces, is often indicative of a unilateral chronic maxillary sinusitis.

Persistent laryngitis and occasionally tracheobronchitis may be associated with purulent post-nasal discharge bathing the larynx particularly during sleep.

Recurring attacks of bronchitis in children are often associated with recurring sinusitis but in these cases the lesion may be regarded as a generalized infection of the whole respiratory tract. The presence of a persistent purulent nasal discharge in children associated with a persistently productive cough usually indicates early bronchiectasis rather than bronchitis due to sinusitis.

Bronchiectasis and sinusitis

Bronchiectasis and sinusitis in children are commonly associated with wax keratosis in the external auditory meatus. Kartagener's syndrome of sinusitis, bronchiectasis and dextrocardia is rare. Fibrocystic disease of the lung may also be associated with sinusitis. The view that sinusitis causes bronchiectasis is not substantiated by the studies of Ormerod (1941) and Hogg (1950).

Bronchiectasis frequently arises in infancy due to a virus infection of the bronchial tree which irreversibly damages the mucosa. The same virus infection may also irreversibly damage the mucosa of the upper respiratory tract and the paranasal sinuses. Consequently, both the upper and lower respiratory tract lesions have the same aetiology and one is not due to the other. A patient may therefore have a bronchiectatic lesion without chronic sinusitis, and chronic sinusitis without bronchiectasis. Numerous observations on children with chronic sinusitis only do not show that bronchiectasis develops from chronic sinusitis. A misunderstanding may arise if the rattling wet cough seen in childhood is not recognized as incipient bronchiectasis, for at this stage no gross local dilatation of bronchi has occurred.

The treatment of the sinusitis should be that which would be offered even if the patient did not have bronchiectasis. The prognosis unfortunately is poor for the sinus becomes readily re-infected by droplet infection from the chest lesion. Before any thoracic surgical intervention is undertaken for bronchiectasis any associated sinus lesion should be treated in an attempt to free the respiratory tract of infection. This should be carefully planned with the thoracic surgeon so that the chest operation is done in the best conditions.

Sinusitis and asthma

Occasionally an asthmatic attack occurs in a patient who develops acute sinusitis. Relief may be rapid after antral lavage. Because of this relationship the paranasal sinuses have withstood many surgical insults without lasting benefit to the patient, although undoubtedly those patients with true chronic sinusitis gain some immediate benefit. The exceptional case is probably an example of bacterial allergy. The nasal and paranasal pathology which exists alongside asthma should be treated as if the patient did not have asthma, and the patient should be told that any surgery to the nose is not primarily to help the asthma. If incidentally treatment of the sinusitis benefits the asthma it should be regarded as a bonus gained.

Focal sepsis

Polyarthritis, tenosynovitis, fibrositis, and certain dermatological conditions are sometimes regarded as being the result of chronic sinusitis. If so, they are probably allergic manifestations. The paranasal sinus disease, if present, should be treated as it needs treatment and not to cure the doubtfully associated lesion. Under no circumstances should an uninfected paranasal sinus be treated in the hope of alleviating a doubtfully associated disease.

References

Asherson, N. (1939). *Journal of Laryngology*, **54**, 691

Bennett, R. J. and Moore, J. R. (1954). *Journal of Laryngology*, **68**, 535

Bordley, J. E. and Bosley, W. R. (1973). *Annals of Otology, Rhinology and Laryngology*, **82**, 696

Bosley, R. J. (1963). *Laryngoscope*, **77**, 60

Cairns, H. (1930). *Journal of Laryngology*, **45**, 385

Cairns, H. and Schiller, F. (1948). *Proceeding of the Royal Society of Medicine*, **41**, 805

Chandler, J. R., Langenbrunner, D. J. and Stevens, E. R. (1970). *Laryngoscope*, **80**, 1414

Dawes, J. D. K. (1961). *Journal of Laryngology*, **75**, 297

Eagleton, W. P. (1926). *Cavernous Sinus Thrombophlebitis.* New York; Macmillan

Falconer, M. A. and Latham, R. W. (1964). *Journal of Laryngology*, **78**, 937

Friedmann, G. and Harrison, M. S. (1970). *Journal of Neurology, Neurosurgery and Psychiatry*, **13**, 225

Goodale, R. L. and Montgomery, W. W. (1958). *Archives of Otolaryngology*, **68**, 271

Goodyear, H. M. (1944). *Annals of Otology, Rhinology and Laryngology, St. Louis*, **53**, 242

Hargrove, S. W. C. (1955). *Journal of Laryngology*, **69**, 709

Hogg, J. C. (1950). *Proceedings of the Royal Society of Medicine*, **43**, 1087

Howarth, W. (1936). *Journal of Laryngology*, **51**, 387

Kinder, P. L. and Leaver, P. K. (1974). *Journal of Laryngology*, **88**, 551

Ludman, H. and Bulman, L. (1976). *Journal of Laryngology*, **90**, 519

Macbeth, R. G. (1949). *Proceedings of the Royal Society of Medicine*, **42**, 284

Macbeth, R. G. (1952). *Journal of Laryngology*, **66**, 18

Macbeth, R. G. (1954). *Journal of Laryngology*, **68**, 465

Ormerod, F. C. (1941). *Journal of Laryngology*, **56**, 227

Reading, P. (1955). *Journal of Laryngology*, **69**, 729

Reid, J. L. and McGuckin, F. (1946). *Journal of Laryngology*, **61**, 273

Runecke, R. D., and Montgomery, W. W. (1964). *Archives of Ophthalmology*, **71**, 50

Skillern, R. H. (1923). *The Catarrhal and Suppurative Diseases of the Accessory Nasal Sinuses.* 3rd ed. Philadelphia; Lippincott

Tamari, M. J. and Bear, S. H. (1953). *Journal of the International College of Surgeons*, **20**, 269

Turner, A. L., and Reynolds, F. E. (1931). *Intracranial Pyogenic Diseases.* Edinburgh; Oliver and Boyd

Wilensky, O. W. (1932). *Archives of Otolaryngology*, **15**, 805

Wilkerson, W. W. (1945). *Laryngoscope*, **55**, 294

Wood, P. H. (1952). *Journal of Laryngology*, **66**, 496

16 Non-healing granulomas of the nose
D F N Harrison

Granulomatous destruction of part or whole of the nose is a well-recognized clinical condition throughout the world, yet if clearly defined conditions such as syphilis or malignant tumour are excluded, there remains a group of patients who, despite conspicuous differences in natural history and clinical behaviour, are usually collected together under the single heading of 'non-healing granuloma'.

Attempts have been made to relate individual specific histopathological features to clinical manifestations and thus subdivide this group into specific entities. This has resulted in confusion due to the difficulty of obtaining representative biopsy material and the comparative rarity of the conditions. Since most patients invariably died accurate diagnosis was, until recently, largely an academic exercise. This is no longer the case, and in-depth studies by Harrison (1974), and by Michaels and Gregory (1977) have clearly demonstrated the need for differentiating two, or possibly three, quite separate diseases within this group.

Wegener's granulomatosis

The condition described by Wegener in 1939 primarily affects the kidneys, lungs and occasionally nose or other parts of the body. Godman and Chung (1954) showed that it was a necrotizing granuloma affecting all parts of the respiratory tract, with generalized focal necrotizing vasculitis involving both arteries and veins usually in the lungs, glomerulitis characterized by necrosis and thrombosis of loops of the capillary tufts, capsular adhesion and subsequent development as a granuloma.

The clinical condition is well defined and although the first manifestation may be seen in the nose, middle ear, pharynx etc., this will invariably be followed by evidence of renal involvement. Onset is often insidious with a non-specific infection of the respiratory tract. Patients complain of malaise, fever or general weakness, symptoms quite out of proportion with an apparently mild chest infection. Occasionally, epistaxis or nasal obstruction may lead to detection of a granulomatous mass—usually on the nasal septum. At this time urine analysis invariably shows the presence of red cells or casts and, untreated, the condition progresses to a fatal outcome from renal failure within six months.

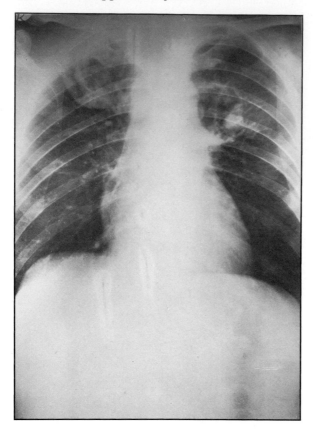

Figure 16.1   X-ray chest of patient with Wegener's granulomatosis to show bilateral apical
cavities

Giant cell granulomas can be found throughout the respiratory tract, and elsewhere there is widespread angiitis indistinguishable from polyarteritis nodosa. This is responsible for the destructive renal lesions and may also be seen on the skin, usually of the arms and legs. Pulmonary lesions are areas of infarction undergoing necrosis and liquefaction with subsequent cavity formation (*Figure 16.1*). Haemoptysis or production of purulent sputum may confuse the diagnosis; one patient was treated for over a week in a chest unit before haematuria and epistaxis occurred! Even in uncontrolled cases the nasal lesions progress slowly, never causing gross destruction. Maximum deformity is usually a septal perforation unless, in ignorance, surgery or radiotherapy has been used as therapy. Patients presenting with granulomatous lesions outside the lungs or kidneys, where biopsy has excluded other pathology, must have urine examination for red cells and casts. Without evidence of renal disease, and despite confident histological examination of non-renal biopsy material, it is doubtful if a definitive diagnosis of Wegener's granulomatosis can or should be made. However, early diagnosis is of paramount importance in the treatment of this condition and renal biopsy may be justifiable in doubtful cases.

Aetiology remains unknown although the list of suggested causes is long and comprehensive. Drug hypersensitivity and autoimmunity enjoy popularity although sophisticated immunological investigations by Shillitoe *et al.* (1974) did no more than suggest future lines of inquiry and the need for prospective studies.

Treatment

The dramatic change in prognosis for patients with Wegener's granulomatosis occurred in the late 1960s when cytotoxic drugs were added to the more conventional corticosteroids. This improvement was due, not to increased immunosuppression or anti-inflammatory effect, but possibly to the two drugs acting at differing points in the immune reaction. Both alkylating agents and antimetabolites are equally effective and it may well be that there is also a direct action on the granulomas by the cytotoxic drug.

Since the lethal destruction occurs in the kidney, long-term survival essentially depends upon control of the disease whilst renal function is relatively unimpaired. This is rarely possible because of delay in diagnosis and the rapidity of destruction of renal tissue. The drug of choice has been azathioprine (Imuran) already widely employed in transplant surgery, skin diseases and other conditions. It is an imidazolyl derivative of mercaptopurine affecting both RNA and DNA. Toxic effects include bone marrow hypoplasia, hepatotoxicity and reduction in host resistance to infection although experience has shown these to be uncommon even with the large doses used in the treatment of Wegener's granulomatosis. It is essential to achieve a maximum daily dosage in the adult of 200 mg as rapidly as possible, certainly within two days. Prednisolone, initially 40 mg/day, is then added and this dosage reduced until the ESR has returned to normal limits. In desperate situations another cytotoxic agent cyclophosphamide may be added in doses of 100 mg/day. A remarkable feature of this regime is the rapidity with which the patient begins to feel better. Even when there is no evidence of clinical change, subjective improvement is dramatic, preceeding a fall in the ESR by several days (*Figure 16.2*).

The toxic effects of these drugs is largely dose-related and every effort must be made

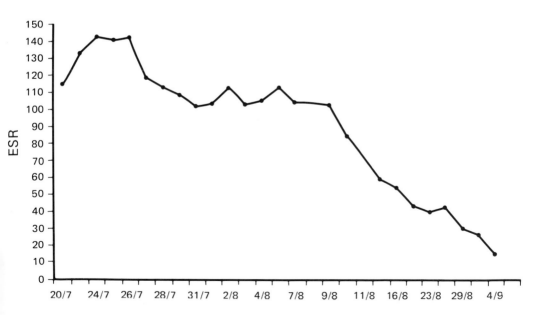

Figure 16.2 Change in ESR following treatment of Wegener's granulomatosis with azathioprine and prednisolone

to reduce daily intake as soon as possible. Assuming that residual renal function is adequate for survival then some improvement in creatinine clearance and blood-urea levels can be expected. Renal biopsy and expert evaluation of renal function will be essential for the purpose of long-term prognosis and possible consideration of renal transplantation. Meanwhile the most reliable guide to dosage appears to be the ESR. Increase in this value will precede recurrence of disease and certainly reduction in dosage in many patients is followed by an increase in ESR, although the significance of this has yet to be tested. The potential dangers of long-term therapy with both cytotoxic and corticosteroid drugs are well documented and these patients must be carefully monitored by people experienced in such problems. In my own experience reduction in dosage is always possible, the patients being more sensitive to loss of corticosteroids than to azathioprine. Only one patient, however, from a group of 32 with Wegener's granulomatosis, has succeeded in abandoning all therapy. Only 16 years old at the time of onset, renal disease was minimal and it is most likely that long-term prognosis depends ultimately on the degree of residual renal impairment.

Long-term follow-up of patients surviving more than two years following diagnosis reveals that death occurs primarily from infection in severely damaged kidneys. No recurrence of the disease had taken place in any patient. Consideration of these long-term survivors for renal transplantation may offer them a prospect of a near normal life expectancy.

Non-healing granuloma

Malignant or non-healing granuloma is completely different in both natural history and prognosis, being essentially a slowly progressing destructive ulceration of the face. Usually beginning in the region of the nose, soft tissues, bone and cartilage are eventually destroyed by a chronic inflammatory reaction. Uncontrolled, death occurs after several years from cachexia or intercurrent infection.

McBride (1897) is usually credited in the English literature with the first description of this condition, though his account appears to have been based on a failure to find any other condition responsible for the facial destruction. In essence it may well be described as a wave of non-specific granulation tissue advancing throughout the face and gradually destroying normal tissue. This behaviour is not dissimilar from that found in malignant tumours in this region and patients are reported as dying from systemic metastasis with a primary lesion confidently diagnosed as a 'non-healing granuloma' (or else one of its many synonyms).

Rate of tissue destruction varies from patient to patient and it is now suggested that all are in fact malignant lymphomas but with varying degrees of immunological control. Michaels and Gregory (1977) found common histological features in ten patients with a clinical diagnosis of 'midline granuloma'—widespread necrosis and atypical cells; collectively termed NACE (necrosis with atypical cellular exudate). The cytological features were such as to suggest a malignant lymphoma and four of these patients had similar metastases in regional lymph nodes. They believe that all are malignant lymphomas but because of considerable necrosis and infection there is difficulty in obtaining adequate representative material.

Local destruction may be extremely slow, with subsequent increase in rate being

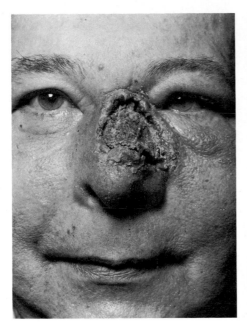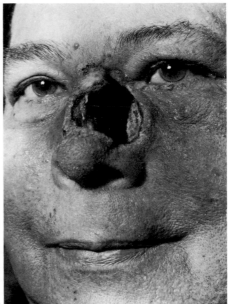

Figure 16.3 Removal of dead bone and skin following radiotherapy for 'midline' granuloma

related to the appearance of a definite malignant lymphoma. Histological proof will then depend upon the experience and viewpoint of the pathologist. Clinically this condition must be considered as malignant, and treatment with radiotherapy is indicated, though many radiotherapists will insist upon histological confirmation of malignancy before giving curative dosage. In theory all cases should receive curative dosage to both primary and possibly regional lymph nodes on the assumption that this is in reality a malignant lymphoma. Undoubtedly, some respond to non-curative dosage, probably substantiating the premise that there are varying degrees of immunological control. Recurrence of local disease, often associated with histological evidence of a substantive malignant lymphoma, is then an indication for increasing radiotherapeutic dosage to curative levels.

It is usually necessary to follow radiotherapeutic control with toilet surgery to remove dead bone or other necrotic tissue. Steroid therapy is never indicated and must be considered as potentially harmful in a condition now considered to be neoplastic (*Figure 16.3*).

Clinically, epidemiologically and histopathologically there is little similarity between non-healing nasal granuloma and the nasal lesions of Wegener's granulomatosis. Local tissue destruction, systemic disturbance and prognosis all differ sufficiently to provide clear differentiation, even if histopathological confusion remains. Early diagnosis and effective therapy is essential in both conditions to prevent extensive destruction or irreversible renal damage. Unfortunately, many patients will continue to be seen initially by the uninitiated, resulting in unnecessary deformities or avoidable deaths.

The increased survival of patients presenting with advanced lesions in lung, kidney and nose, when treated with cytotoxic and steroid drugs, and the singular lack of success when this regime is unwisely applied to patients with non-healing granuloma of the nose, has widened the diagnostic and credulity gap between these two conditions. Both conditions must now be considered as eminently curable providing diagnosis is both early and substantive.

References

Godman, G. C. and Chung, J. (1954). 'Wegener's granulomatosis: pathology and review of literature', *Archives of Pathology*, **58**, 522

Harrison, D. F. N. (1974). Non-healing granulomata of the upper respiratory tract', *British Medical Journal*, **4**, 205

McBride, P. (1897). Case of rapid destruction of the nose and face,' *Journal of Laryngology*, **12**, 64

Michaels, L. and Gregory, M. M. (1977). 'Pathology of 'non-healing (midline) granuloma', *Journal of Clinical Pathology*, **30**, 317

Shillitoe, E. J. *et al.* (1974). 'Immunological features of Wegener's granulomatosis', *Lancet*, **1**, 281

Wegener, F. (1939). 'Über eine eigenartige rhinogene Granulomatose mit besonderer Beteiligung des Arteriensystems und der Nieren', *Beiträge zur Pathologischen Anatomie und zur Allgemeinen Pathologie*, **102**, 36

17 Tumours of the nose and sinuses
D F N Harrison

Tumours arising within or involving the nasal cavity and related paranasal sinuses were recognized in the time of Hippocrates who distinquished between hard and soft tumour, but believed that treatment only shortened the patient's life! Many of these were probably simple nasal polypi and not neoplasms, for a tumour by our present definition is 'an abnormal mass of tissue, the growth of which exceeds and is uncoordinated with that of normal tissues and persists in the same excessive manner after cessation of the stimuli which evoked the change'.

Tumour Registeries pay little attention to benign tumours in the nose and sinuses but, accepting that malignant neoplasms of all types make up only 3 per cent of cancers involving the upper respiratory and alimentary tracts and less than 1 per cent of all malignancies, it is apparent that nasal and sinus tumours are uncommon. Individual reports of personal or institutional series of patients, although inadequate for calculating true incidence rates, are valuable when presenting relative incidence figures and results of treatment. Such sources of information are essential when writing a comprehensive survey of this complex problem providing that it is appreciated that both aetiological factors and true incidence figures will vary throughout the world. As yet there is no generally accepted clinical or pathological classification for tumours arising in or around the nasal cavity and paranasal sinuses. A wide variety of both benign and malignant tumours occurs within this region and the close anatomical relationship between nasal passages and adjoining sinuses results in rapid spread from one to the other. Despite this, considerable variations in incidence, histology and behaviour of the many tumours found in both areas necessitate consideration of each as a separate entity.

Tumours of the nasal cavity

Apart from those tumours which arise from mesenchymally-derived structures, most benign or malignant tumours develop from:

(1) pseudostratified columnar epithelium;

(2) squamous epithelium;

(3) melanocytes;

(4) olfactory neuroepithelium (Michaels and Hyams, 1975).

The majority of tumours have an epithelial origin and if these are considered as one group then those with non-epithelial origin can be considered separately. Within such a division each anatomical site can be considered separately.

Epithelial tumours

The basic cellular pattern of the nasal epithelium is pseudostratified columnar epithelium. Benign papillary adenomas are common and since their cilia are usually atrophic, may be diagnosed as rhinosporidiosis. Ciliated and mucous cells may, however, be seen in the papillary carcinoma, the mucus-secreting form being most commonly found in the ethmoid and associated with inhalation of irritant particles of wood dust, nickel or tobacco snuff (Acheson *et al.*, 1968). Such tumours have little tendency to metastasize, being locally invasive. This condition will be discussed in detail when considering paranasal sinus tumours.

Apart from the nasal vestibule, squamous epithelium is only found in the nose secondary to chronic irritation, as in snuff or cocaine inhalers, or with tumour formation. Vestibular papillomas are similar to those found growing from squamous epithelium elsewhere in the body and should be removed by local excision. Benign septal papilloma—keratinizing, exophytic with a broad base—must also be removed with a surrounding area of normal mucosa to prevent local regrowth. Of more interest and the source of some controversy is the inverted papilloma or Ringertz tumour. Arising almost exclusively from the lateral wall of the nose or occasionally the maxillary sinus, the tumour grows rapidly, filling the nasal cavity with firm red or grey masses. Always unilateral, extension into the ethmoid and maxillary sinuses occurs in at least 60 per cent of cases. Symptoms are similar to those found with nasal polypi though pressure absorption of surrounding bone is common. An incidence of around 2 per cent of all nasal and sinus tumours is quoted although Suh *et al.*, (1977) saw only 57 patients within 30 years. There is a male predominance of approximately 5 to 1 and three-quarters of the patients are between 40 and 70 years of age.

Clinical appearance is typical and histological examination shows epithelial inversion into underlying stroma instead of growing outwards as in other papillomas. The surface of the neoplasm is covered by alternating layers of squamous and columnar epithelium, this tumour being sometimes described as a transitional cell papilloma (*Figure 17.1*). There is a marked tendency for local recurrence, irrespective of methods of treatment, although it has been suggested that this simply represents regrowth of residual tissue following inadequate removal. There is also a small but definite incidence of coincidental malignancy (2 per cent) and malignant transformation (5–13 per cent) (Osborn, 1970; Hyams, 1971). The marked difference in behaviour of these tumours may be related to their origin from the Schneiderian membrane which is derived from ectoderm rather than endoderm like the remainder of respiratory epithelium. The risk of associated or subsequent malignancy together with the near-certainty of local regrowth after simple intranasal avulsion indicates that this tumour must be removed by thorough intranasal or transantral ethmoidectomy. Rapid or persistent growth indicates a need for lateral rhinotomy. It should not be necessary to stress the need for histological examination of all tissue removed, although no prediction as to the likelihood of recurrence or malignant change can be expected, for epithelial atypia is common. Recurrence rates of 71 per cent have been reported after local transnasal removal (Trible and Lekagul, 1971), reducing to only 13 per cent after lateral rhinotomy.

Radiotherapy has no part to play in the non-malignant nasal papilloma.

Squamous carcinoma

Almost 90 per cent of identifiable primary malignant tumours arising within the nasal cavity are squamous cell carcinomas. Most arise from the ethmoidal and maxillary sinuses which make up much of the lateral wall or when arising from the nasal epithelium rapidly extend to involve these sinuses.

Squamous carcinoma of the nasal vestibule occurs predominantly in men over the age of 60 years. Extension into columella, nasal floor or upper lip indicates local aggressiveness and is frequently associated with metastasis to facial or parotid lymph nodes. Very small tumours can be excised but primary therapy is usually with radiotherapy giving a 5-year cure rate of over 75 per cent. Uncontrolled local or metastatic disease indicates a need for radical resection with consequent problems in effective reconstruction.

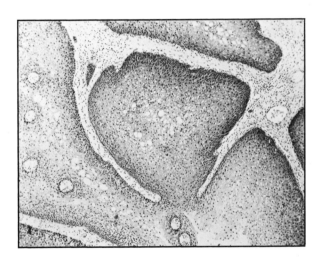

Figure 17.1 Transitional cell papilloma. (×65) reduced to three-fifths on reproduction

Squamous carcinoma arising from septal mucosa is uncommon, with only 97 verified cases in the literature (Weimert, Batsakis and Rice, 1978). Most are found on the anterior part of the septum close to the mucocutaneous junction, producing septal crusting and bleeding. There is a marked predominance of males, most being over the age of 50 years, although one case is reported in a 23 year old woman. The tumour may be papillary or sessile but is invariably well differentiated, although the degree of differentiation does not appear to correlate with likelihood of metastasis or prognosis. Experience of management of these tumours is limited but early cancers of the nasal septum are probably best treated by external radiation or radium needle implants. Advanced tumours need a combination of radiotherapy with wide surgical excision such as rhinectomy (*Figure 17.2*). Over 10 per cent of reported cases developed metastatic deposits in the facial or parotid lymph nodes either unilaterally or bilaterally. Prophylactic neck dissection is therefore of little value and neck dissection is reserved for patients with clinical evidence of lymph node involvement. Prognosis is related to size of tumour at diagnosis and the presence of metastases. Five-year cure rates exceeding 50 per cent are unlikely.

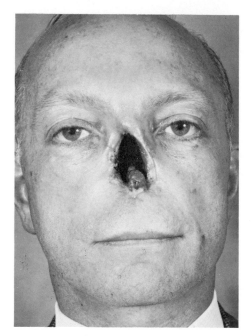 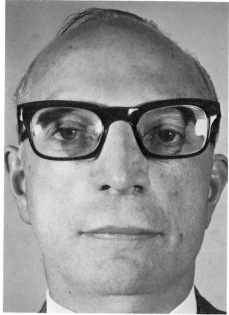

Figure 17.2   These photographs illustrate the excellent cosmetic result obtained with a well-made nasal prosthesis

Malignant melanoma

Until 1974 when melanin was demonstrated within the dentitic cells of the stroma covering nasal septum and turbinals, there was doubt as to whether primary malignant melanomas occurred within the nasal cavity. Isolated cases with proven nasal malignant melanoma were explained away as secondaries from undetected primaries, ignoring the rarity with which such secondaries are found in patients dying from melanomatosis.

Benign tumours of melanocytes are extremely rare in the nasal cavity but about 1 per cent of all malignant melanomas may arise from the mucosal lining of the nose. Approximately one quarter of these come from the septum, the remainder presenting as polypi or tumours growing from the turbinals (Harrison, 1976b) (*Figures 17.3* and *17.4*).

Most patients are over the age of 50 years at diagnosis although patients as young as 15 years have been seen. There is no significant sex predominance and the usual presenting symptoms are nasal obstruction and epistaxis. Not all tumours are pigmented and amelanotic lesions may be misdiagnosed as anaplastic carcinoma or malignant lymphomas unless intracytoplasmic pigment is sought. Absence of pigment does not influence subsequent prognosis for an amelanotic primary can produce pigmented metastatic deposits. When planning the treatment regime, it is important to recognize the near-impossibility of carrying out a truly radical excision. However, with this disease—and possibly adenoid cystic carcinoma—the eventual outcome may be related as much to the patient's immunological competence as to the effectiveness

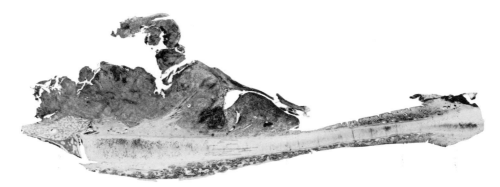

Figure 17.3 Histological section (× 3) of nasal septum to show a malignant melanoma. Note that disease is present at lower end of surgical specimen. All nasal mucosa should be removed in this condition

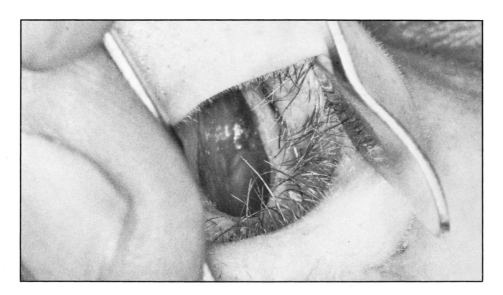

Figure 17.4 Malignant melanomatous polyp right nasal passage

of the surgical procedure. Since radiotherapy appears to have little effect on this tumour, apart from delaying surgery, the best management appears to lie in removing as much tumour as possible by a lateral rhinotomy or rhinectomy (*Figure 17.5*). In most instances this is a mucosal disease and it is technically possible to remove the nasal lining intact except for the cribriform plate area. If involved the nasal septum is removed completely and the whole lateral wall of the nose should be included in the specimen, since it is not only impossible to differentiate amelanotic areas from normal mucosa but oncologically unsound to leave potentially dangerous tissue *in situ*. If regional metastases are present or develop, then individual lymph nodes must be removed, but there is no evidence to support a policy of prophylactic or curative radical neck dissection with a primary arising from nasal mucosa.

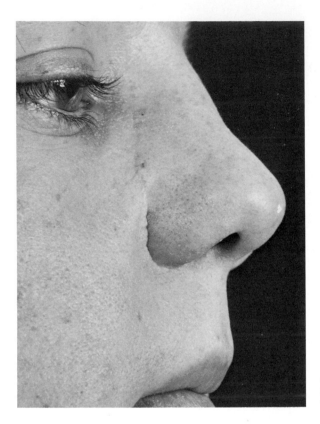

Figure 17.5 Right lateral rhinotomy in a boy of 17 years. Note the good cosmetic result

The purpose of this regime is to alleviate the patient's nasal symptoms and by removal of the large part of the tumour to allow the host immunological defences to destroy residual or metastatic disease. Systemic chemotherapy would appear undesirable because of the risk of immunosuppression but measures designed to produce non-specific immunostimulation, such as intralesional BCG have been advocated although unsuccessful in my experience.

Prediction of long-term survival is difficult, being largely unrelated to the size of the primary tumour. Few patients present with detectable systemic disease diagnosed by melanin in the urine but following excisional surgery many may develop melanomatosis. More fortunate patients, even when inaccessible tumour has been left *in situ*, will have no further trouble although follow-up must continue indefinitely. The remainder develop local disease without gross regional or clinically detectable systemic metastasis. They remain in a state of symbiosis with their tumour until an immunological challenge, such as influenza, alters the balance with consequent melanomatosis.

Large series of patients show a loss each year but three-year survival figures of 50 per cent can be expected, falling to 30 per cent at five years (Harrison, 1976b)

Olfactory neuroblastoma

Neurogenous tumours of the nasal cavity and sinuses make up 3 per cent of malignant tumours found in this area. They may arise from the central nervous system, peripheral nerves and ganglia or the olfactory region. The first record of an olfactory neuroblastoma was in 1926 (Berger and Luc, 1926) and by 1972 only 130 cases had been reported. Recently the incidence appears to be increasing, possibly because of improvements in histological diagnosis such as fume-induced fluorescence (Judge and McGavran, 1976). This tumour is neuroectodermal in origin and may arise from the cribriform plate or the olfactory area in the lateral wall of the nose. It occurs in any age group, from 8–80 years, without any clear sex predominance. Although composed of varying proportions of neuroblasts or the differentiated neurocyte there is no evidence that either has a measurable effect upon prognosis. There is little purpose in dividing this tumour into subgroups, since all components are present to varying degrees in all tumours.

Nasal obstruction with headache and epistaxis are common symptoms. The tumour is usually visible in the nose, being polypoidal, reddish-grey in colour and extremely vascular. Tomography invariably shows some degree of bone destruction, as with most malignant tumours in this area, but biopsy utilizing electron microscopy and fluorescence techniques will confirm the diagnosis. Assays of urinary catecholamines, including the metabolites dopamine and 3-methoxy-4-hydroxy mandelic acid (VMA), are useful in monitoring local recurrence. Regional or systemic metastases can be expected in 25 per cent of patients but local control over five years can be obtained in 33 per cent by a combination of curative radiotherapy followed by lateral rhinotomy for lesions confined to the lateral nasal wall. Craniofacial resection is reserved for tumours on the cribriform plate.

Non-epithelial tumours

All mesenchymal tissue can be the seat of origin of both benign and malignant tumours, though the latter make up no more than 10 per cent of all malignancies arising in the nasal cavity and paranasal sinuses.

Vascular tumours can be found in all parts of the nasal cavity, the commonest being the capillary haemangioma or 'bleeding polyp' of the septum. Growing as a pedunculated mass from the anterior end of the septum the tumour is rare before puberty. Nasal obstruction and, when ulcerated, epistaxis are the most common symptoms. Excision must be accompanied by a cuff of surrounding mucoperichondrium to avoid local recurrence.

Cavernous haemangiomas occur more frequently on the lateral nasal wall, particularly from the turbinals. In the young they are frequently called hamartomas although this term should strictly be reserved for lesions where there is definite evidence of developmental anomaly, either actual malformation with tissue excess already present at birth or an unborn tissue anomaly which manifests itself by excessive growth before puberty. When small, these tumours can sometimes be excised after preliminary cryosurgery. Extensive lesions are uncommon and may require both radiotherapy and radical surgery.

The malignant counterpart of the benign haemangioma is the angiosarcoma, usually differentiated by its tendency to invade bone and metastasize. Local control is difficult and long-term survival is reported as less than 10 per cent. Juvenile angiofibroma (Harrison, 1976) is now well established as a benign tumour, possibly a hamartoma, arising from the posterior nose and should strictly be included in this chapter. Traditions, however, die hard and many still consider this as originating within the nasopharynx.

Some mention must be made of the haemangiopericytoma, an uncommon vascular tumour believed to be derived from the pericyte, a cell whose processes surround the endothelial cells of capillaries. More commonly found in the thigh or retroperitoneum, 25 per cent occur within the head and neck in adults within the sixth and seventh decades of life. Symptoms are those of nasal obstruction and epistaxis, diagnosis being made at biopsy. Differential diagnosis will include adenoid cystic carcinoma, olfactory neuroblastoma and anaplastic carcinoma. If readily accessible the tumour should be removed but most recorded cases have received radiotherapy as first therapy. Only a small number of patients with this tumour in the nasal cavity have been treated, an overall five-year cure rate of 50 per cent being generally quoted for combinations of radiotherapy and surgery (Compagno, 1978).

Cartilaginous tumours

All forms of cartilaginous tumours are rare, Kilby and Ambegaokar (1977) finding only 128 cases in the literature arising from the sinuses and nasal cavities. Fifty per cent were thought to arise from the ethmoids and nasal cavity with a further 17 per cent from the nasal septum. Endochondromas, pure cartilaginous tumours, grow slowly and are described as being smooth, firm and lobulated. Sex distribution is equal and nasal chondromas have been recorded as early as eight months and as late as 70 years. 'Impure' endochondromas contain other tissues and may be designated as fibrochondromas, angiochondromas etc. Differentiation from malignant chondrosarcomas is not always easy either clinically or histologically.

Local excision is effective with small nasal tumours but in many recorded cases indications are that malignancy may occur after repeated local removals. Large tumours should therefore be removed radically at the first attempt.
Irradiation is of little value and is usually used when the disease is beyond surgical cure.

Peripheral nerve tumours

Slow-growing benign tumours of the nerve sheath are found throughout the body. Recognized as a well-established clinical entity, they must be differentiated from other solid, non-vascular masses in the head and neck. Some doubt has been expressed, however, regarding the histological terminology of these tumours although they are readily separated clinically. The outer membrane of the nerve sheath is the neurilemma and the inner is the sheath of Schwann (or neurolemma). Schwannomas are solitary encapsulated masses attached to or involving a nerve. Neurofibromas are non-encapsulated, multiple and in 10 per cent of patients are said to undergo malignant change. This is, of course, an over-simplification but in the nose most of these tumours will be solitary Schwannomas and should be removed by means of a lateral rhinotomy approach (*Figure 17.6*). Malignant nerve tumours are both rare and lethal.

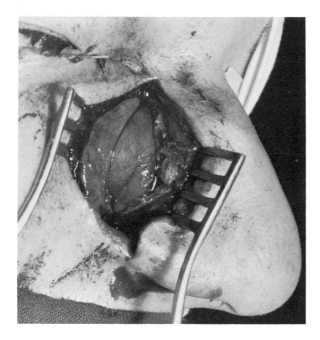

Figure 17.6 Intranasal neuro-fibroma revealed by a lateral rhinotomy exposure

Nasal gliomas are not really tumours in the specific sense; they are benign, congenital masses presenting in the nose and must be differentiated from other nasal tumours. It is likely that they arise in the same manner as encephalocoeles but the meningeal connection may have closed. Found in both sexes, about 60 per cent are extranasal, 30 per cent intranasal, the remainder being combined defects (Karma, Rasanen and Karja, 1977). Most appear after birth and being firm, grey and not pulsatile may be mistaken for a nasal polyp. If the meningeal connection is patent (as in 80 per cent of patients) avulsion will be followed by a cerebrospinal leak.

Extranasal tumours may be found in the midline or to one side. The nose is often broadened and the lacrimal duct compressed. Intranasal tumours cause nasal obstruction and feeding problems. Unfortunately, tomography does not always show the deficiency in the skull base and it is usually impossible to differentiate these lesions with certainty from meningocoeles or encephalocoeles. Histologically, they are composed of neuroglial cells, mainly astrocytes, interlaced with fibrous and vascular connective tissue. Growth is slow and recurrence after inadequate removal is not an indication of malignancy for, in essence, these are really composed of brain tissue with significant gliosis—not really gliomas. Pre-operative biopsy is unnecessary and potentially harmful. In most patients a diagnostic craniotomy permits inspection and closure of any bony defect followed by removal of the extracranial portion of the mass. This should be done during childhood, between five and ten years, before facial growth has been affected by the enlarging tumour.

Malignant lymphoma

Less than 10 per cent of malignant tumours arising within the nose and paranasal sinuses are malignant lymphomas.

Non-Hodgkin lymphomas are now divided into diffuse and nodular varieties, the latter having a more favourable prognosis (Sofferman and Cummings, 1975). Reticulum-cell sarcoma is replaced by diffuse, histiocytic and stem-cell types but when confined to the nose carries an expected five-year survival rate of at least 70 per cent. When these tumours arise within the paranasal sinuses the symptoms are indistinguishable from squamous carcinoma. In the nasal cavity, however, their granular appearance combined with local tissue destruction may lead to a diagnosis of non-healing granuloma.

Surgery is limited to obtaining biopsy material–confirmation of diagnosis being followed by thorough clinical examination to exclude systemic disease. This will include a marrow biopsy together with whole-body lymphangiography. Treatment is with radiotherapy to the local lesion and regional lymph nodes although coincidental or post-radiation multidrug chemotherapy is essential with systemic disease and may be advised in less extensive tumours.

Nasal and sinus lymphomas rarely occur before 40 years of age, are usually found in the region of the ethmoid and seldom metastasize to the cervical lymph nodes. Despite good recorded five-year survival figures, late recurrence after more than seven years has been recorded.

Over 75 per cent of extra-medullary plasmacytomas are found in the region of the head and neck, most being in the nose, paranasal sinuses and nasopharynx. Approximately 10 per cent of head and neck plasmacytomas occur in multiple sites although it is possible that some primary tumours are in fact manifestations of undiagnosed diffuse myelomatosis.

Symptoms of the localized disease are those common to many nasal tumours: obstruction, epistaxis and the presence of a bulky friable mass. Most patients are over the age of 40 years, diagnosis being made from examination of biopsy material. Differential diagnosis from sarcoidosis or malignant lymphoma may be difficult. Immunofluorescence studies may be helpful in demonstrating the monoclonal character of the immunoglobulin (Ig) produced by plasmacytoma.

Treatment of localized tumours is by radiotherapy although maximum regression may not occur for three months. At this time surgical removal of residual disease may be considered. The possibility of the development of multiple myeloma requires regular screening for at least two years after radiotherapy. Local recurrence may occur many years after treatment although a five-year salvage rate of 50 per cent is reported.

A wide variety of relatively uncommon tumours arise from the mesenchymal tissues of the nasal cavity and related sinuses. The most frequently found soft-tissue sarcomas are embryonal rhabdomyosarcomas and neurofibrosarcomas. In each prognosis is related primarily to:

(1) histological features of the tumour with particular respect to differentiation;
(2) size of the lesion;
(3) presence of invasion of bone, blood vessel or nerve; or
(4) metastatic disease in regional lymph node or systemically.

Symptoms are those common to most large tumours in this region, consisting of nasal obstruction, epistaxis, discharge, facial pain and swelling. Diagnosis is by biopsy.

Conventional therapy, whether it be by radical excision or radiotherapy alone, carries a risk of 80 per cent local recurrence and combination therapy, perhaps with the addition of chemotherapy, has certainly increased the long-term survival rates for childhood rhabdomyosarcomas, although not producing such favourable results in adults (Gorfert *et al.*, 1977). Leiomyosarcomas are rarer and appear to be better differentiated, occasionally being diagnosed as benign. Probably arising from nasal or sinus blood vessels, radical excision is rarely possible and a 75 per cent incidence of local recurrence after surgery is reported. These tumours are only minimally radiosensitive (Dropkin, Tang and Williams, 1976).

In general the majority of nasal tumours, whether benign or malignant, produce similar symptoms. Expansion of the nasal framework occurs with any intranasal mass allowed to grow. All need biopsy for specific diagnosis. Involvement of paranasal sinuses is unfortunately common, thereby complicating treatment and, as with other head and neck tumours, early diagnosis is essential.

Tumours of the paranasal sinuses

Benign non-odontogenic tumours are uncommon within the paranasal sinuses representing less than 20 per cent of all malignancies found in this region.

Benign epithelial tumours are rare, usually being found accidently, and the commonest benign tumours arise from mesenchymal tissue. Access to the paranasal sinuses is limited resulting in dependence on clinical and radiological assessment for early diagnosis.

Osteoma

Benign osteogenic tumours of slow growth can be found in at least 1 per cent of all patients having routine radiology of the frontal sinuses. These tumours occur almost exclusively in the bones of skull and face, being most frequent on the lingual aspect of the mandible. Statistics vary greatly as to the frequency within the paranasal sinuses but 70 per cent frontal, 25 per cent ethmoid and 5 per cent for maxillary and sphenoidal sinuses appears to be generally acceptable (*Figures 17.7* and *17.8*). There is considerable difficulty in determining the site of origin of large osteomas and Handousa (1952), reporting on a modest 35 patients, recorded site of origin in relation to the various skull bones as determined by the histological appearance of the tumour after removal. They may be 'ivory', composed of hard compact bone; 'spongy', where

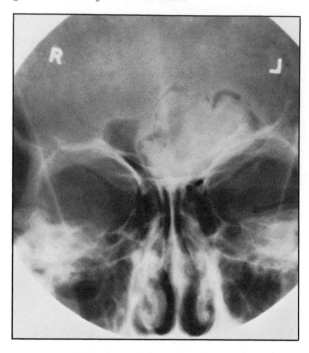

Figure 17.7 X-ray showing osteoma filling the left frontal sinus

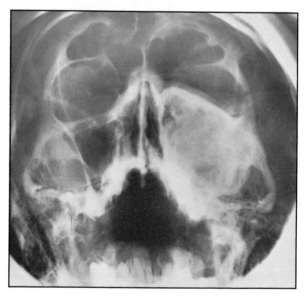

Figure 17.8 Radiological appearance of a cancellous osteoma of the left maxilla

a cortical plate surrounds mature cancellous bone with a lamellar structure; or a mixture of the two. With increasing age of the tumour there is a decrease in osteogenesis. Diagnosis is usually made between 15 and 35 years but in Arab countries both incidence and growth rate appear to be increased.

Theories of origin are many, including embryologic, infectious and traumatic factors. The higher incidence in males is said to favour nonspecific trauma. Persistence of embryonal periosteum in areas where endochondral and membrane bones meet would explain the frequency with which osteomas occur at the junction of ethmoidal and frontal sinuses. There is certainly an ethnic variation though no reliable evidence as to variations in site and histological appearance.

Growth is usually slow, symptoms being related either to extension of tumour to surrounding tissues or pressure on related sensory nerves. Secondary mucocoeles are reported from obstruction to the fronto–nasal duct.

Sphenoidal sinus osteomas are rare but produce headache and eventually orbital involvement (Mikaelian, Lewis and Behringer, 1976). Most osteomas are attached only at one site—usually by a narrow pedicle. Removal is surgical and relatively easy with small tumours. However, symptoms and diagnosis are usually related to tumours large enough to fill the sinus or expand into adjoining areas.

Fragmentation may be necessary to remove large masses of bone (*Figure 17.9*), care being taken in the frontal sinus to avoid damage to exposed dura or uninvolved fronto–nasal duct. Regrowth in the young patient may occur if the site of origin is not completely removed. This is commonly in the vicinity of centres of primary or secondary ossification.

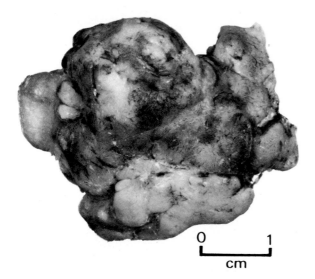

0   1
cm

Figure 17.9 Complete osteoma removed from frontal sinus showing lobulated shape

Devic and Bussy (1912) recognized that some patients have a triad of lesions consisting of soft-tissue masses, bone lesions and multiple colonic polypi. This condition is now called Gardener's syndrome and is inherited as an autosomal dominant trait characterized by a pleitropic single gene representing only one of a group of conditions known collectively as hereditary pre-malignant adenomatous colonic polyposis. Multiple osteomas of the skeleton, particularly jaws, skull and long bones are common, as are other mesenchymal and epithelial defects. Most authorities believe that virtually 100 per cent of the colonic polypi will become malignant and early colectomy is essential.

Fibro–osseous disease of the maxilla

Until the concept of fibrous dysplasia in single bones was conceived around 1940 most fibro–osseous lesions in the jaws were regarded as benign tumours and given such names as ossifying fibroma, fibrous osteoma or, indeed, any of the 35 synonyms used at that time.

In essence, fibro–osseous lesions cover a group of conditions where normal bone is replaced by collagen, fibroblasts and varying amounts of osteoid tissue. Such masses may vary from extensive disfiguring tumours to small virtually unnoticed localized swellings (*Figure 17.10*). Most patients with jaw tumours do not have the diffuse polyostotic lesions of Albright's syndrome nor the skin lesions and precocious puberty.

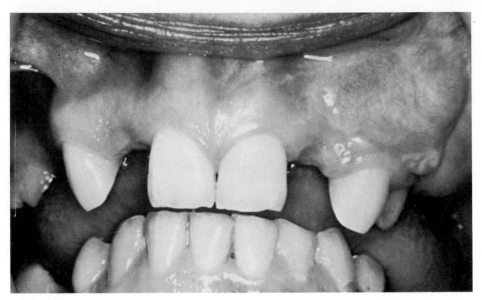

Figure 17.10   Expansion of the left upper alveolus in a woman of 32 years with fibro–osseous dysplasia

Classically, most jaw lesions appear within the first two decades with unilateral facial swelling, deformity of the alveolar margin and occasionally loosening of teeth. The swelling is bony, hard, diffuse and painless. In most cases the greatest expansion has occurred by 30 years of age by which time growth has ceased and a decision regarding surgical paring of excess bone can be made. Involvement of the orbit with proptosis is unusual but might indicate early surgical intervention (Ramsey, Strang and Frazell, 1968).

Radiological appearances are variable, depending upon relative amounts of connective tissue to bone, but they may help to differentiate these benign tumours from osteogenic sarcomas. Histological examination of biopsies, which themselves may not be representative, show a mixture of fibrous and osseous tissue ranging from active fibromas at one end of the spectrum to a mature osteoma at the other end. Unless these patients are irradiated malignancy does not occur and most should be left alone until growth has ceased.

Osteosarcoma of the maxilla

Despite being the commonest primary malignant tumour of bone, osteosarcoma is rare, with a quoted incidence of about one case/100 000 population/year. Most occur in the long bones with less than 7 per cent in the jaws. Average age on diagnosis is usually given as around 30 years although a recent report by Windle-Taylor (1977) quoted a figure of 50 years.

Rapid growth of the tumour, frequently with nasal obstruction, pain and epistaxis, leads to early diagnosis except in rare patients with pre-existing Paget's disease or fibrous dysplasia. Apart from biopsy, radiology probably provides the most useful information as to the extent of tumour involvement. Not only standard views but axial and basal polytomography together with CAT scanning should be used to assess the limits of bone destruction. Pulmonary metastases are uncommon initially although a frequent cause of death.

Malignant supportive tissue in the maxilla is capable of producing cartilage, osteoid or even mature bone in varying amounts within the same tumour. Prognosis, however, is unrelated to whether the tumour is called a chondrosarcoma or osteosarcoma and the eventual outcome will depend upon the feasibility of local resection of tumour. Radiotherapy appears to be ineffective although frequently used in the hope of avoiding major jaw resection in young patients. There is some suggestion that adjuvant chemotherapy may assist in reducing the risk of systemic metastasis in long bone sarcoma and if the primary maxillary osteosarcoma is resectable then this modality would seem to be of some value.

Prognosis for long-bone sarcoma is given as 5–23 per cent five-year survival. Small numbers of patients with sarcoma of the maxilla may expect a five-year survival rate of 25 per cent (Windle-Taylor, 1977), although Livolsi (1977) quotes a figure less than 20 per cent.

Definitive surgery should include the whole maxilla with clearance of pterygoid region and usually orbit. As with malignant melanoma small amounts of residual tumour may not influence the eventual outcome, for the patient's immunological competence may play a major role in long-term control.

Ameloblastoma

Previously termed adamantinoma, the ameloblastoma occurs more frequently in the mandible than in the maxilla representing less than 0.1 per cent of all sinus tumours. Site of origin remains in doubt although the epithelial debris of Malassez in the peridontal membrane as well as the epithelial lining of follicular cysts have been suggested. Histological appearances are variable and may be confused with basal cell or adenoid cystic carcinoma.

Tumours start in cancellous bone, and grow slowly by extension into marrow spaces producing bone resorption. Invariably they become larger than is suggested by radiological assessment and surgical removal must be radical to prevent local regrowth. Essentially this is a benign tumour and radio-insensitive. However, growth is both slow and progressive necessitating early and thorough removal.

Differentiation between other slow growing bony tumours of the maxilla, such as osteoblastoma (Chatterji, Purohit and Bikaner, 1978) and osteoclastoma must be made by biopsy.

Myxomas

Stout (1948) published the first extensive review of myxomas defining them as true mesenchymal tumours which do not metastasize nor include chondroblasts, myoblasts or other recognizable tissue. Kirchow had noted their resemblance to the mucinous substance of the umbilical cord in 1871. They are benign connective tissue tumours, uncommon in the head and neck but common in the heart. Most prevalent in the third and fourth decades, equal in sex incidence and invariably isolated, they present as a soft indolent mass. Pain and loosening of teeth may occur in the jaws, growth is usually slow and may suddenly increase, producing very large tumours (Stout 1948). Macroscopically, the surface is slimy, grey and gelatinous, consistency varying with the fibrous content. There is doubt as to whether the capsule is rudimentary, for infiltration is common and radical removal essential—a local recurrence rate of 25 per cent is reported (Zimmerman and Dahlin, 1958), most within the first two years.

Differentiation from malignant tumours such as liposarcoma, with areas of myxomatous degeneration, is important, and separation from benign connective tissue tumours is only possible on biopsy. It is doubtful if a malignant myxoma exists, for local recurrence is invariably a feature of inadequate local excision (Caanalis, Smith and Konrad, 1976).

Lymphoma of the upper jaw

Since 1958, when Burkitt (1958) drew attention to the fact that the jaws were frequently affected by the multifocal tumour seen in certain African children, it has been appreciated that jaw lymphomas have a well-defined geographic distribution. However, the natural history and behaviour may vary within different countries and ethnic groups although each tumour originates around developing odontogenic tissue, attacking surrounding osteoid and soft tissue (Kummoona, 1977). Although predominantly a tumour of childhood, the Burkitt lymphoma may occur at any age and if untreated is fatal. Invariably multifocal, retroperitoneal and visceral involvment can be found, even when the jaw tumour is the presenting symptom. In the African, it had been suggested that predominantly jaw tumour cases have a better prognosis but this is not so in patients from the Middle East where maxillary lesions are highly fulminating. Surgery in all cases is limited to the obtaining of tissue for biopsy and, in marked contradistinction to the cases reported from Uganda, response to cytotoxic therapy is poor. Patients, reported from the USA, show similarities to the African group with occasional spontaneous remission with an estimated 25 per cent long-term survivors.

The maxilla is involved in at least 50 per cent of patients in high-risk endemic areas of Africa dropping to below 15 per cent in low-risk areas such as North America. Highest incidence is said to be at three years becoming rare after the age of 15 years. It is likely that this uncommon tumour is related to viral infections in susceptible ethnic groups and is distinctive from other lymphomas.

Carcinoma of the paranasal sinuses

Malignant tumours arising from the mucosal lining of the paranasal sinuses are uncommon, representing less than 15 per cent of all neoplasms of the upper respiratory tract. Over 80 per cent are squamous carcinoma, with about equal numbers of adenocarcinoma and adenoid cystic tumours. The intimate relationship between nasal passage and sinuses is largely responsible for the ease with which such tumours spread from one sinus to another, and it also increases the technical difficulties of radical surgical excision.

Classification

The purposes of classification are many but primarily serve to facilitate exchange of information between treatment centres and to aid oncologists in planning therapy. Sites such as the paranasal sinuses can only be visualized radiologically unless the tumour has extended outside surrounding bony walls. Consequently, diagnosis is usually late (on average six months following first significant symptom) and accurate delineation of tumour extent difficult. Despite this, there is a common value in the usage of most systems of classification providing that inherent weakness is appreciated and accepted.

The commonest site within the paranasal sinuses for the development of neoplasia is the maxillary antrum. It has long been appreciated that tumours situated in the postero–superior part of this sinus, defined by Ohngren (1933) as being above an imaginary plane extending from the medial canthus to the angle of the mandible, carry a worse prognosis than those situated antero–inferiorly. The reason for this, ignoring variations in histology which are not included in most systems of classification, are related to the difficulties of resecting disease from those structures intimately related to this part of the maxillary sinus—such as orbit or pterygoid region.

Tumours also present later in this region and will be more extensive when diagnosed. In practice this system was over complicated but has been incorporated into the American Joint Committee (AJC) system of 1976—with all its deficiencies (Harrison, 1978).

A more realistic classification, covering the whole upper jaw, was suggested by Lederman (1970). Two parallel lines are drawn across a frontal section of the skull, the upper line passing through the orbital floor and the lower through the floor of the antra. These lines are supplemented by two vertical lines extending down from the medial orbital wall on each side of the nasal floor.

The vertical lines separate ethmoid and nasal fossa from maxillary sinus—the nasal septum separates ethmoid and nasal fossa into right and left sides. Three regions are delineated—suprastructure, mesostructure and infrastructure (*Figure 17.11*). Although not perfect, nor entirely accurate because of the difficulty in determining clinically the true extent of all except the smallest tumours, this is the only system covering the whole upper jaw.

Harrison (1978) has critically examined the various classification systems in common use with particular reference to their practicability and inherent weaknesses. All are clinically orientated, being dependent upon the expertise and integrity of individual clinicians. Their underlying purpose is to obtain homogenous, statistically equivalent groups of patients for the purpose of assessing, evaluating and comparing various therapeutic methods.

Aetiology

A previous history of chronic sinusitis is unlikely to be of more significance in the production of sinus cancer than is chronic ear disease in carcinoma of the middle ear.

TNM classification

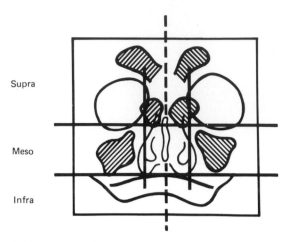

Supra

Meso

Infra

REGIONS AND SITES

Superior Region (Suprastructure)
    Ethmoid labyrinth
    Frontal sinus
    Sphenoid sinus (without nasopharyngeal involvement)
    Olfactory portion of nasal fossa i.e. above middle turbinal

Middle Region (Meostructure)
    Lateral—maxillary antrum
    Medial—the respiratory portion of the nasal fossa
    Vestibule of the nose
    Nasal septum
    Lateral nasal wall (including inferior turbinate)

Inferior Region (Infrastructure)
    Floor of antrum
    Floor of nose
    Tumours involving simultaneously
    Hard palate and antrum
    Hard palate and floor of nose
    Dental tumours

Figure 17.11   Proposed TNM classification (Lederman)
for neoplasms of the nose and paranasal sinuses

However, the high incidence of adenocarcinoma of the paranasal sinuses in woodworkers was first noted by Macbeth (1965). In his region of the country 49 per cent of sinus cancers were adenocarcinomas, most arising from the ethmoidal labyrinth and in patients under the age of 60 years. The relationship of this particular tumour to exposure to certain wood dust has now been substantiated, although the delay time between exposure and carcinogenesis may be lengthy. A three-year survival figure of 50 per cent is reported for treatment by radiotherapy followed by radical excision. Five- and ten-year figures may, however, show a considerable drop in these rates (Saunders and Ruff, 1976).

The unusually high incidence of antro-ethmoidal cancer in the Bantu of South Africa has been blamed on the use of home-made carcinogenic snuff. Starting in the ethmoid, diagnosis is rarely made before the disease is advanced. It is interesting to note that the woods used by the Bantu to incinerate herbs to mix with their snuff or to light fires by the Kenya Highlanders (who develop nasopharyngeal cancer) are similar to those used by many wood machinists in the past.

Symptoms

Unhappily, early symptoms are rare, depending as they do on the primary site and extension of the tumour. *Table 17.1* illustrates the frequency with which the various manifestations may present and illustrates symptoms of late disease. Occasionally, an early tumour fortuitously situated close to naso-lacrimal duct or infraorbital nerve may produce significant symptoms. Most patients, however, are not diagnosed until penetration of surrounding bony walls has occurred, producing swelling of face, proptosis or epistaxis.

Table 17.1   Symptoms in 648 cases of carcinoma of the paranasal sinuses and nasal cavity from 1940–1964

Nature or site	*Percentage as initial symptom*	*Total percentage*
Pain	17.4	40.9
Nasal obstruction	19.6	36.4
Purulent nasal secretion	15.7	30.6
Symptoms from the oral cavity	10.0	15.3
Dental symptoms	3.7	7.9
Swelling on cheek	11.3	33.6
Sanguineous nasal secretion	8.2	25.9
Ocular symptoms	4.6	18.2

Symptoms referable to oral cavity, such as palatal swelling (*Figure 17.12*), pain or loosening of teeth, may lead to referral to a dentist with risk of delay in diagnosis. Similarly, ocular paresis, proptosis or epiphora may take the patient to the ophthalmic surgeon.

Swelling of the cheek, unless due to obvious inflammation in skin or related teeth, must be viewed as a highly suspicious finding in any age group. Pain is usually described as persistent and dull and occasionally associated with areas of paraesthesia or anaesthesia.

Neoplasms arising in the ethmoid air-cells or involving the nasal passages rapidly produce nasal obstruction and epistaxis. The patient rarely ignores such symptoms although diagnosis may still be delayed.

Diagnosis

Earlier diagnosis should lead to earlier treatment and in general a better prognosis. The majority of patients with paranasal sinus cancer have symptoms for at least six months before a diagnosis is reached. Any patient showing ulceration or friable granulation tissue in the nasal cavity must have a biopsy taken and, in most cases, examination under general anaesthesia to determine the true extent of disease. Most cases are all too obvious when first seen and it is essential that any patient in whom there is the slightest suspicion of neoplasia should be completely investigated including the removal of the whole mucosal lining of the maxillary antrum for histological examination.

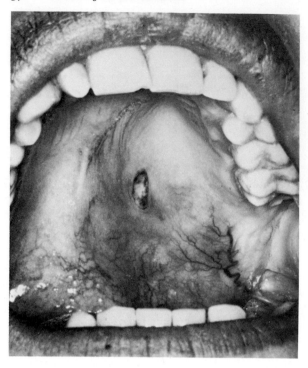

Figure 17.12 Swelling of the palate with central ulceration in a patient with carcinoma of the left maxillary antrum

Radiological evidence of bone destruction is present in over 60 per cent of sinus cancers (*Figure 17.13*) and polytomography is essential to determine as far as possible the extent of bone loss (*Figure 17.14*) although this is invariably greater than expected. Opacity of the maxillary sinus necessitates lavage. This may produce a blood-stained fluid with tumour fragments. A clear lavage does not indicate absence of neoplasm and exploration of the maxillary sinus is essential if there is the slightest suspicion. Fibre-optic inspection of the sinus cavity via the inferior meatus has not as yet proved reliable. Normal lymphatic drainage of the maxillary antrum and ethmoids is first to the retropharyngeal lymph nodes and then to the upper deep cervical and submandibular nodes. Since the former cannot usually be palpated, metastases to the primary nodes may not be uncommon. However, cervical lymph node involvement is unusual even if there is extension of tumour to regions possessing a rich lymphatic supply, such as facial skin, alveolar buccal sulcus or pterygoid musculature. Although extension of tumour outside the mucosal lining of the paranasal sinuses is common the actual extent is often difficult to determine with accuracy. This not only affects the final staging of the disease but also ignores the histology of the primary tumour. Variations in natural history have already been commented upon regarding adenocarcinoma. Adenoid cystic carcinomas, which arise from minor salivary glands, tend to grow insidiously along perineural lymphatics and may thus have extended well outside the determinable margins of the tumour. However, there appears to be some degree of immunological tolerance to this tumour, for solitary pulmonary metastases may remain of constant size for many years. Despite the most aggressive therapy, five-year salvage rates of less than 10 per cent are usual.

Although uncommon, more than 50 authenticated cases of frontal sinus carcinoma

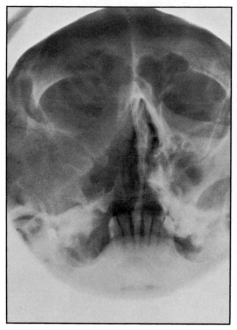

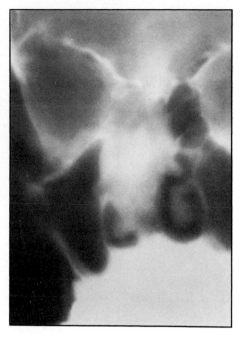

Figure 17.13   Radiological appearances of an advanced neoplasm of the right maxillary antrum showing destruction of the bony roof, medial and posterolateral walls

Figure 17.14   Polytomography of an ethmoidal carcinoma indicating extension through the nasal septum to involve cribriform plate and ethmoids on the opposite side. The maxillary antra appear clear

have been reported many presenting initially as mucocoeles. Bone destruction is usually greater than expected, as is sclerosis.

Confusion with ethmoidal neoplasms extending into the frontal region or primary tumours of the orbital lobe of the lacrimal gland is likely but combination treatment of radiotherapy and radical surgery will be required irrespective of aetiology. Prognosis is poor (Robinson, 1975).

Treatment

Failure to cure paranasal sinus cancer is primarily failure to eradicate extension of tumour outside the sinus bony walls. Regional lymph node metastases are uncommon, between 3 and 5 per cent, and even less present with systemic metastases. It is extension of tumour to orbital apex, cribriform plate, posterior ethmoidal cells, pterygoid region and nasopharynx which results in disease left *in situ*. Consequently, it is such extensions which must be determined initially and classified accordingly. Bony erosion within the limits of potential excision, such as the anterior orbital floor, are less serious if treated radically and even facial skin may be successfully excised if care is taken to ensure adequate margins of resection. Removal of the cribriform plate area, as described by Ketcham *et al.* (1973), can be effective, providing involvement is minimal and tumour has not reached the optic chiasma.

No system of classification as yet considers the histological nature of the neoplasm although this will certainly affect long-term prognosis. It is certainly true that malignant lymphomas and anaplastic tumours respond best to radiotherapy but neither surgery nor radiotherapy alone has proved to be of great benefit in the management of malignant tumours in this region.

The purpose of pre-operative radiotherapy is to reduce the bulk of the tumour and viability of any undestroyed cells. This reduces or eliminates the risk of local recurrence following secondary surgery. In practice a curative course of telecobalt therapy is given to the whole upper jaw including the orbit. Four to six weeks later the surgical excision is performed; this depends upon the age and general condition of the patient and the site and extent of the original tumour. The minimum for maxillary sinus disease will be a partial maxillectomy although most patients require total maxillectomy, often combined with clearance of orbital contents. Palatal fenestration, now both archaic and inaccurate, no longer plays a serious role in sinus cancer.

If removal of the eye is indicated the eyelids may be preserved since they are rarely involved. Primary closure soon leads to a skin-lined socket aiding the wearing of a prosthesis (*Figure 17.15*).

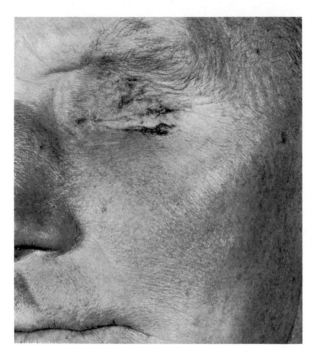

Figure 17.15 Primary closure following removal of orbital contents utilizing both eyelids minus lash margins and tarsal plates

Disease limited to the ethmoidal labyrinth is best treated by pre-operative radiotherapy followed by lateral rhinotomy and total ethmoidectomy in all cases (Harrison, 1977). Craniofacial resection may be indicated if disease remains on the cribriform plate. This formidable procedure has proved most successful in specially skilled hands and must now be considered an integral part of the management of ethmoidal cancer. Unfortunately, radical surgical excision is limited by anatomical considerations such as the skull base. Similarly radiotherapeutic dosage is restricted by close proximity to bone and brain. Most patients will die from failure to control local disease and variations in treatment regime such as surgery followed by radiotherapy or combinations including chemotherapy, are now under trial seeking improvement on the generally accepted maximum five-year cure rate of about 30 per cent.

Surgical procedure

Paleopathological evidence suggests that neoplastic disease existed in the upper jaw in earliest times, being found in pre-Christian Nubian skulls.

Probably the first successful total maxillectomy—for osteosarcoma—was carried out by Joseph Gonsol of Lyons in 1827. Moure (1902) of Bordeaux described his lateral rhinotomy in 1902 and these two operations have provided the mainstay of sinus cancer surgery to date.

Lateral rhinotomy

It is unfortunate that many surgeons are reluctant to utilize this procedure being unaware of the excellent exposure that can be obtained with little or no post-operative deformity. Classically, the skin incision extends from below the inner extremity of the eyebrow, down the side of the nose as far as the anterior nares. However, the upper limit need reach no further than the medial canthus without loss of exposure and produces an almost invisible scar. Retraction of the soft tissues lays bare the nasal bone, ascending process and much of the anterior surface of the maxilla. Removal of all or part of these bones enlarges the operative field enabling complete removal of the lateral wall of the nose with exposure of maxillary antrum, orbital contents and sphenoidal sinus (*Figure 17.16*).

Bleeding is rarely a problem and, even after previous irradiation, primary healing is assured. If it be necessary to remove the orbital contents then the skin incision is extended to the medial canthus and into the conjunctival sac. Primary closure of the eyelids completes the repair.

Total maxillectomy

Detailed accounts of this procedure are to be found in most textbooks concerned with operative surgery of the head and neck. Unfortunately, some of these descriptions appear to ignore many practical considerations concentrating primarily on problems of applied anatomy.

(a) The Weber–Fergusson incision is commonly used to expose the facial surface of the maxilla. Post-operative oedema of the lower eyelid is minimized by placing the transverse incision close to the lid margin although some surgeons prefer to extend a lateral rhinotomy incision up to the eyebrow rather than use this transverse extension. Their claim that this gives improved access to the fronto–ethmoid region is untenable since experience show that involvement of the ethmoidal labyrinth invariably necessitates removal of orbital contents. Since there is rarely a need to remove both

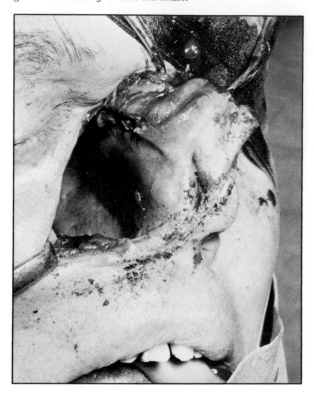

Figure 17.16 Reflection of the whole right side of nose illustrating the excellent access of lateral rhinotomy

eyelids, evisceration may be performed by exposing the orbital margin through the conjunctival sac and carrying out an extraperiosteal dissection.

(b) It is common practice to use controlled hypotensive anaesthesia for this operation although case selection must rest in the hands of the anaesthetist. Bleeding is then minimal and ligation of the maxillary artery is only required when troublesome haemorrhage is encountered in the pterygoid region. The anterior ethmoidal artery can be ignored and pressure will control bleeding from the orbital apex following exenteration.

(c) Section of the zygomatic bone and intra-orbital rim can be carried out with electric or Gigli saw. There is rarely room to use the former instrument in the mouth when dividing the hard palate. A chisel is both effective and quick but must be directed just lateral to the midline in order to enter the nasal passage rather than the septum. The same instrument serves to separate the posterior end of the pterygoid plates from the maxillary tuberosity. It is my practice to dissect out these bones after removal of the maxilla since this avoids much troublesome bleeding from the alveolar branches of the maxillary artery. Where the maxilla has been weakened by malignant erosion the use of chisels may result in uncontrolled fissure fractures. The electric saw avoids the complication and should be used wherever possible.

(d) Considerable apprehension may be felt by both surgeon and patient that total maxillectomy is inevitably followed by sinking of the eye.

The lower part of the fascia bulbi (Tenon's capsule) is thickened and connected to both medial and lateral cheek ligaments to form a sling upon which the eyeball rests. This suspensory ligament (of Lockwood) will prevent dropping of the eye following removal of the orbital floor providing the periosteum and its medial and lateral attachments are undamaged. However, re-inforcement can be provided by a sling from the temporalis muscle fixed medially to the exposed orbicularis oculi muscle.

(e) A split-skin graft may be used to cover the raw skin surface although this is undesirable if there is any doubt as to extension of tumour through the anterior maxillary wall. It is absolutely essential that a prosthesis be introduced into the palatal defect at the end of the operation. This not only avoids post-operative contracture but enables the patient to eat a normal diet without soiling the operative cavity. Fixation is rarely a problem and at a later date this heavy temporary prosthesis is replaced by a light permanent prosthesis (*Figure 17.17*) resulting in minimal cosmetic disability.

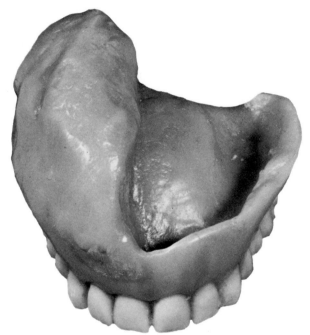

Figure 17.17 Permanent prosthesis used after total maxillectomy

Partial maxillectomy

Anything less than complete removal of the whole maxilla is a partial operation, the term hemimaxillectomy being quite meaningless.

Consequently, partial maxillectomy may cover procedures varying from simple alveolectomy to removal of palate, alveolus and anterior wall of maxilla. Since these operations are performed perorally there is no external deformity and the immediate fitting of a prosthesis minimizes post-operative disability.

Palatal fenestrations were originally performed for the purpose of making an inspection window into the maxillary antrum following radiotherapeutic treatment of antral neoplasms (*Figure 17.18*). If the term is used in its literal sense, i.e. removal of one half of the palate, the resulting bony defect is totally inadequate. In practice the alveolar margin and lateral wall of the nose are included in the bony removal in order to produce an easily visible cavity and to avoid leaving the potentially dangerous

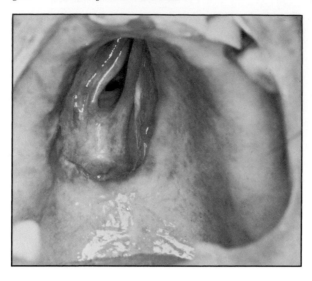

Figure 17.18 Palatal fenestration—illustrating the restricted view of the interior of the maxillary antrum

ethmoidal labyrinth. There seems little sense in the continuing usage of these all-embracing titles for complicated operations since the term 'partial maxillectomy' adequately covers all variants, particularly when accompanied by an accurate account of the actual procedure.

Metastatic carcinoma in the paranasal sinuses

The possibility of a metastasis to the nose or paranasal sinuses is rarely part of the clinical differential diagnosis because of the far greater probability of primary neoplasia. Metastatic tumours to this region are rarely recognized but this may be due to the fact that complete skeletal surveys are not routine in patients with bone metastasizing cancers.

However, there are three primary sites of neoplasia which metastasize with some frequency to the maxilla. Foremost is the renal carcinoma, followed by breast and lung. The clinical signs will be similar to those found in primary sinus cancer and the age incidence will not differ markedly, except in lung cancer which affects a somewhat younger age group. The marked vascularity of secondary renal carcinoma results in epistaxis being a frequent symptom and it is not uncommon for this metastasis to be detected before the primary tumour is suspected. Apart from renal carcinoma, the prognosis for patients with secondary neoplasia in the sinuses is the same as for carcinomatosis and diagnosis is made histologically rather than clinically. However, renal carcinoma is unpredictable in behaviour and only 15 per cent present with classic symptoms of haematuria, pain and a palpable mass. Treatment prior to metastasis gives a five-year survival of over 60 per cent but this drops to about two-year average survival once distant spread is discovered. Despite this, if the maxillary sinus is the only detectable metastasis then removal of primary and radical resection of the secondary has resulted in an occasional long-term survival (Bernstein, Montgomery and Balogh, 1966).

References

Acheson, E. D., Cowdell, R. H., Hadfield, E. H. and MacBeth, R. G. (1968). 'Nasal cancer in woodworkers in the furniture industry', *British medical Journal*, **2**, 587

Berger, L. and Luc, R. (1926). 'L'esthesioneuro epithelioma olfactif', *Bulletin Pour Etude Cancer*, **15**,504

Bernstein, J. M., Montgomery, W. W. and Balogh, K. (1966). 'Metastatic tumours to the maxilla, nose and paranasal sinuses', *Laryngoscope*, **76**, 621

Burkett, D. (1958). 'A sarcoma involving jaws in African children', *British Journal of Surgery*, **46**, 218

Canalis, R. F., Smith, G. A. and Konrad, H. R. (1976). 'Myxomas of the head and neck', *Archives of Otolaryngology*, **102**, 300

Castro, El, B., Lewis, J. S. and Strong, E. W. (1973). 'Plasmacytoma of paranasal sinusis and nasal cavity', *Archives of Otolaryngology*, **97**, 326

Chatterji, P., Purohit, G. N. and Bikaner, I. N. (1978). 'Benign osteoblastoma of the maxilla', *Journal of Laryngology*, **92**, 337

Compagno, J. (1978). 'Haemangiopericytoma-like tumours of the nasal cavity', *Laryngoscope*, **88**, 460

Devic, C. and Bussy, E. (1912). 'Un cas de polypose adenomatense generalisee a tout l'intestine', *Archives des maladies de l'appareil digestif et de la nutrition*, **6**, 278

Dropkin, L. R., Tang Chik Kwun and Williams, J. R. (1976). 'Leiomyosarcoma of the nasal cavity and Paranasal sinuses', *Annals of Otolaryngology*, **85**, 388

Gorfert, H., Lindberg, R. D., Sinkovics, J. G. and Ayala, G. (1977). 'Soft tissue sarcoma of the head and neck after puberty', *Archives of Otolaryngology*, **103**, 365

Handousa, A. B. (1952). 'Primary benign neoplasms of the nose', *Journal of Laryngology*, **66**, 421

Harrison, D. F. N. (1976a). 'Juvenile postnasal angiofibroma—an evaluation', *Clinical Otolaryngology*, **1**, 187

Harrison, D. F. N. (1976b). 'Malignant melanomata arising in the nasal mucous membrane', *Journal of Laryngology*, **90**, 993

Harrison, D. F. N. (1977). 'Lateral rhinotomy: a neglected operation,' *Annals of Otorhinolaryngology*, **86**, 756

Harrison, D. F. N. (1978). 'Critical look at the classification of maxillary sinus carcinoma', *Annals of Otolaryngology*, **87**, 1

Hyams, V. J. (1971). 'Papillomas of the nasal cavity and paranasal sinuses. A clinicopathological study of 315 cases', *Annals of Otology, Rhinology and Laryngology*, **80**, 192

Judge, D. M. and McGavran, M. H. (1976). 'Fume-induced fluorescence in diagnosis of nasal neuroblastoma', *Archives of Otolaryngology*, **102**, 97

Karma, P., Rasanen, O. and Karja, J. (1977).

'Nasal Glioma', *Laryngoscope*, **87**, 1169

Ketcham, A. S. Chretien, P. B., Van Buren, J. M., Howe, R. G., Beazley, R. M. and Herdt, J. R. (1973). 'The ethmoid sinuses–a reevaluation of surgical resection', *American Journal of Surgery*, **126**, 469

Kilby, D. and Ambegaokar, A. G. (1977). 'The nasal chondroma, *Journal of Laryngology*, **91**, 415

Kummoona, R. (1977). 'Jaw lymphoma in Middle East children', *British Journal of Oral Surgery*, **15**, 153

Lederman, M. (1970). 'Tumours of the upper jaw: natural history and treatment', *Journal of Laryngology*, **84**, 369

Livolsi, V. A. (1977). 'Osteogenic sarcoma of the maxilla', *Archives of Otolaryngology*, **103**, 485

MacBeth, R. G. (1965). 'Malignant disease of the paranasal sinus', *Journal of Laryngology*, **74**, 592

Michaels, L. and Hyams, V. J. (1975). 'Objectivity in the classification of tumours of the nasal epithelium', *Postgraduate Medical Journal*, **51**, 695

Mikaelian, D. O., Lewis, W. J. and Behringer, W. H. (1976). 'Primary osteoma of the sphenoidal sinus', *Laryngoscope*, **86**, 728

Moure, E. J. (1902). 'Traitment des tumors malignes primitives de l'ethmoide', *Revue de Laryngologie, Otologie et Rhinologie*, **23**, 401

Ohngren, L. G. (1933). 'Malignant tumours of the maxillo–ethmoid region, *Acta Otolaryngolica*, *Supplement*, **19**, 1

Osborn, D. A. (1970). 'Nature and behaviour of transitional tumours in the upper respiratory tract', *Cancer*, **25**, 50

Pahor, A. L. (1977). 'Extramedullary plasmacytoma of the head and neck, parotid and submandibular salivary glands', *Journal of Laryngology*, **91**, 241

Ramsey, H. E., Strong, E. W. and Frazell, E. L. (1968). 'Fibrous dysplasia of the craniofacial bones', *American Journal of Surgery*, **116**, 542

Robinson, J. M. (1975). 'Frontal sinus cancer manifested as a frontal mucocoele', *Archives of Otolaryngology*, **101**, 718

Saunders, S. H. and Ruff, T. (1976). 'Adenocarcinoma of the paranasal sinuses', *Journal of Laryngology*, **90**, 157

Sofferman, R. A. and Cummings, C. W. (1975). 'Malignant lymphoma of the paranasal sinuses', *Archives of Otolaryngology*, **101**, 287

Stout, A. P. (1948). 'The tumour of primitive mesenchyme', *Annals of Surgery*, **127**, 706

Suh, Kv-W., Facer, G. W., Devine, K. D., Weiland, L. H. and Zujko. R. D. (1977). 'Inverted papilloma of the nose and paranasal sinuses', *Laryngoscope*, **87**, 35

Trible, W. M. and Lekagul, S. (1971). 'Inverting papilloma of the nose and paranasal sinuses', *Laryngoscope*, **81**, 663

Weimert, T. A., Batsakis, J. G. and Rice, D. H. (1978). 'Carcinomas of the nasal septum', *Journal of Laryngology*, **92**, 209

Windle-Taylor, P. C. (1977). 'Osteosarcoma of the upper jaw', *Journal of Maxillary and Facial Surgery*, 5, 62

Zimmerman, D. C. and Dahlin, D. C. (1958). 'Myxomatous tumours of the jaws', *Orological Surgery*, 11, 1069

18   Facial pain

Philip H Golding-Wood

'Every pain has its distinct and pregnant signification if we will but search carefully for it.' (John Hilton.)

Pain is known and feared by all, but the subjective experience is impossible to define. We all know that differences in pain thresholds may enlarge the moderate discomfort of one individual to 'agony' in another. More than differences in threshold are involved, however, as any clinician with battle experience knows. Severe wounds are commonly accepted in war without much evidence of pain; yet the man who can seemingly tolerate an extensive shell wound with composure, may next minute evince the usual discomfort at an inept venepuncture.

Patients whose sole complaint is one of pain in or about the face are as frequently referred to the otorhinologist as to the neurologist or dental surgeon. These various disciplines are here united, for there is but a single common pathway for pain and the phenomenon of referred pain is nowhere so highly developed as in the trigeminal system.

The various cranio–facial structures must be reviewed as interdependent functioning systems, not as constituent parts of anatomy isolated from one another by departmental barriers. Certainly the detection of some abnormality in the nose, sinuses or ears is likely to prove easier than the assessment of its relevance to the patient's complaint.

These problems must often be resolved almost entirely from the patient's history, but in taking this, the clinician's aim must be to develop rapport as well as to elicit details of the complaint. The patient is always emotionally involved but remains the only source of information as to the nature and quality of his pain. So the patient's reaction to pain may seriously impair his ability to relay its nature to the clinician, and he is likely to be a poor interpreter. Many individuals have difficulty in describing symptoms clearly whilst those with identical lesions may use entirely different terms. Others, from previous inconclusive diagnostic attempts, have become depressed and preoccupied with symptoms and are thus clinically almost indistinguishable from those with functional ailments. Casual but astute observation of the patient's mannerisms is essential. Mannerisms such as facial expression, jaw clenching or hand movements may be as informative as spoken words.

The more excitable and apprehensive the patient, the more difficult matters become, yet it remains essential to evaluate the patient as a whole. The psychic element of pain is always important; either in its role in confusing the diagnosis and localization of a lesion, or as a factor modifying pain and disability.

A complaint of facial pain may be both puzzling and stubborn. Frequently it demands repeated assessment but it remains a never failing source of fascination. Small wonder that Oliver Wendell Holmes declared: 'If I wished to show a student the difficulties of practice, I should give him a pain in the face to treat'.

The neurophysiology of facial pain

Somatic pain indicates some pathological irritation of pain receptors whose impulses travel in discrete afferent pathways. What the patient describes as pain is not merely a sensation, however, but one that is accompanied by an aversive feeling, tone or emotion that makes him try to avoid it.

Unlike all other affective states, such as elation or sorrow, pain is always peripherally projected to some part of the body, although such reference may lack precision, as in otalgia or facial pain of dental disease or nasal disorder.

Facial pain has a special emotional significance, for it is the face that mostly expresses our emotional feelings and, in women especially, the face is particularly important in sexual attraction.

The central pathways of pain

Pain sensation from most facial structures reaches the brain stem via the sensory root of the trigeminal nerve. It is estimated that one-third of its 140 000 fibres are small-diameter pain afferents.

On entering the pons, the pain fibres turn downwards away from other sensory afferents and descend in the postero–lateral aspect of the pons, medulla and upper cervical cord as the spinal tract of the trigeminal. Within this nucleus fibre rearrangement occurs, approximating to an upside-down representation of the facial areas; the ophthalmic fibres below and the mandibular fibres at the upper pole of the nucleus (*Figure 18.1*).

Extratrigeminal pain fibres from other orocranial areas travel variously in the nervus intermedius of the facial, the glossopharyngeal, vagus and upper cervical dorsal roots. All these pain afferents also join the spinal trigeminal tract, which thus constitutes the 'pain nucleus' of the head.

The central axons of cells in this 'pain nucleus' travel upwards in the brain stem as the bulbothalamic tract. These fibres ascend both crossed and uncrossed, so pain arising from any facial site is projected to both cerebral hemispheres.

Above, the bulbothalamic tracts terminate in the postero–ventral nucleus of the thalamus, just medial to the spinothalamic termination of pain fibres from elsewhere in the body. From the thalamus the pain impulses are simultaneously projected to four other parts of the brain, each providing a specific component to the patient's total experience of pain. These projections are as follows:

Perceptual projection   Perceptual projection to inferior paracentral (sensory) cerebral cortex provides anatomical localization of a painful stimulus and possibly its nature.

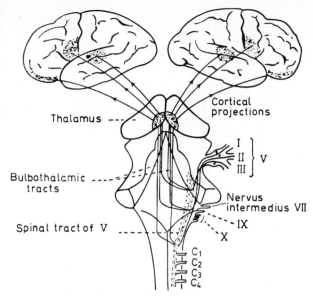

Figure 18.1 The central connections of trigeminal pain afferent fibres. (Pain fibres from facial, glossopharyngeal, vagus and upper cervical nerves also connect with the spinal tract of the trigeminal and are similarly projected)

Emotional projection These fibres, passing to the orbital surface of the frontal lobes, provide the specifically emotional element to pain. It is the fibres of this system that are divided in such neurosurgical operations as orbitofrontal leucotomy. Such an operation leaves the patient still aware of something amiss but he no longer complains that it hurts him.

Memory projection This fibre projection passes to the memory storage system in the temporal lobes, whereby the patient builds up his memory of past, painful experiences.

Visceral reflex projection Fibres from thalamus to subjacent hypothalamic nuclei provide the visceral nervous reflexes, the endocrine changes, and the respiratory effects that may accompany painful stimulation.

Influence of the reticular system

As is well known, tolerance to pain varies greatly, not merely between individuals, but also in a particular patient depending on his mood, concentration on other matters, drug medication, etc. These fluctuations in pain intensity appear to be determined by the influence of the brain-stem reticular system on the cerebral projection system already outlined (*Figure 18.2*)

Collaterals of the bulbothalamic tracts connect with cells of the brain stem reticular system, whose upward discharge to nearly all areas of the cerebral cortex constantly enhances the prevailing awareness of environment and sensory experience, including pain. Many factors increasing this reticulo–cortical activity may thus intensify awareness of pain; as for example emotional tensions from domestic discord, personal anxiety or the action of drugs such as caffeine.

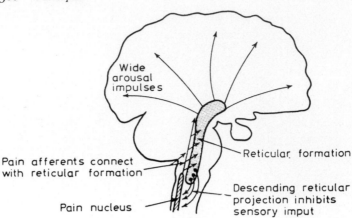

Figure 18.2   Diagram to show the reticular formation and its influence
on pain sensation

Conversely, the reticular cells have also a descending system of discharge to
presynaptic terminals of sensory pathways to the brain stem and these exert an
inhibiting effect. By this means the normal flow of afferent impulses through sensory
systems can be reduced even to the point of preventing their arrival as may occur in
hypnosis. Drugs such as chlorpromazine increase the inhibiting reticular discharge
and this may reduce awareness of pain without diminishing the patient's general
alertness.

Pain receptors

Pain receptors are fine, free-branching axons of a primary afferent neurone. These
receptors are particularly abundant in the cutaneous layers and mucous membranes,
and next in periodontium and periosteum. After these they are distributed in order of
decreasing prevalence in arteries, ligaments, joint capsules, tendons, fascia and
connective tissue septa of muscle. The density of this innervation determines the local
sensitivity to pain.

How pain receptors are stimulated, however, remains uncertain. Skin receptors
seem to evoke immediate pain by mechanical stimulation. Injury also causes local cell
destruction and the liberated enzymes may produce inflammatory peptides such as
bradykinin, histamine, 5-hydroxytryptamine and acetylcholine. It is now suggested
that prostaglandin E1 sensitizes the pain receptor to the action of these chemical
mediators. This effect may explain the action of peripherally acting analgesics such as
aspirin, for this inhibits prostaglandin synthetase, thus preventing the formation of
prostaglandins.

Two kinds of small-diameter afferent nerve fibres are known to conduct pain
impulses:

(1) Myelinated A fibres, 1–4 μm in size, that conduct at 5–15 m/s.
(2) Unmyelinated C fibres, 0.5–1 μm in size, that conduct at 0.5–2 m/s.

These differences in fibre size and conduction speed are associated with differences in the type of sensation. Thus two basically different kinds of pain can be distinguished; a fast and a slow.

Fast and slow pain

Fast pain transmitted by A-type fibres is essentially sharp in nature and the patient reacts to such stimulation in a fraction of a second. It travels in well-defined, long-fibred, central pathways. Skin, mucosa, cornea and ligaments have many fast pain fibres, so pain from these is generally sharp in nature.

Slow pain transmitted by C fibres takes several seconds for it to become consciously felt. It is usually interpreted as an ache (toothache is typical). It often arises in lesions which are expanding under pressure. Apical dental abscesses, intramedullary bone lesions etc. are characteristic.

The essential characteristics of these two basic types of pain are given in *Table 18.1*.

Table 18.1

	Fast superficial pain	*Slow deep pain*
Speed of conscious recognition	Rapid	Slow
Sensation	Sharp	Dull ache
Subject localization	Good	Poor
Typical excitatory stimulus	Stretch	Expansile pressure
Throbbing	Absent	May occur
Diurnal behaviour	Seldom affected	Often worse at night
Predominant tissues	Skin, cornea, muco-cutaneous junctions	Bone, periosteum, tooth, muscle
Tenderness	Well localized	Poorly localized
Referral	Infrequent	Frequent
Radiation	Often	Usual

The peripheral distribution of pain afferent fibres of face and head

Skin

The accepted cutaneous distribution of such fibres within the branches of the trigeminal and upper cervical nerves follows an almost constant pattern, as indicated in *Figure 18.3*. Personal experience, however, suggests that the dermatome of the second trigeminal division requires subdivision. The upper part of this dermatome, supplied by the zygomatico–facial and zygomatico–temporal nerves, is not made analgesic by resection of the maxillary nerve at the foramen rotundum. The implications of this are discussed in Chapter 20.

Cornea

The cornea possesses only pain-sensitive fibres which join the long ciliary nerves from the nasociliary branch of the ophthalmic division.

Within the mouth

The teeth and periodontal membranes, the oral mucosa as far back as the uvula, and the tongue anterior to the circumvallate papillae are all innervated by trigeminus. The glosso–pharyngeal nerve supplies the posterior third of the tongue, the mucosa covering the inferior faucial region, tonsils and adjoining larynx, together with the mucosa of the middle ear and the eustachian tube.

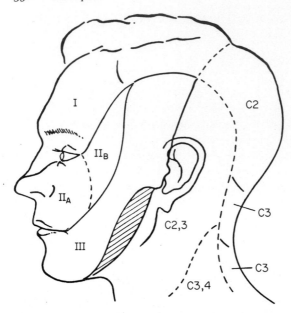

Figure 18.3   The facial dermatomes. The shaded area shows the variable boundary between the third division of trigeminal and the upper cervical nerve area. Only part A of the second division of trigeminal is rendered analgesic by resection of the second division alone. (Modified from Haymaker and Woodhall)

External auditory meatus and tympanic membrane

The trigeminal innervation appears confined to a variable area of the anterior wall of the auditory meatus and drum. In the development of the middle ear, the fifth, seventh, ninth and tenth cranial nerves all participate with considerable overlap, and consequently definitive areas attributable to any one nerve can hardly be expected. The concha of the ear and posterior wall of the external meatus have additional pain afferent innervation from the vagus, which also contributes afferent fibres to the pharyngeal mucosa and the posterior part of the tongue. Some pain afferents from the concha also join the facial nerve and run centripetally in its nervus intermedius root.

Gate-control theory

The gate-control theory of Melzack and Wall (1965) provides an important step forward in our understanding of pain. They proposed that pain is not due to activity occurring exclusively in specific pathways, but rather, that it results from activity in several interacting neural systems each with its own specialized function (*Figure 18.4*).

The gate is situated anatomically in the cells of the substantia gelatinosa which caps the dorsal horns throughout the spinal cord and is equally closely associated with the spinal tract of the trigeminal. This modulates the afferent patterns before they

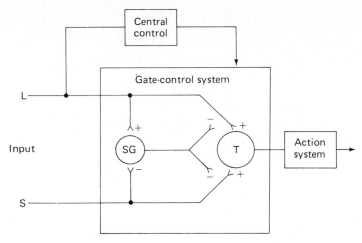

Figure 18.4 Diagram of the Gate-Control Theory. Large diameter fibres (L) project to the substantia gelatinosa (SG) and the first central transmission (T) cells. The substantia gelatinosa exerts an inhibitory effect on afferent fibre terminals, this is increased by (L) fibre activity and decreased by small fibre (S) activity. The (T) cells project the summated excitatory or inhibitory impulses to the action system. Note that gate control is also influenced by central control mechanisms

influence the first central transmission (T) cells. The T cells activate neural mechanisms responsible for the perception of, and response to, pain. The signal that triggers this action system occurs when the input to the T cells reaches a critical level. This level is determined by the afferent barrage already modulated by substantia gelatinosa activity. This, in turn, is determined by the relative balance of activity in large diameter (L) and small diameter (S) fibres. Activity in large fibres tends to inhibit transmission (closes the gate), whilst small fibre activity tends to facilitate transmission (opens the gate). The transmission from T cells to higher centres occurs not only through the spino–thalamic tracts but is also transmitted centrally in the dorsal columns. This sensory information, after processing in the central control mechanisms, can influence the gate by way of descending tracts.

The gate-control theory would seem to explain much that was hitherto puzzling in post-herpetic neuralgia. Noordenbos (1968) found a disproportionate loss of large fibres from nerves following infection with herpes zoster. This leaves the unopposed action of small fibres on T cells, a wide-open gate, and pain which may be caused by non-noxious stimulae such as light touch.

It has long been apparent that the traditional teaching that there are but two independent pathways of tracts and nuclei by which sensory signals reach the brain, is far too simplistic a view. There are more tracts and nuclei and they interact; nuclei do not just relay signals, they are concerned in processing information and they work in different ways; they are all under descending control from higher levels.

The essence of the gate-control theory is a segmental interaction between large and small fibre inputs working on a reciprocal basis, so that when large fibre activity predominates, peripheral access to tract cells connected with pain is relatively barred. Conversely, a predominance of small fibre inputs swings the gate further open and allows more peripheral access.

This theory requires that impulses in fibres that are not nociceptive as judged by electrical recording may, firstly, cause pain, and secondly, prevent or reduce it. In healthy subjects the hypothesis of pain from impulses in non-nociceptive fibres appears false, at least in respect of the larger myelinated fibres, for no electrical stimuli to such fibres evoke pain.

The gate-control theory has been criticized by many neurophysiologists primarily because one half of the proposed reciprocal mechanism, i.e. the facilitation of peripheral access to tract cells by small fibre activity, could not be demonstrated. The origins of these and other apparent contradictions remains to be found, but may depend on differences between experimental and chronic pathological pain. That such differences exist is only too apparent to those who have observed such states as causalgia or phantom limb pain. In certain states with chronic pain and particularly in the hyperaesthesia associated with partial lesions of peripheral nerves, every sort of nerve fibre appears to contribute to the sensation of pain.

Whatever its present inadequacies, the gate theory remains a useful working hypothesis and it provides a physiological basis for mechanisms previously thought purely psychological, such as attention and the obliteration of one sensation by another. It may well provide some basis for understanding the relief of pain sometimes procured by acupuncture or transcutaneous electrical stimulation.

The psychological aspects of facial pain

Any severe or prolonged pain immediately evokes psychological factors. Their importance depends upon the past emotional experiences of the individual and the particular situation surrounding the pain. There is no distinct line between somatic and psychogenic pain, few pains being primarily one or the other.

The young infant who receives ample warmth, nourishment and love from his mother and this largely through his mouth, starts with a good emotional basis. The mother with emotional problems, however, is apt to convey an ambivalent message of love and hate to the child which confuses not only this early relationship but all subsequent ones.

As the face is so important in our communication with others, it is often involved in difficulties with our own self concept. Thus facial pain may be a cry for help!

The child who seldom obtains attention except by crying with pain, becomes conditioned to expect attention when pain is again experienced in later life. Should this expectation fail, the demand for attention increases. So a demanding patient who is not satisfied with all that we are able or willing to give, is bred. As doctors, we react in our own individual ways to these excessive demands and a good doctor–patient relationship may easily be lost.

Those who primarily associated pain with punishment may later almost welcome pain because of its ability to relieve guilt. Guilt, which is far more burdensome than pain, may be due to unacceptable thoughts or acts. In others pain may substitute for a normal grief reaction and thus reduce the feelings of loss, especially if there were unacceptable ambivalent feelings towards the lost person.

Pain frequently becomes a most useful somatic symptom. The patient wanting to be accepted by his doctor talks of somatic pain rather than of painful emotional experiences. The doctor, with limited time, generally prefers to concentrate on the somatic pains rather than the complicated emotional problems. We end up with two individuals talking around a subject that neither wishes to deal with directly. This brings the risk that the surgeon, out of frustration, may perform a potentially destructive procedure in an attempt to relieve the patient of pain that primarily originates in the psyche.

Facial pain may persist long after it should on the basis of organic pathology. The individual may here interpret the damaged face as damaged self. The result is anxiety expressed as pain. The anxiety stems from the patient's fear that his distorted face will lead to rejection by family, friends or workmates. Surgery cannot relieve these painful anxieties. Relief comes only when the patient is able to express his anxiety and receive reassuring answers to his questions from the significant individuals in his life.

Penman (1954) gave cogent reasons for concluding that 'curable' pain should be relieved promptly. Pain present for more than six months in a neurotic individual may become too valuable in his interpersonal relationships to be given up. For such individuals the pain becomes an old friend and one to be lived with. It seems the pain serves an emotional need and relieves the patient of the distress of anxiety or depression. Such pain can become a prop that sustains the patient against his inadequacies in other directions of life, whether these be marital, sexual or in work. Such a prop must be recognized for what it is, for its removal will not benefit the patient.

Psychogenic factors may magnify any form of physical pain. We all see patients whose subjective disability is grossly excessive in comparison with the somatic lesion. We must constantly compare the magnitude of the patient's subjective symptoms with the objective evidence of disease. Thus a patient may claim he has been unable to bite solid food for months or years. Should we find neither atrophy of relevant muscles, nor loss of radiographic density of the mandible, the major problem is certainly psychic. Equally it is important to compare the amount of pain experienced by direct examination of an allegedly tender area with that which can be evoked by similar palpation made apparently accidentally whilst the patient's attention is distracted elsewhere.

The existence of psychic pain, however, does not eliminate the presence of genuine somatic disease. One's thought processes must not be disconnected the moment a psychic pain-creation pattern is found to exist!

The kind of pain

The patient with real somatic pain seldom has difficulty in saying what kind of pain he has (i.e. whether it is sharp, burning, an ache, etc.). Those with psychic pain cannot do so. The more specific the questions, the more vague the answers become. Such pains are often described as simultaneously sharp, aching and burning; or they can be throbbing and sharp. Frequently such pain is described as 'pulling' or 'drawing' or 'tight'. Equally it is often claimed to be constant. Alternatively the patient's well-nourished appearance contrasts with his complaint of severe pain that has almost prevented sleep for months.

Behaviour

Not all psychological pain can be recognized by its bizarre behaviour. The emotionally crippled patient may once have had a genuine somatic pain in the same region. There is some memory as to how this behaved and perhaps traces of residual signs. Superficially, the symptoms conform to a typical somatic pattern but if the doctor is both perceptive and specific in question and on examination, clues may emerge. Thus the time scale of the history may be important. A strained muscle or ligament may hurt for a number of weeks, it cannot be still hurting two to three years later.

The patient may complain of numbness in addition to pain in the face. The numbness may involve several peripheral nerves and not conform to the anatomical pattern expected. Widespread hyperaesthesias and/or wide radiation patterns of pain are typical of a pronounced psychic element, but there is a diagnostic pitfall. Some normal people regularly develop similar transformations of ordinary somatic pain but will respond promptly and normally to the treatment proper for their somatic lesion.

Personality patterns

In atypical neuralgias Friedman (1964) showed that frequently there was a history of the initial pain occurring at the time of a significant event in the patient's emotional life. He found the response to pain determined by the patient's emotional state and behaviour pattern. The personality patterns most commonly seen were characterized as ambitious, perfectionistic, or over-conscientious. Some had difficulty in sexual adjustment. Others appeared masochistic, the pains representing repressed forbidden sexual wishes or warnings related to these. The pains seemed to provide punishment for attempts to gratify these wishes. He noted that pain may be symbolic of repressed rage or anger and that, for some patients, pains were symptoms of anxiety or depression.

Psychiatric syndromes

Pain, particularly in the face, may be the presenting feature in several major psychiatric syndromes the recognition of which is all-important.

Depression
The pain masks an underlying depressive illness that is much less apparent than when pain is not present. If looked for, however, the hallmark symptoms of depression will be found and the diagnosis can be made. A loss of interest in all aspects of life and body functions becomes apparent. Specifically we need to look for difficulty in sleeping, loss of appetite, loss of weight, loss of sexual desire and ability, self neglect, fatigue and apathy, pessimism, worry and difficulty in concentrating. Psychiatric assessment and treatment is essential for the patient's loss of interest otherwise frequently leads to loss of interest in life itself; suicide may result.

Conversion hysteria
There has been unnecessary confusion over this term but essentially it denotes a conversion of anxiety into a somatic symptom without discernible physiologic change.

Consequently these patients seem relatively free from anxiety or depression. Whilst a somatic symptom may occur in persons of any personality type, it is most frequent in those with a hysterical personality. This is characterized by vanity, egocentricity, dramatization, demanding ways, dependency, immaturity and shallowness. This personality is more frequently seen in women and the most common symptom of conversion hysteria is pain, generally in the face.

The risk here is that the pain of conversion reaction is treated as an organic illness because of the relative absence of anxiety or depression. Where there is lack of organic pathology to explain the somatic symptoms, particularly pain, psychiatric consultation is often indicated.

Hypochondriasis

Symptoms and particularly pain, can be produced or aggravated purely through the hypochondriac's obsessive concern about bodily functions. Hypochondriasis varies from the mild concern generally seen where the cause of the symptoms is obscure, to a severe degree that borders on psychosis. The approach depends upon the severity of the emotional illness but frequently a thorough medical examination and subsequent reassurance is all that is required. In this state, pain is frequently the tension headache due to muscle spasm secondary to anxiety. This pain is most frequently in the occipital, temporal or frontal regions but may occur in the face itself. Associated pains in the back, belly or legs are not uncommon.

The motivationally disabled

These patients are effectively disabled by pain that is psychologically generated. The disability which may prevent them from working or running a family, probably followed a somatic injury or disease that seemed to behave normally. Objectively this lesion evolved, responded to treatment and healed. The subjectively conscious symptoms, however, did not subside; they persisted and ultimately became completely refractory. Whereas the individual with a healthy motivation wants to get well at both conscious and subconscious levels of his mind, the motivationally disturbed patient is at odds within himself. Consciously he sincerely wants to be well but subconsciously he needs, wants and attains the opposite. These unfortunate patients are certainly not malingering. They believe they are physically ill but mentally well. Some psychic problem at subconscious level seems to create the disability in order to solve some inner conflict.

Clinically the variations of motivational disability seem infinite, yet they present well-defined contrasts with physical disability. Several common situations are summarized below. If only they could be cured as easily as they can be recognized!

The patient who subconsciously feels inadequate

These patients have a deep-seated belief that they are inferior beings in respect of their performance at work or at home, sexually or in their ability to earn or compete. This self-judgment may be grossly in error or be entirely true. Being physically disabled provides an escape from the need to perform adequately and this without any associated stigma.

At conscious level these patients want to get well and will do anything that seems to offer a reasonable chance of help. Their sincerity is demonstrated by the number of treatments and operations to which they will submit. In contrast, the malingerer will rarely submit to surgery!

The patient who has lost the major purpose in life

This is often a woman whose children have grown up and have lives and homes of their own and whose husband is too busy with work to give her much time. It may be a man who lacks hobbies but who has been retired; or a still active man who has lost interest in work and has little interest in anything else.

The anxious patient

Pain is normally accompanied by anxiety. For most this is merely the understandable fear of the unknown, of cancer or other dread disease. Such patients accept well-reasoned reassurance and relax visibly when told that they do not have cancer or whatever else they feared.

In others, anxiety is a pathological trait so severe as to be disabling. These pathologically anxious patients remain so, despite all reasonable reassurance. They have an inexhaustible and repetitive supply of questions. They search for absolute guarantees and certainty. Such patients, in whom muscle tenderness is often prominent, require special care in management. An exhaustive investigation, undertaken largely in the hope of reassuring the patient, is likely to have the reverse effect!

Management of the motivationally ill

These patients reject any suggestion that there is a psychic component to their disability. This threatens them with facing the stigma of personal inadequacy, that is only avoided by the physical illness. Whilst by one device or another they can be made to see a psychiatrist, this is most unlikely to help. One essential condition for successful psychotherapy is the patient's conscious belief that he needs it and his conscious participation in it. These patients will usually defend with their lives, either literally by suicide or symbolically by a psychosis, the concept that they are physically and not psychologically ill. Their sole objective in seeing a psychiatrist is to prove their mental health, not to have their emotional clockwork fixed, for they believe this is as good as anyone's.

A fundamental error and one that I have made, is to confront the patient with one's own conviction that the source of his pain and disability arises within the mind. The patient will defend himself at all costs from conscious awareness of these facts. In the effort to convince himself rather than us of the genuineness of his disability, he will get worse.

This syndrome of motivational disorder may accompany unresolved third-party legal liability. Here it is desirable that this liability be resolved in the earliest practicable manner. Such achievement is usually followed within six months or so by a return to work or other acceptable function, no matter whether the resolution of the liability was advantageous to the patient or not.

Iatrogenic disease

The essence of psychic pain is that it represents a disguised although verbalized appeal for help. At the same time, the symptom can be used to thwart help, should it not relieve the patient's poorly communicated emotional anguish.

Those who will openly accept the fact that they have emotional difficulties and that these may relate to their pain can often be helped by an understanding and reassuring regime, perhaps combined with psychotherapy.

Inept handling, however, may lead to iatrogenic disease just as surely as complications may follow the knife, or side effects the medication. The anxious doctor attempting to relieve his own anxiety by carrying out endless examinations and treatments merely instils these very anxieties in his patients. The doctor who, from anxiety or desire for self-gratification, cannot bring himself to discharge the patient but continually brings him back for review, all too readily engenders dependence in his patient. This can progress even to the point that the patient loses his individuality and ability to function as a healthy member of society.

Beware the patient who comes to you as the 'last resort' having already seen many other clinicians. On occasion, one can achieve a genuine triumph by dealing successfully with something hitherto overlooked. It is long odds, however, that this patient's history reveals a psychological need to be disabled. It is certainly possible by well-intentioned treatment to rid the patient of presenting complaints but only by replacing them with others that are worse.

A typical story is that the patient's problem has defied all previous attempts at diagnosis and treatment. The latest doctor has made a new diagnosis and starts appropriate treatment, perhaps performs an operation. Next day the patient appears cured. The triumph is short-lived. Three months later the patient has returned to his original state perhaps with new symptoms provided by the latest treatment of his soma. Too late the doctor realizes that the patient has a tongue that is hinged in the middle and wags at both ends, particularly to his own detriment.

Classification

Excluding local lesions evident on routine examination, cases presenting as facial pain may be classified as follows:

Neural pain

(a) *Primary neuralgias*
   Trigeminal neuralgia
   Glossopharyngeal neuralgia
   Tympanic neuralgia
(b) *Secondary neuralgias*
   Pressure involvements of trigeminal or glossopharyngeal nerves
   Dental neuralgias
   Nasal neuralgias
   Baro–sinusitis
   Traumatic lesions
   Cervical neuralgias
(c) *Central lesions*
   Post-herpetic neuralgia
   Disseminated (multiple) sclerosis
   Brain-stem lesions
   Thalamic lesions
(d) *Distant referred pain (from coronary insufficiency)*

Ocular pain

Glossodynia

Muscle and joint pain

(a) Myofascial triggers
(b) Painful myospasm
(c) Cervical myalgia
(d) Temporo–mandibular joint disorders
(e) Bruxism

Vascular pain

(a) Periodic migrainous neuralgia
(b) Temporal arteritis

Atypical facial neuralgias

The primary neuralgias

Almost confined to the elderly, the primary neuralgias (trigeminal and glossopharyngeal) are clear-cut entities. They are characterized by brief paroxysms of severe,

stabbing pain within a definitive neural area. Pain is often precipitated by sensory stimuli. Periods of pain-free remission occur, but are followed by inevitable recurrence at shorter intervals.

The severity of pain frequently defies description and may bring the patient to self-destruction.

Although diagnosis should not be difficult and definitive treatment is highly effective, too many patients still spend several years in a fruitless search for relief.

Trigeminal neuralgia (Tic douloureux)

This condition, almost confined to the over 60s, is characterized by brief paroxysms of severe stabbing pain, within some part of the trigeminal area. Periods of remission may follow a short series of paroxysms but inevitably the pain returns. As the free intervals grow shorter and the paroxysms more frequent, whilst spreading to wider trigeminal areas, the patient's distress becomes terrible indeed.

Electron microscopy now reveals hitherto unsuspected nerve cell and fibre changes (Beaver, 1967; Kerr 1967). Proliferative and disorganized changes occur in the myelin sheath surrounding some extremely tortuous and hypertrophied axons. Clumps of abnormal Nissl's substance may occur in some of the Gasserian ganglion cells.

Clinical recognition depends on the pain being unilateral, trigeminal, short, sharp, sudden and severe. These attacks are generally precipitated by sensory stimuli and remain unassociated with any sensory or motor loss. Although bilateral involvement is known, it is almost never concurrent, and for practical purposes tic douloureux is unilateral and does not cross the midline.

Almost always the pain initially affects either the second or third division, spreading only later to the first division. It is exceptional for the pain to start in or around the eye. Between short paroxysms of pain, the patient is free of any discomfort.

Sharp stabs of excruciating pain cause the patient to wince and avoid any precipitating factors. Touching the face, especially about the nostrils or near the mouth, as in washing, shaving, or brushing the teeth, may trigger off an attack. Loud noises or cold winds may have the same effect, but pain rarely disturbs sleep.

The pain tends to start in certain foci and spreads in certain directions. It never affects diffusely the entire territory of the nerve or even one division. Commonly the pain starts in the upper gum later spreading towards the orbit, the ear or downwards to the chin.

Most patients conform exactly to the above criteria but a careful history may reveal some unusual features, for the picture is never as clear-cut in the clinical setting as in the textbook. Uncommon features that may co-exist with typical spasms are:

(1) Prolonged burning or aching pain.
(2) Precipitating factors may be absent.
(3) Pain may extend to the neck or posterior scalp.
(4) Spontaneous hyperaesthesia may occur.

The less classic the picture, the more essential the use of non-permanent peripheral nerve section to assess the role of trigeminal denervation. Diagnosis demands complete lack of either motor or sensory loss. The presence of either implies a structural lesion of the trigeminal nerve, evoked perhaps by pressure of acoustic neurinoma, intracranial aneurysm, invasion by naso–pharyngeal carcinoma or Gasserian tumour.

Despite the clarity of the symptoms many patients are still denied prompt diagnosis. Most patients with long-standing tic douloureux have had at least some type of useless intra-oral surgery. There have generally been several useless dental extractions, based solely on the patient's conviction that first one, and then another, sound tooth was responsible. The paranasal sinuses also are still too often subjected to unwarranted surgery.

Differential diagnosis

Dental pain from a carious tooth can closely mimic tic douloureux. This possibility must be remembered and, at least in younger patients, the teeth carefully examined with percussion and thermal tests and suitable dental radiographs.

Pain similar to tic douloureux can be due to myositis of the temporal or masseter muscles. Pain may be paroxysmal but is generally more continuous than in tic douloureux. It is aggravated by eating and drinking and is often relieved by local heat. Diagnosis depends on deep palpation of the temporal and masseteric muscles, revealing a discrete myositic nodule, pressure upon which promptly reproduces the patient's pain. Radiant heat, massage, and local anaesthetic infiltration into the nodule relieves. This entity, which also presents signs of jaw joint disorder, is frequently overlooked.

Rarely, a space-occupying mass within the middle or posterior cranial fossa may present a picture almost identical with the idiopathic neuralgia. Whenever atypical features are found, full investigations are desirable, lest one treats the pain and misses the tumour.

Treatment

Carbamazepine   The introduction of carbamazepine (Tegretol) appeared to transform therapy. It remains of great value but the earlier enthusiasm has waned with the recognition that drug resistance and toxicity are prone to develop over the years (Taylor, 1966). Almost specific in its effect, carbamazepine rapidly relieves some 80 per cent of patients. A small dose, 100 mg thrice daily, is gradually increased as required to a maximum of 200 mg six times daily. This drug, which is undoubtedly toxic, is best taken with meals to avoid gastric distress. Dizziness, diffuse erythematous rashes, jaundice or leucopenia may occur. Fatal aplastic anaemia has been reported but the risks appear substantially less than the admittedly small risks of intracranial surgery in expert hands.

Phenytoin (Epanutin)   Alone this drug is effective in only 20 per cent of cases but it is well tolerated in doses of 300–400 mg daily. A combination with carbamazepine may relieve pain at non-toxic levels where neither drug alone will do so.

Peripheral neurectomy   Avulsion of peripheral branches of the trigeminal nerve within the trigger zone gives prompt relief but the pain recurs in about a year. This appears to be due to nerve regeneration but revision operation has seldom proved equally successful.

Trans-antral resection of the maxillary nerve at the foramen rotundum has, in my previous experience, been uniformly followed by recurrence in about 18 months. The possible role of blocking the foramen rotundum is considered further in Chapter 20.

Despite these limitations, peripheral neurectomy certainly retains a place prior to sensory root section and may be all that is required to allow some elderly sufferers to live out their lives in comfort.

For first division pain the incision is made through the unshaven eyebrow, seeking out not only the obvious supra-orbital and supra-trochlear nerves, but also the infra-trochlear branch and any lateral infero-lacrimal twig.

Alcohol injections of peripheral branches have generally been abandoned as less effective and far more trying than open neurectomy.

Gasserian ganglion injection   Preferably under radiographic control, a needle is inserted through the foramen ovale into the Gasserian ganglion. Whilst a few experts such as Penman have obtained results almost rivalling those of sensory root section, most found the ready diffusibility of alcohol gave an unacceptable risk of corneal anaesthesia and later ulceration. Replacement of hypobaric alcohol with hyperbaric 5 per cent phenol-in-glycerin has given great improvement in control. This injected into the rootlets is painless and in a cooperative patient the injection can be stopped before corneal anaesthesia supervenes. The reported results are impressive and recurrent pain will yield to further injection.

Root section   Since its introduction by Frazier in 1901, sensory root section in the middle cranial fossa has been accepted as the safest, most certain way to obtain long-standing relief. The results in thousands of reported cases were reviewed by White and Sweet (1969). In expert hands, the mortality is less than 1 per cent. Early relief is almost invariable but up to 15 per cent have eventual return of attacks. This seems due to the sensory fibres being cut too close to the ganglion, thus a few ganglion cells remain attached to their central processes and their peripheral ends can regenerate. Such operation is now confined to patients unresponsive to carbamazepine or intolerant of effective dosage. Wherever possible, differential section is employed to spare the ophthalmic fibres and possible keratitis.

The otologist should be aware of the temporary middle-ear effusion and deafness that may follow middle fossa operation and of the facial paralysis that occasionally occurs. Atrophic ulceration of the ala nasi is an unusual sequel of trigeminal denervation. Initially, intense alar paraesthesiae evoke compulsive rubbing or scratching. The skin becomes dusky red and a slowly progressive ulceration occurs. In most recorded cases, treatment by cervical sympathectomy is followed by rapid healing.

The main complication of this operation, however, is the occurrence of a continuous pain quite different from the original paroxysms and occurring throughout the anaesthetic area. This anaesthesia dolorosa, an intractable and highly unpleasant burning and tingling sensation in the numbed face, renders some 10 per cent of those submitted to root section permanently miserable. To a large extent, however, it can be avoided by excluding from root section those who tolerate only poorly the effects of temporary denervation by peripheral neurectomy. It is desirable that such be used first.

Intracranial decompression of trigeminal pathways   The techniques of Taarnhoj (1952) and of Pudenz and Shelden (1952) that were deliberately designed not to produce severe sensory loss, have nevertheless yielded protracted periods of relief of pain. The technique is essentially one of neurolysis of the ganglion and its root fibres in Meckel's cave. They do not produce total anaesthesia and thus nearly obviate the risk of keratitis and severe paraesthesia, but they are followed by a relatively high incidence of recurrence.

Intramedullary trigeminal tractotomy   This preserves the sense of touch and position and avoids the complications that may follow sensory loss. It has no risk of paralysing the muscles of mastication, but may be followed by ataxia. It should rarely be the initial surgical procedure. It finds a place in the rare (3 per cent) cases of bilateral neuralgia, when it is vital that the patient retains sense of touch and position on at least one side of the jaw and tongue.

Radiofrequency gangliolysis   This is a refinement of earlier methods of electrocoagulation. A needle electrode with a thermistor tip is inserted percutaneously through the foramen ovale under radiographic control. A short-acting anaesthetic (Brevital or nitrous oxide–oxygen) is intermittently used and the patient awoken for testing at repeated intervals. The needle's position within the sensory root fibres is checked by electrical stimulation. The tip of the 2-mm electrode is heated to 70–100 °C for successive periods of 30–60 s and the patient reawoken to test the extent and degree of sensory loss. Repositioning the electrode and further checks on physiological responses prior to further episodes of coagulation, enables the pain to be relieved without total anaesthesia of the skin. Touch and position sense are usually preserved, for the larger myelinated axons are more heat-resistant than the smaller pain afferents.

By this means mortality has been almost eliminated. The motor root is usually preserved and risks of corneal ulceration or severe paraesthesae almost eliminated. Unfortunately 20 per cent of patients experience recurrent pain within a year and more do so later. Although the procedure can be repeated effectively the high risk of recurrence is likely to debar it from becoming the treatment of choice.

Glossopharyngeal neuralgia

This is similarly intermittent, agonizing paroxysmal pain of identical quality to trigeminal neuralgia, from which it varies in its location about the faucial area, and/or within the ear.

Paroxysms of stabbing pain start in the base of the tongue and faucial region on one side and often radiate into the ear. They are provoked by swallowing, talking and coughing. Whilst each bout of pain rarely lasts more than a minute or two, they may recur frequently for some hours or even days at a time, during which time the patient may be unable to swallow even his own spittle. Cutaneous trigger zones are unusual, but may occur over the auricle or tragus.

Conversely pain deep in the ear, paroxysmal and unbearable, may occur alone. Whilst between attacks, merely touching the ear may induce pain, with its onset there is often an irresistible urge to dig a finger into the ear as deeply and forcibly as possible. Such pain appears limited to the tympanic branch of the glossopharyngeal, the so-called 'tympanic plexus' neuralgia.

It is clear that glossopharyngeal neuralgia need not involve all branches simultaneously, any more than trigeminal neuralgia may affect all divisions.

The typical picture is so characteristic that the diagnosis is seldom difficult, despite its rarity. It may, however, be confused with trigeminal neuralgia in patients with pain in the region of the tragus or deep to the angle of the jaw. Typical glossopharyngeal neuralgia, however, may be temporarily relieved by cocainization of the glossopharyngeal area of the throat.

It must also be differentiated from secondary glossopharyngeal neuralgia, due to adjacent lesions such as acoustic neurinoma or other tumour involving the nerve (Cohen, 1937) or irritation by an elongated styloid process (Asherson, 1957). In these cases, the pain, although it may initially be subject to exacerbation, eventually becomes more aching in type and continuous.

Medical treatment of glossopharyngeal tic

Although less successful than with trigeminal neuralgia, carbamazepine (Tegretol) at times proves similarly effective, failing which surgical treatment is mandatory.

Surgical treatment of glossopharyngeal tic

There are several different approaches, the proper choice of which is indicated by individual circumstances.

The intracranial   A unilateral, posterior fossa craniotomy is used for section of the glossopharyngeal rootlets, together with the nervus intermedius and upper vagal rootlets, for pain occasionally persists if the latter are not included. This operation is the only certain means of ensuring permanent relief; but though risks are low, they are inevitably greater than in alternative procedures, which thus have a place.

Infratemporal avulsion of glossopharyngeal nerve   The nerve may be avulsed in the neck following its exposure either through the tonsillar bed (Wilson and McAlpine, 1946) or by an external cervical approach (Shaheen, 1963). Either procedure relieves pain in the throat at minimal risk but neither precludes subsequent recurrence of pain in the ear.

The intratympanic (Golding-Wood, 1962)   Intratympanic resection of the tympanic branch of the ninth cranial nerve, with or without the chorda tympani, may suffice to relieve at least aural pain, and in a case reported by Kersley (1965), also pain in the throat.

In a peripheral resection such as this the possibilities of later recurrence must be accepted, despite long periods of relief now obtained in a large proportion of the few cases known. Nevertheless, the minimal risk justifies the initial use of this method in any case associated with aural pain.

Secondary neuralgias

In general, the secondary neuralgias are symptomatic of disturbance of the nerve by neighbouring pathology or local trauma.

In the early stages paroxysmal pain may occur but, even so, these exacerbations are more prolonged than those of tic douloureux. Later, these paroxysms tend to merge into the more or less continuous pain that is so characteristic of the secondary neuralgias. Paraesthesiae may occur, and skin sensitivity is often altered, either hypersensitivity or partial analgesia being common.

Although frequently dental in origin, the secondary neuralgias are a widely varied group, and appropriate treatment depends on the cause of the individual case.

Pressure involvements of trigeminal or glossopharyngeal nerves

In acoustic neuroma

Such pain is rarely paroxysmal, but on occasions intermittent pressure from an acoustic tumour may simulate either tic douloureux or glossopharyngeal neuralgia.

Suspicion arises where either type of pain is associated with ipsilateral deafness. In such an event, loss of the corneal reflex is a cardinal finding.

In nasopharyngeal carcinoma

Trigeminal pain may be an early, indeed the solitary, presenting symptom of nasopharyngeal carcinoma. It may affect any division or more than one. Initially the pain may occur in violent paroxysms, but these tend later to become a permanently smouldering pain. The pain is frequently associated with ophthalmoplegia, especially when it is the first division that is involved for this is by intracranial spread. The third division becomes involved by extracranial spread; the second division equally by either route.

In lesions of the jaws

Antral neoplasms are generally painless at first, but when eroding the posterior wall of the antrum may give severe pain, sometimes paroxysmal initially. Metastatic carcinoma of the jaws generally gives pain, and severe third division trigeminal pain may be the initial presentation of mandibular metastasis. Dental cysts, odontomes, etc. only give pain if infected or pressing directly on the nerve.

In intracranial aneurysm

Trigeminal pain is a classic sign of saccular aneurysms of the intraclinoid part of the carotid artery that later may burst into the cavernous sinus. Either first or first and second divisions may be affected. The pain, which may be sudden in onset, is severe and continuous. It tends to be followed rapidly by numbness, ophthalmoplegia and frequent visual impairment. A bruit over the neck and orbit is typical, arteriography is confirmatory and common carotid ligation relieves.

In elongated styloid process

In 4 per cent of the population the styloid is grossly enlarged, palpable through the pharyngeal wall and visible in antero–posterior radiographs. Only a few such cases produce symptoms, generally experienced as a dull, intermittent or persistent pain in the ear, neck or pharynx, aggravated by swallowing.

This may first appear as local pain, persisting months after a tonsillectomy. At times the pain may be so severe and paroxysmal as to simulate glossopharyngeal neuralgia (Asherson, 1957).

Occasionally a long styloid process becomes fractured, producing severe pain on turning the head. These cases are best relieved by excision of the styloid process.

Dental neuralgias

Just as dental caries is the commonest disease of man, so dental conditions are the commonest cause of facial pain. Pain mostly arises from the pulp space or periodontal membrane becoming infected from dental caries, or involved in pressure resorption from a neighbouring unerupted, impacted tooth.

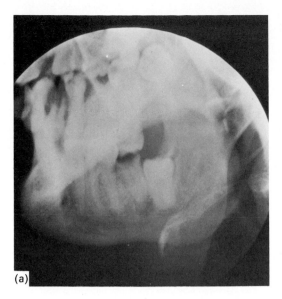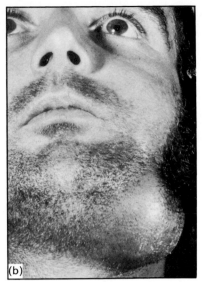

(a)

(b)

Figure 18.5   (a) and (b) Periapical abscess with large submandibular swelling arising from the second lower molar tooth

Pulp space infections
Infection mostly invades the pulp space via a carious cavity. Pulpitis is characterized by poorly localized pain. The affected tooth is sensitive to thermal change, but not to percussion, unless the periodontal membrane has been involved by apical extension of infection. Acute infections give severe, throbbing pain, often intermittent and frequently more severe at night. In chronic infection, the pain is less intense, dull and aching in quality, but still intermittent and frequently paroxysmal (*Figure 18.5a and b*).

Periodontal infections
In contrast to pulpitis, the pain of periodontal infection is constant, not paroxysmal. It is generally well localized and the affected tooth is sensitive to percussion. Although the pain may vary with temperature variations, the marked thermal sensitivity of pulpitis does not occur. The gum adjacent to the affected tooth may be slightly swollen, congested and tender.

Whilst in many instances it is obvious that the patient has toothache, the affected tooth may be other than he suspects. At other times, the dental cause of pain may be far from obvious and is only revealed by painstaking examination.

Visual inspection and probing will reveal surface caries, but cavities between adjacent teeth or recurrent caries underneath a sound surface restoration, will be revealed only by suitable radiographs. A lateral oblique film of the mandible is no substitute for good dental films, which should routinely include intra-oral films of the upper and lower jaws, and a posterior bite wing film. Wherever evidence of caries exists, signs of chronic pulp space infection must be sought.

Each tooth should be tapped to exclude periodontal trouble, and then checked with both hot and cold stimuli, particularly those with large amalgam fillings. An effective method is to touch each tooth alternatively with a heated ball of base plate gutta percha, and with a cotton-wool probe dipped in ice water. Even healthy teeth may give some transient reaction to such thermal stimuli, but one with a diseased pulp will give an acute paroxysm of pain.

Dental neuralgias are common, and may closely simulate other entities. This mimicry in trigeminal neuralgia has already been mentioned. An interesting example was reported by Tinn (1947), where pain closely simulating tic douloureux of the second and third divisions, but in fact due to an acute pulpitis of a maxillary premolar, was detected only by the thermal responses of the affected tooth.

Whilst dental pain is commonly referred to another tooth, often in the opposing jaw, it is but rarely referred across the midline. This can occur, however, and Mollison (1944) reported a case of severe otalgia reflexly produced by a carious lower premolar of the opposite side, extraction of which gave immediate relief.

Purely neuralgic pain of dental origin most commonly results from chronic pulpitis, apical periodontitis or from unerupted impacted teeth. The patient may complain of paroxysmal shooting pain in any of several facial areas; fronto-nasal, naso-labial, maxillary, mandibular, hyoid or in the tongue. Once the possibility is suspected, the pain may, by its location, indicate at least the approximate position of the affected tooth (*Figure 18.6*). Similarly, the type of pain may indicate pulp or periodontal infection.

Unerupted, impacted teeth

The third molars are notoriously prone to incomplete eruption, and those in the lower jaw particularly, to malposition and impaction. Nevertheless, the mere presence of an unerupted ectopic or impacted tooth does not imply that it is the cause of pain.

The inferior dental nerve lies very close to the developing roots of the third mandibular molar, malposition of which is a frequent cause of pain, experienced as third division neuralgia or otalgia (*Figure 18.7*).

With the unerupted third lower molar, pain mostly arises from the pressure of developing roots against the nerve. Symptoms thus occur at 16–20 years of age, but are seldom accompanied by local pain about the tooth in question. Alternatively the

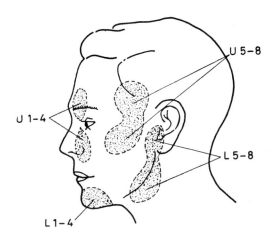

U 5-8

U 1-4

L 5-8

L 1-4

Figure 18.6   Diagram to show how the site of referred pain may indicate the approximate position of affected tooth

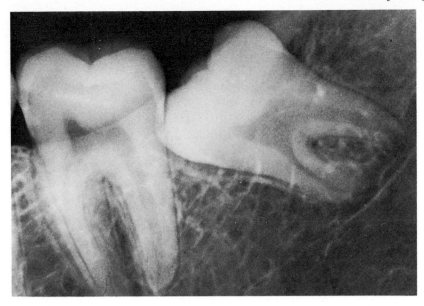

Figure 18.7   An impacted wisdom tooth evokes pain by pressure on the roots of the adjacent molar

unerupted tooth becomes twisted into a horizontal position, its crown producing painful pressure-erosion of the posterior roots of the second molar. This is revealed by x-rays, confirmed by local anaesthetic block and cured by extraction.

Post-extraction neuralgia

Local and/or neuralgic pain may follow any dental extraction or simpler restorative root-canal procedure. Most cases can be treated quite simply if the condition is diagnosed early, but many complicated histories have started from a simple so-called 'dry socket'. Incomplete extraction or local osteitis explains many; in others there is direct injury to the nerve trunk.

The latter is most commonly seen in extraction of the third mandibular molar, where the mechanism of injury seems well established. The injury occurs from pressure with the extraction forceps as these are being deeply settled into position. The cancellous bone is relatively malleable, and is thus readily crushed down without the use of extreme force, into the inferior alveolar canal. The same can happen if chisels or elevators are incautiously used in the deeper dissection required for the removal of impacted or unerupted wisdoms. The ensuing pain is generally accompanied by some sensory disturbance about the mental foramen, either paraesthesia or analgesia. Generally the pain ceases after a number of weeks, and sensory changes previously noted clear up. Rarely, the tooth roots are incurved below the inferior alveolar canal so that the nerve is enclosed by them, and in such a condition, lasting nerve damage necessarily follows extraction. Since the outline of the inferior alveolar canal is usually well delineated on x-ray, the patient can be warned prior to extraction of this risk and its attendant sensory loss. In fact patients adapt well to the sensory diminution, but are frequently annoyed by the early symptoms of nerve regeneration, inducing tingling 'pins and needles'.

Rarely, a persistent neuralgia may follow an apparently uncomplicated dental extraction, as described by Behrman (1949). In such an event, the pain generally starts after an interval of a few days and is at first localized about the site of extraction, which may remain persistently tender. Later, the pain may spread to involve the entire gum, even the entire jaw on the affected side. Whilst occasionally paroxysmal, the pain is generally continuous though often prone to considerable fluctuation in intensity. Behrman's cases were but transiently or not at all relieved by either trigeminal or sympathetic denervation. The author, however, has met several cases conforming exactly to this clinical pattern, mostly after extraction of an upper canine or premolar. In each of these, transantral section of the maxillary nerve at the foramen rotundum gave consistent relief, enduring through several years of follow-up.

The edentulous jaw

The fact that the jaw appears edentulous and healed does not exclude dental pain arising from retained roots or unerupted teeth.

In the lower jaw, the alveolar resorption that follows loss of the teeth may later precipitate pain. After years of continuous use of complete dentures, resorption may progress to the point that the mental foramen is traumatized by the base of the prosthesis. Intermittent pain and paraesthesiae over the distribution of the mental nerve follow. Women seem particularly prone to this, possibly through their feminine reluctance to be seen edentulous, even though the simple removal of their dentures would relieve distress.

The diagnosis is simple enough, but the prosthetic correction can be difficult. If this is not solved, avulsion of the inferior dental nerve at the mental foramen should relieve the pain.

Galvanism

Severe pain within the mouth can occur from galvanism induced by the juxtaposition of dissimilar metals in a recent dental restoration. Such pain may be accompanied by local ulceration.

Nasal neuralgias

Our knowledge of nasal pain derives from two main sources:

(1) Clinical observations of the pain correlated with the exact site of the pathological lesion in the nose or sinuses.
(2) Experimental investigation of direct painful stimulation of the walls of the nose and the sinuses in human subjects (*Figures 18.8, 18.9* and *18.10*).

The nasal mucosa is found to be sensitive to pain and to cold but is unresponsive to touch or to warmth. Even light touch elicits pain of a surprising intensity and a characteristically disagreeable quality. It remains purely localized and tends to be diffuse.

The exciting stimulus in painful nasal affections is generally pressure from congestion and oedema of the mucosa. In the sinuses pressure changes may follow occlusion of the sinus ostium. The effect of positive pressure within the maxillary sinus

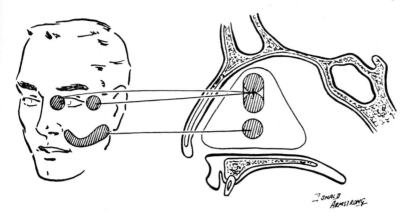

Figure 18.8 Diagram of areas of reference of pain from experimental stimulation of nasal septum. (After McAuliffe, G. W., Goodell, H. and Wolff, H. G.)

has been studied experimentally in man by inflating a balloon introduced into the sinus through a fistulous opening resulting from the extraction of an upper molar. It has been found that:

(1) Pressure of 20 mmHg gave a sensation of fullness.
(2) Pressures of 50–80 mmHg for 2 h gave moderate pain with associated engorgement of the turbinate, anaesthesia of which abolished the pain.
(3) Pressure of 200 mmHg gave immediate severe pain.

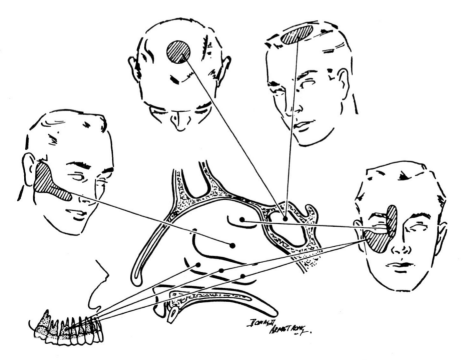

Figure 18.9 Diagram of areas of reference of pain from stimulation of the turbinates and the sphenoidal sinuses. (After McAuliffe, G. W., Goodell, H. and Wolff, H. G.)

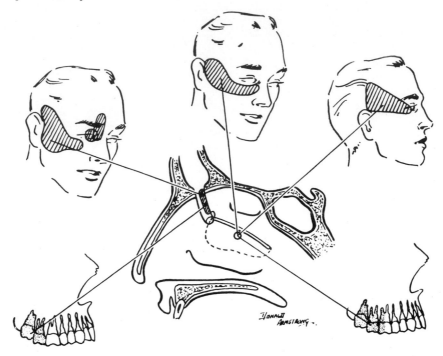

Figure 18.10   Diagram of areas of reference of pain from stimulation of the frontal sinus, fronto–nasal duct and the ostium of the maxillary sinus. (After McAuliffe, G. W., Goodell, H. and Wolff, H. G.)

Sinus pain may be experienced locally or referred to the peripheral distribution of either ophthalmic or maxillary divisions of the trigeminal. As the trigeminal innervation of the paranasal sinuses is overlapping and sometimes redundant, pain arising from within the sinuses often assumes bizarre and varied patterns. This is the more evident as referred pain is almost as common as localized pain.

Whilst many patients are specifically referred to the rhinologist on the assumption that their headaches are due to sinus disease, this seldom proves to be the case. Certainly acute frontal sinusitis gives intense pain localized about the affected sinus and showing its characteristic periodicity. Pain is seldom so marked in the acute infection of other sinuses and when present may frequently be referred.

From the ethmoidal sinuses pain is frequently referred to the frontal area, between the eyes or to the parietal region.

From the maxillary sinuses, the pain is usually infra-orbital, but may be referred along the zygoma or be described as a diffuse toothache in most of the maxillary teeth of the affected side. Some patients, however, present with pain in one tooth only. Pain from the sphenoidal sinus is often referred to the vertex or to the occipital region. Alternatively it may be frontal or bitemporal or radiate widely over the mastoids and neck. In other cases, it is felt behind the eyes and it may give rise to a burning pain at the junction of hard and soft palate.

Pain arising from sinusitis is almost always aggravated by stooping and relieved by steam inhalations. That arising from the sphenoid sinus is apt to be worse at night. It is typically severe and deep-seated. Whilst a wide variety of pains and headaches have

occur alone. Should this be for the first time and without obvious provocation, or should it continue despite nitroglycerine, then diagnosis can be difficult. The difficulty may be increased by the resting ECG being normal. Exercise tests that would probably show some characteristic abnormality are likely to be too hazardous.

Ocular disorders

Only about 4 per cent of headaches are associated with ocular disorders. Eye strain produced by efforts in accommodation may give rise to local discomfort and frontal headache generally associated with close work. This occurs in ocular muscle imbalance or through refractive error, especially in hypermetropes.

In acute iritis and in acute glaucoma pain is experienced chiefly in the eye, but may spread over the area supplied by the ophthalmic division of the trigeminal nerve. The associated visual impairment will indicate the cause.

Glossodynia

Beyond its label this pain in the tongue tends to remain an enigma, except when due to local irritation, apthous lesion, anaemia or gonadal hormone involution. With macrocytic anaemia the tongue is red; with iron deficiency states, pallid and coated white. Gonadal deficiency also gives atrophy of the papillae and desquamation of the surface epithelium. Ulceration is a frequent complication unless the condition is relieved by appropriate hormone therapy.

Chronic pain in the tongue without physical signs must be suspected to be psychogenic; especially if it does not respect anatomical boundaries and does not interfere with eating or sleeping, or if the patient is post-menopausal.

Muscle and joint pain

Myofascial triggers

Under conditions not yet understood, muscles may develop a myofascial trigger which, when stimulated by stretching, forceful contraction, pressure or thermal change, can elicit pain. The pain may be local but is more commonly referred, hence its location does not identify its source. Such pain has a dull aching quality that is prone to vary in intensity from day to day. Spontaneous remissions may occur.

In a classic paper, Travell and Rinzler (1952) showed that many spatial patterns of pain are associated with such trigger points, the nature of which seems to vary from fibrous nodules to mere areas of abnormal physiological activity. Pressure upon them, however, evokes pain felt not only locally but over the whole area of reference (*Figure 18.11*).

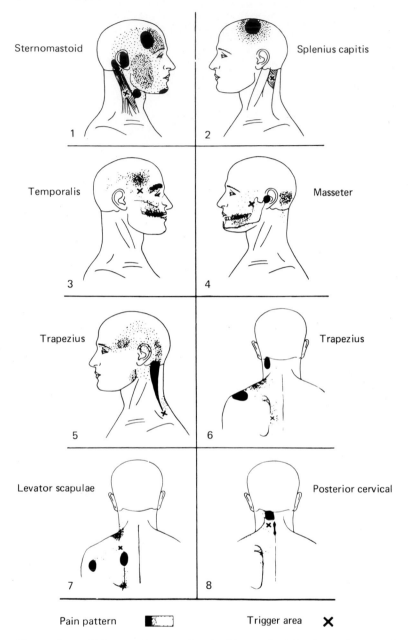

Sternomastoid

1

Splenius capitis

2

Temporalis

3

Masseter

4

Trapezius

5

Trapezius

6

Levator scapulae

7

Posterior cervical

8

Pain pattern ▨▭   Trigger area ✕

Figure 18.11   Trigger points associated with myofascial pain syndromes of the head and neck. (After Treavell and Rinzler, 1952)

    Short-acting local anaesthetic injection of such a trigger point often produces relief of pain that may last days, weeks or even months. Similarly brief intense stimulation of the trigger area by dry needling or transcutaneous electrical stimulation may have the same effect. This so-called 'hyper-stimulation analgesia' resembles the effects of acupuncture.

Painful myospasm

Muscle spasm often occurs reflexly to provide protective splinting to a damaged intervertebral or jaw joint. Similarly occlusal disharmony may result in muscle spasm. Such muscle spasm gives rise to both pain and dysfunction. The pain results from ischaemic irritation of intramuscular perivascular plexuses, the dysfunction from muscle shortening. This painful myospasm often occurs in a masticatory muscle and may be secondary to another source of deep pain within the trigeminal area.

Cervical myalgia

Headache, almost regardless of its source, is apt to give reflex spasm of the posterior cervical muscles, particularly the trapezius. Anxiety and emotional tension are especially provocative and it not uncommonly supervenes in chronic sinusitis. Prolonged effect leads to the formation of spastic nodules in the muscles concerned which thus become tender trigger points and a source of secondary pain. Irrespective of other aetiology the presence of cervical myalgia must be looked for in headache. It may be an important factor in the production of a vicious cycle of headache— spasm—headache and hence the persistence of headache despite the removal of its primary cause.

Radiant heat and massage will often suffice for relief although established trigger points may require appropriate measures.

Temporo–mandibular joint disorders

The pain receptors associated with the jaw joint are confined to the joint capsule, the intra-articular retrodiscal pad of fat and the articular surfaces. Whilst clinicians have long been aware of pain produced by disordered articular surfaces, they have been met by the denial, by anatomists, of any nerve supply to the articular surface of any joint. Such nerves exist, however, and penetrate to the articular cartilage (Miller and Kasahara, 1963). Pain often arises from capsular stresses, largely evoked by a combination of dental malocclusion, emotional tension, and spasm of masticatory muscles. Whilst arthritic change may occur as part of some general condition, most cases are due to some intra-oral cause and are relieved by its correction.

Symptoms commonly arise in young women with a full dentition. Here, pain seems mostly due to changes in occlusion during the formative years, acquired faulty habits of mastication, or occlusal defect associated with incomplete eruption of the third molar. Alternatively, symptoms may arise in middle age when loss of molar teeth results in loss of vertical dimension, over-closure of bite, alteration of the head of the mandible in the articular fossa and diminution of the posterior joint space. In others, badly designed dentures may give trouble by increased vertical dimension or incorrect occlusion giving displacement on closure.

In 80 per cent of these patients such symptoms as pain about the joint accentuated by jaw movement, clicking, locking or trismus and tenderness over the joint, point obviously to a jaw joint disorder. In the remaining 20 per cent, however, joint symptoms may be wholly lacking, the symptoms being limited to pain in or about the

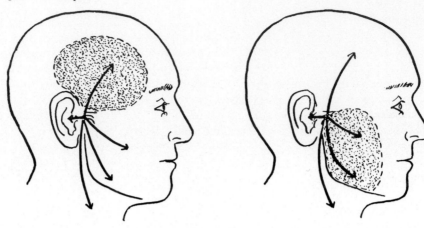

Figure 18.12   Diagrams to show the variable distribution of pain in temporo–mandibular joint disorder. In addition to pain radiating to ear, temple, maxilla, mandible or neck, there may be painful reflex spasm of either temporal or masseter muscle (shaded areas). Similar pain from muscle spasm may occur in dental disorder and in bruxism

ear (Costen's syndrome) or spreading widely over the face. These patterns of pain vary enormously, the pain spreading up to the temple, forwards along the maxilla or mandible, or downwards into the neck. This unusual radiation of pain is due to reflex spasm, especially of the temporal or masseteric muscles (*Figure 18.12*).

Every case of cervico–facial pain not otherwise accountable, must be examined to exclude jaw joint dysfunction. Particular heed is paid to:

(1) The range of movement of the mandible.
(2) The relation of clicks and/or pain to jaw movement.
(3) The teeth present and the dental spaces.
(4) The type of occlusion and bite (in over-closure, there is initial incisor contact before the molars meet).
(5) Radiographs of the jaw joints. Trans-cranial, lateral, oblique views are taken, with the jaws both wide open and closed. Such x-rays may reveal osteoarthritis by roughened articular surfaces or lipping; or show changes in joint shape related to occlusal function.

There are four main syndromes of masticatory pain:

(1) Jaw joint arthropathy
Joint symptoms such as clicking or locking on chewing or talking precede pain generally by months. Later secondary referred pain may occur and the widespread character of masticatory pain comes to dominate and obscure the picture.

(2) Jaw joint pain–dysfunction syndrome
Here the sudden onset of painful jaw movement is accompanied by myospasm of the masticatory muscles and the clinical picture depends on which muscles are in spasm. With unilateral spasm of the elevator muscles, mouth-opening becomes restricted and the jaw deviates to the painful side. Occlusal derangements are often important.

Where loss of molars has induced over-closure, prosthetic correction to raise molar occlusion to the level of incisor contact prevents retrusive condylar displacement. If normal occlusion can be restored so that the teeth grind freely in all directions without locking or bumping, pain is rapidly relieved. The vast majority of jaw joint disorders can be relieved by suitable dental measures. Perhaps 5 per cent require joint surgery—meniscectomy or condylectomy.

(3) Masticatory myalgia
Pain from some other source within the trigeminal area may induce painful spasm of the masticatory muscles and induce discomfort on chewing or other jaw movement. Thus this condition resembles the above except that a history of the initial primary pain will be absent.

(4) Myofascial triggers giving pain about the jaw joint
Such triggers are generally found in the sternomastoid. A history of neck complaint preceding pain in the jaw joint area (or ear) is important. Local anaesthetic block to the sterno–mastoid trigger will provide diagnostic relief.

Bruxism

This interesting and not uncommon dysfunction of the temporo–mandibular joint is produced by habitual and constant grinding of the teeth that proceeds even during sleep. The constant grinding produces the characteristic and marked attrition of the opposing dental surfaces. The result is loss of vertical dimension and posterior displacement of the condylar head and thus features of temporo–mandibular joint disorder. Bruxism must be suspected if the pain is more severe in the morning or awakens the patient at night. Ward finds the commonest cause of bruxism to be intestinal irritation, especially worms.

Temporo-mandibular pain from sexual play
This variety of articular pain is generally bilateral and almost confined to young women in late adolescence. Prolonged and excessive tongue protrusion in deep kissing, clumsily performed, results in unusual compression of the fat pad behind the jaw joint, with mechanical irritation of its rich supply of pain fibres. Treatment here requires nothing beyond simple analgesics, local procaine infiltration of the fat pad and suitable instruction in the art of osculation.

Vascular pain

Episodic, painful distension of the facial vessels is responsible for facial pain of an entirely different character from the neuralgias. The anatomical patterns assumed by this type of pain become understandable only when related to the arterial distribution and not to the neurological dermatomes of the face. These patterns vary, for they can extend over the entire distribution of the external carotid artery, or be limited to a single division of one branch (*Figure 18.13*).

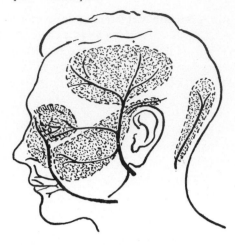

Figure 18.13 Diagram to show the principal sites of vascular pain and their relation to the superficial arteries of the head. (After Wyke)

   In the past, failure to recognize the primary vascular source of pain has led to a great variety of named syndromes by clinicians working in different fields. These syndromes have been variously designated, and are still known as:

> Sphenopalatine neuralgia
> Sluder's lower-half headache
> Ciliary neuralgia
> Vidian neuralgia
> Petrosal neuralgia
> Histamine cephalgia
> Cluster headaches
> Autonomic faciocephalgia

   These syndromes vary in detail, and are not entirely synonymous, but all seem embraced by the single term, 'periodic migrainous neuralgia'.

Periodic migrainous neuralgia

Although little-known, this syndrome is easily recognized. The patient is most often a young or middle-aged man whose history is characteristic. He is subject to recurring, often nocturnal, paroxysms of intense throbbing pain in or about the eye, spreading to the temple or side of the face. The pain, always strictly unilateral, is clearly defined and consistent in the individual. These paroxysms of pain last from half an hour to two hours, and recur daily, generally with the regularity of an alarm clock, commonly at about 2 a.m. After recurring once or even several times in 24 h for some weeks, there is sudden freedom, seldom lasting less than six months, sometimes much longer. Wide radiation of the pain over the scalp to behind the ear and even into the neck is common. Sooner or later these attacks recur, and they often show a seasonal incidence.
   Always violent in its intensity, the pain is intolerable when lying down and the patient is driven to pace the room. During the attack, the affected eye is commonly red

and watering and the nose is blocked on the same side. Later, a copious watery rhinorrhoea often heralds regression of pain.

During an attack, the face is often flushed on the affected side, the temporal arteries being dilated and tender. Pain can temporarily be relieved by ipsilateral carotid compression. Occasionally, there is a ptosis and hyperhydrosis on the affected side.

Treatment

Ergotamine tartrate is highly effective, more so than in migraine. It is given in customary dosage, either by mouth or by self-injection, twice or thrice daily or on retiring in purely nocturnal cases. Ergotamine is continued for the average duration of each bout or until there is no relapse on withdrawal. Treatment is then suspended until the next bout begins.

Some cases, however, are resistant to ergotamine, but will generally respond to methysergide (Deseril), given prophylactically in divided doses totalling 6–12 mg daily. Unfortunately, however, methysergide has recently been inculpated in the development of retroperitoneal fibrosis. Whilst not absolutely contraindicated, its use is now justified only when the condition is refractory to other treatments and the patient's distress warrants the risk involved.

Surgical treatment

Both the rationale and efficacy of surgery remain subject to dispute, for the long periods of spontaneous remission render assessment of operative results difficult.

Petrosal neurectomy and sphenopalatine ganglionectomy with resection of the maxillary artery have both proved remarkably effective at least for long periods of time. This parasympathetic pathway provides not only the vasodilator impulses but probably also the afferent pain pathway for pain impulses from superficial blood vessels.

Temporal arteritis

Although the name suggests a localized pathology, this disorder is now recognized to be a generalized disease of the arteries of the head and neck. The ophthalmic and retinal arteries are particularly liable to attack. Pathologically, it is a granulomatous arteritis characterized by disintegration of the internal elastic lamina and chronic inflammatory cellular infiltration of the tunica media. This process may produce gradual arterial occlusion and/or thrombosis on which the clinical effects depend.

Almost confined to the elderly, it is a self-limiting disorder. It burns itself out in a few months but is apt to leave blindness in its wake.

Initial pain and tenderness generally occur in the scalp, spreading to involve the face and jaws. The pain is constant, often with sharp exacerbations or aggravation by chewing. This pain, interfering with sleep and accompanied by general malaise, precedes the development of headaches by several weeks. The superficial temporal arteries are generally swollen, nodular and tender with diminished pulsation.

Blindness in one or both eyes has occurred in over 50 per cent cases. Due to ischaemia of the retina or optic nerve, it is frequently abrupt and may precede other signs, but generally occurs one to three months later.

The carotico–vertebral and cerebral arteries are frequently involved but considerable stenosis can occur here without symptoms. Cerebral symptoms occur only when the vascular supply is reduced to a critical level.

Diagnosis may be suspected by the nature of the pain and the appearance of the temporal artery. It is confirmed by arterial biopsy which may be conclusive even when the vessels appear clinically normal. The ever-present risk of blindness forbids waiting for the result of arterial biopsy. Given a high ESR, steroids (40–60 mg prednisolone daily) should be started immediately and continued for six months in lower maintenance dosage. Vision is protected by steroid therapy started prior to the onset of visual symptoms. Head and facial pains subside. Biopsy of the temporal arteries still remains essential for pathological proof.

Atypical facial neuralgia

When the definitive pathological entities so far considered have been eliminated, there remain patients whose pain defies analysis and remains intractable to analgesics or other therapeutic measures such as nerve blocks, sinus operations, dental interventions or peripheral neurectomies.

This mixed collection comprises the atypical facial neuralgias, the characteristics of which may be listed as follows:

(1) The pain is deep. It is frequently described in vivid terms that suggest painful pressure, or merely as dull, aching, gripping, boring, throbbing, burning, etc.
(2) It tends to be most evident about the maxillary region, but shows no limitation to any area supplied by a single nerve.
(3) The pain tends to be continuously present for weeks, months or years, but severe exacerbations may occur.
(4) External stimuli, movements or other activities of the patient neither precipitate nor aggravate the pain.
(5) The pain may be unilateral, but with time it tends to spread across the midline.

These patients are commonly women, middle-aged, edentulous and haggard. As their condition is ill-understood and refractory it is facile to label them neurotic. Certainly there are a proportion who reveal characteristics of depressive psychosis with evident agitation, and their sleep characteristically disturbed. Others seem but poorly adjusted to life, with poor records of work or social relationship, and the onset of pain can perhaps be related to an intense emotional conflict. Such patients may benefit from psychiatric assistance and antidepressive drugs.

In most cases, however, the experienced observer is left with an impression of some pathophysiological form of disturbance, however much this may defy definition. These patients go from clinic to clinic, seeking relief that does not come. They will submit readily enough to any measures suggested, although their experience denies them much hope of relief.

It is all too easy for the surgeon to consider some form of neurectomy, sensory or autonomic, but for the patient's sake the temptation is to be resisted. An induced anaesthesia dolorosa will add merely another burden to their miserable lives in which drug addiction too commonly occurs.

All the doctor can offer is oft-repeated, sympathetic discussion of their complaint which may carry them along. Ultimately, this strange condition, after resisting every form of treatment, may sometimes clear spontaneously.

Acupuncture

Acupuncture represents the distillation of 5000 years of empirical observation by the Chinese.

The inquiring Western medical mind is at first baffled and appalled by a bizarre profusion of acupuncture points associated with an ancient conceptual system of meridians which carry Yin (spirits) and Yang (blood). It must, however, be remembered that the system of 12 bilateral meridians running from the chest to the distal parts of the limbs or head was developed many centuries before there was any true anatomical or physiological knowledge. Viewed simply as a system of geographical body notation to locate hundreds of possible acupuncture points, it remains superb.

Classical Chinese acupuncture with its listed combinations for using different spots in different diseases and a variety of times, places, suns and moons for their application, is a remarkable collection of antique mythology. Present medical interest has at least established that despite the damage wrought by quacks prepared to capitalize on human suffering, acupuncture can no longer be dismissed as propaganda, hypnosis or twaddle.

If relevant acupuncture points are organized upon a basis of pain syndromes, their number is fairly small. Workers in modern pain clinics can function effectively using about 50 points. At these loci, fine needles are inserted most often for about 2 cm, after which they may be twirled, vibrated or stimulated electronically.

By such means, and not only among the Chinese, a state of profound analgesia has frequently been induced so that even major surgery can be carried out in some totally awake patients who may chat amiably with the doctor throughout the operation.

The diverse location of acupuncture needles to induce analgesia is perplexing in terms of our traditional concepts of a discrete segmental organization of the nervous system. Melzack, Stillwell and Fox (1977) think it conceivable that acupuncture analgesia is a special case of hyperstimulation analgesia. They suggest that trigger points and acupuncture points, although discovered independently and labelled differently, represent the same phenomenon. They believe that stimulation of either point could bring increased input to the central biasing mechanism in the brain-stem reticular formation which would close the gates to inputs from selected body areas.

As yet, however, we have but fragmentary knowledge of acupuncture analgesia and many questions remain unanswered. It is no panacea and as yet direct comparison with well-established methods is impracticable. Nevertheless, acupuncture promises to find a place in the treatment of some painful musculo–skeletal disorders, psychosomatic diseases, in post-operative pain and in dentistry. The researches it has stimulated seem likely to provide clues about pain mechanisms generally.

References

Alling, C. C. (1968). *Facial Pain.* Philadelphia; Lea and Febiger

Asherson, N. (1957) *Journal of Laryngology and Otology,* **71,** 453

Beaver, D. L. (1967). *Journal of Neurosurgery,* **26,** 138

Behrman, S. (1949). *British Dental Journal,* **86,** 197

Burton, C. (1976). *Postgraduate Medicine,* **59,** 105

Campbell, J. (1955). *Dental Practitioner,* **5,** 175

Cohen, H. (1937). *Journal of Laryngology and Otology,* **42,** 527

Dudley Hart, F. (1974). *Treatment of Chronic Pain.* Lancaster; Medical and Technical Publishing Co.

Engel, G. L. (1959). *American Journal of Medicine,* **26,** 899

Erickson, T. C. (1936). *Archives of Neurology and Psychiatry,* **35,** 1070

Freidman, A. P. (1964). *Oral Surgery,* **18,** 730

Gerson, G. R., Jones, R. B. and Luscombe, D. K. (1977). *Postgraduate Medical Journal,* **53** (Suppl 4), 104

Glaser, M. A. and Beerman, H. A. (1938). *Archives of Internal Medicine,* **61,** 172

Godtfredson, E. (1947). *Proceedings of the Royal Society of Medicine,* **40,** 131

Golding-Wood, P. H. (1962). *Journal of Laryngology and Otology,* **76,** 683

Gordon, G. (Ed.) (1977). 'Somatic and Visceral Sensory Mechanisms', *British Medical Bulletin,* **3,** No. 2

Hankey, G. J. (1962). *Proceedings of the Royal Society of Medicine,* **55,** 787

Hansen, R. M. (1968). *Laryngoscope,* **78,** 1164

Hilding, A. C. (1943). *Annals of Otology, Rhinology & Laryngology, St. Louis,* **52,** 817

Holmes, T. H., Goodell, H., Wolff, S. and Wolff, H. G. (1960). *The Nose.* Springfield, Ill: Thomas

Hutchins, H. C. and Reynolds, O. E. (1947). *Journal of Dental Research,* **26,** 3

Jefferson, G. (1938). *British Journal of Surgery,* **26,** 267

Kenyon, F. E. (1976). *British Journal of Psychiatry,* **129,** 1

Kerr, F. W. L. (1967). *Journal of Neurosurgery,* **26,** 151

Kersley, J. A. (1965). *Journal of Laryngology and Otology,* **79,** 734

Knight, G. (1963). *Lancet,* **1,** 6

Knighton, R. S. and Dumke, P. R. (1966). *Pain.* Boston; Little, Brown and Co.

McAuliffe, G. W., Goodell, H. and Wolff, H. G.

(1945). *Association for Research into Nervous and Mental Diseases, Research Publications,* **23,** 185

Melzack, R. (1973). *The Puzzle of Pain.* London; Penguin Education

Melzack, R. (1975). *Pain,* **1,** 357

Melzack, R., Stillwell, D. M. and Fox, E. J. (1977). *Pain,* **3,** 3

Melzack, R. and Wall, P. D. (1965). *Science,* **150,** 971

Miller, M. R. and Kasahara, M. (1963). *Anatomical Record,* **145,** 13

Mollison, W. M. (1944). *Proceedings of the Royal Society of Medicine,* **37,** 179

Nathan, P. W. (1976). *Brain,* **99,** 123

Noordenbos, W. (1968). In *Pain.* Ed. by Soulaviac, A., Cahn, J., and Charpentier, J. London and New York; Academic Press

Penman, J. (1954). *Lancet,* **1,** 633

Pilling, L. F., Brannick, T. L. and Swenson, W. M. (1967). *Canadian Medical Association Journal,* **97,** 387

Shaheen, O. H. (1963). *Annals of Otology, Rhinology and Laryngology, St. Louis,* **72,** 873

Sluder, G. (1927). *Nasal Neurology, Headaches, and Eye Disorders.* London; Kimpton

Sternbach, R. A. (1975). *International Journal of Psychiatric Medicine,* **6,** 63

Stookey, B. and Ransohoff, J. (1959). *Trigeminal Neuralgia.* Springfield, Ill; Thomas

Sweet, W. H. and Wepsie, J. G. (1974). *Journal of Neurosurgery,* **39,** 143

Szasz, T. S. (1957). *Pain and Pleasure: A Study of Bodily Feelings.* New York; Basic Books

Taylor, J. C. (1966). *Journal of Neurology, Neurosurgery and Psychiatry,* **29,** 478

Tinn, C. A. (1947). *British Dental Journal,* **82,** 189

Travell, J. and Rinzler, S. H. (1952). *Postgraduate Medicine,* **11,** 425

Wall, P. D. and Taub, A. (1962). *Journal of Neurophysiology,* **25,** 110

Warren, F. Z. (1976). *Handbook of Medical Acupuncture.* New York; Van Nostrand Reinhold Co.

White, J. C. and Sweet, W. H. (1969). *Pain and the Neurosurgeon. A forty-year Experience.* Springfield, Illinois; Thomas

Wilson, C. P. and McAlpine, D. (1946). *Proceedings of the Royal Society of Medicine,* **40,** 82

Wolff, H. G. (1963). *Headache and other Head Pain* (2nd Ed.) London; Oxford University Press

Wyke, B. D. (1968). *British Journal of Hospital Medicine,* **1,** 46

19 Trans-ethmoidal hypophysectomy
Stephen H Richards

Historical

The pituitary gland may be removed by a trans-cranial or by an extra-cranial route. In the extra-cranial approach the pituitary fossa is entered from below and of necessity the surgeon has to operate through the sphenoid sinus. There are, however, many different ways in which the sphenoid sinus may be entered and these various routes, together with their inventors, are listed in *Table 19.1*.

Table 19.1

Technique	Inventor
Trans-nasal	Schloffer (1907)
	Kocher (1909)
	MacBeth (1961)
Sublabial trans-septal	Cushing (1912)
Trans-septal	Hirsch (1911)
	Cushing
	Bateman (1963)
Trans-palatal	Preysing
Trans-ethmoidal	Chiari (1912)
	Nager (1940)
	Angell-James (1967)
Trans-antral	Hamberger (1960)

Schloffer (1907) was the first to perform a trans-sphenoidal removal of a pituitary tumour. In order to gain access he split the nose in the midline and then proceeded to remove the whole of the nasal septum and the turbinates (excenteration nasi). This approach was modified by Kocher (1909) who, after splitting the nose in the midline, proceeded to carry out a submucous resection of the nasal septum thereby gaining access to the rostrum and to the sphenoid sinus. Both the above methods gave rise to disfuguring nasal scars which were avoided by Cushing (1912). He used a sublabial route to gain access to the nasal septum which he then removed submucosally as in Kocher's method.

Hirsch (1911) also approached the sphenoid sinus through the nasal septum but used a purely endonasal incision as described by Killian for the submucous resection operation. The trans-nasal route was later revived by Macbeth (1961) who avoided disfigurement by raising the nasal skeleton as an osteoplastic flap. The trans-septal route was used by Bateman (1963) who used the trans-septal approach in association with the trans-ethmoidal.

Preysing approached the septum through the hard palate and this route was at first adopted by Nager (1940). These trans-nasal and trans-septal procedures have the advantage of keeping the surgeon strictly in the midline and the operation is therefore less likely to endanger laterally-placed structures such as the oculomotor nerves and the cavernous sinuses. Also they afford a good view of the diaphragma sellae and of any supra-sellar extension of the tumour. The distance from the pituitary gland, however, is considerable and the surgeon has to operate through a long narrow tunnel.

In 1912 Chiari described the trans-ethmoidal approach through an external ethmoid incision and this approach gives a much wider access by a shorter route. It was later adopted and perfected by Nager (1940) and by Angell-James (1967) and is the approach most commonly used by present-day hypophyseal surgeons (Williams, 1974; Dalton, 1974; Richards, Thomas and Kilby, 1974).

The trans-antral route was practised and advocated by Hamberger *et al.* (1960). The antrum was entered through a sublabial antrotomy and the sphenoid sinus approached by removing the ethmoid cells through the antrum. Although giving a good wide access to the pituitary fossa, the route is a long one requiring a good deal of extra-sphenoid surgery and bleeding is often severe.

From 1909 to 1935 Harvey Cushing performed no less than 171 trans-sphenoidal hypophysectomies with considerable success and a low mortality. He then however gave up the trans-sphenoidal operation in favour of the trans-frontal operation and this route has since been favoured by neurosurgeons. Cairns (1936) and Henderson (1939) however advocated the continued use of the trans-sphenoidal operation in certain cases. The advantage of the trans-frontal route is that it enables the surgeon to deal more directly with a large supra-sellar extension of the tumour. Also it is less likely to lead to such complications as meningitis and CSF rhinorrhoea. It is however a much more formidable procedure for the patient and carries the extra risk of an intracranial operation. The main disadvantage is that the pituitary fossa itself is not directly visible by this route and it is not possible to deal adequately with extensions of the tumour into the sphenoid sinus or into the clivus (*Figure 19.2*). It remains nevertheless the operation of choice in those patients who have a large supra-sellar tumour.

Indications for operation

During the past 25 years the indications for hypophysectomy have undergone a considerable change. Previously, partial removal of the gland in order to relieve the pressure effects of a pituitary tumour was all that was possible or desirable. Total removal of the gland with a view to reversing endocrine disorders such as acromegaly and Cushing's disease would almost certainly have resulted in the death of the patient from steroid deficiency. During the decade 1950 to 1960 the development of systemic

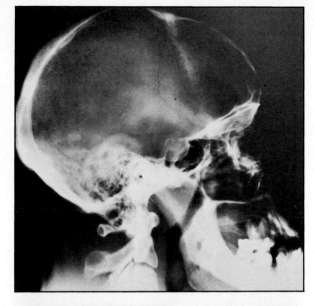

Figure 19.1 Lateral radiograph of skull in patient with acromegaly showing the protruding jaw and prominent supra-orbital ridges

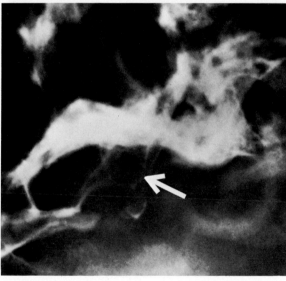

Figure 19.2 Same patient as *Figure 19.1* showing enlarged pituitary fossa with bone erosion in the clivus due to extension of the tumour (marked with arrow)

steroids and of a versatile operating microscope made total hypophysectomy possible.

At the present time the indications for hypophysectomy are as follows:

Acromegaly

Some of the most consistent and gratifying results of hypophysectomy are obtained in this condition. Operation is indicated where there is clinical evidence of acromegaly and where the resting growth hormone level is 15 ng/100 ml or greater and which

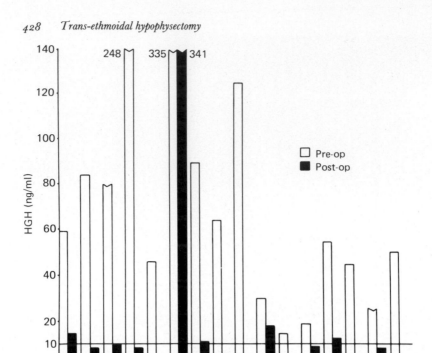

Figure 19.3   Fasting serum growth hormone levels in 16 acromegalics before and after trans-ethmoidal hypophysectomy

Table 19.2   Shoe size in eleven consecutive cases of acromegaly

Patient	Before operation	6 months or more after operation
BJ	7 Broad	6 Broad
SH	7 Broad	5½ Broad
VW	10 Broad	9½ Broad
UM	7 Broad	6½ Normal
IMD	6 Broad	5 Normal
MED	7 Broad	6 Broad
ES	7 Broad	6½ Broad
BW	9 Broad	8½ Broad
WS	10 Broad	9 Broad
EC	No change	
MM	6 Broad	5½ Broad
KS	9 Broad	9 Broad (now very loose)

does not suppress on taking 50 g of glucose by mouth. Even where the symptoms of the disease are mild, operation is indicated, otherwise the patient's life expectancy after the age of 30 is considerably diminished (Fraser, 1970).

Pre-operative skull x-rays show enlargement of the pituitary fossa and all cases should have a pre-operative pneumonencephalogram to exclude the presence of a supra-sellar extension. Provided such a supra-sellar extension is not excessively large it can be removed satisfactorily by the trans-sphenoidal approach as it tends to prolapse caudally once the main tumour mass in the fossa has been removed.

Following operation the growth hormone levels return to normal or near normal (*Figure 19.3*) and the clinical features are reversed (*Table 19.2*). Soft-tissue shrinkage occurs during the course of a few weeks or months but bone changes such as regression of the protruding jaw take many years and continue to improve for ten years or more. It is not yet possible to state whether the improvement is permanent, but in the author's series the patients who have had surgery ten years or more before the time of writing have remained in clinical remission and still have growth hormone levels which are within normal limits.

Cushing's disease

Hypophysectomy is indicated where biochemical and radiological investigations indicate that the disease is of pituitary rather than of suprarenal origin. To establish the diagnosis it is necessary to evaluate plasma cortisone levels, 24-h 17 ketosteroid output, circulating ACTH levels and to perform radiological studies of the adrenals and of the pituitary fossa. The pituitary fossa is usually radiologically normal and shows enlargement in only 10–20 per cent of cases (Salassa *et al.*, 1959).

After operation there is a dramatic improvement in the patient's appearance (*see Figure 19.4*) with loss of weight and a lowering of blood pressure. In the author's experience the number of non-respondents to surgery is larger than following hypophysectomy for acromegaly. This may be due to wrong diagnosis, failure to

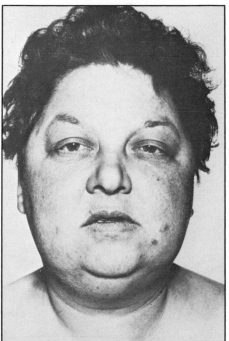 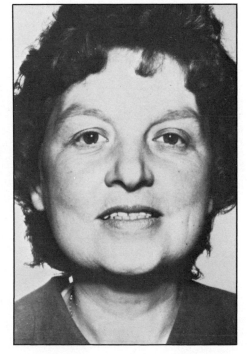

Figure 19.4   Patient with Cushing's disease before (left) and six months after (right) transethmoidal hypophysectomy

remove the complete gland or because there is an extra-sellar source of ACTH production. The removed gland does not in all instances contain the basophil adenoma but shows so-called Crooke's changes in the cells (Crooke, 1935).

Breast cancer

The initial enthusiasm for hypophysectomy in the treatment of advanced breast cancer has now waned but it is still employed in certain cases. Early workers in this field found that hypophysectomy gave temporary symptomatic relief to approximately two-thirds of all cases (Angell-James, 1967). In the author's series of patients, where results were assessed by an independent panel, only 15 per cent showed objective and measurable evidence of tumour regression. Furthermore, this occurred only in those cases where there was biochemical evidence of total hypophysectomy (*Table 19.3*). The life expectancy of these patients was not improved (Roberts, 1970).

Table 19.3   52 consecutive cases of hypophysectomy for breast cancer (Roberts, 1970)

	No. of cases	*No. of remissions*
Complete ablation	42	16
Incomplete ablation	10	0

Most surgeons, radiotherapists and oncologists have now accepted that the results of surgery for the relief of advanced breast cancer are not sufficiently superior to those of chemotherapy to justify the additional discomfort of operation. In the post-menopausal female with bony metastases, however, trans-ethmoidal hypophysectomy is still the most effective method of affording relief of pain but the surgeon should make every effort to ensure total removal of the gland.

Diabetic retinopathy

Many workers have demonstrated that hypophysectomy successfully halts the advance of diabetic retinopathy (Angell-James, 1967). The operation is indicated in those cases where there is a florid proliferative retinopathy which does not respond to other forms of therapy. Recent advances in photo-coagulation have however considerably reduced the number of cases for which hypophysectomy is required. Removal of the pituitary gland in severe diabetic subjects is not without its disadvantages in that they become liable to sudden and severe episodes of hypoglycaemia which are difficult to control.

Chromophobe tumours

Until the present decade it has been customary to treat these tumours conservatively and to embark on surgery only when pressure effects (usually those involving the optic pathways) become evident. At this stage the tumour would have been large with a substantial supra-sellar extension needing a trans-cranial approach for removal.

It is now becoming increasingly clear that chromophobe adenomas should be operated upon at an earlier stage for the following reasons. Firstly, it is relatively easy to effect complete removal of the tumour when it is small, whereas this is difficult and often impossible when it is large. Secondly, chromophobe tumours tend to expand suddenly, especially during pregnancy to produce a rapid onset of blindness (Falconer and Stafford-Bell, 1975). Thirdly, it is now recognized that these tumours are capable of producing endocrine changes, notably amenorrhoea and galactorrhoea in females (Forbes-Allbright syndrome) or impotence in males.

Since the assay of prolactin has been possible it has been recognized that some chromophobe tumours produce hyperprolactinaemia (Childs *et al.*, 1975). A patient with symptoms of diminished gonadal activity, radiological evidence of even minimal enlargement of the pituitary fossa and hyperprolactinaemia should probably have a surgical exploration of the pituitary gland by the trans-sphenoidal route. In these cases the tumour may be small and no more than 2 or 3 mm in diameter. When such a small adenoma is encountered it is clearly possible and desirable to remove it, leaving the major portion of the gland intact. This procedure is usually successful in restoring a normal menstrual cycle, reducing the circulating prolactin levels to normal, and in many instances, normal pregnancies have ensued (Dolman *et al.*, 1977).

Carcinoma of the prostate

Results of hypophysectomy for this condition have proved disappointing. Out of 14 cases treated, Angell-James (1967) found there was remission of disease in only two patients and in these two the period of remission did not exceed six months. Patients are usually referred for this operation only when stilboestrol therapy ceases to be effective, but when this stage is reached the tumour is apparently no longer capable of being restrained by hormonal measures.

Miscellaneous

In addition to the above, the trans-sphenoidal operation is a useful approach by which to explore unexplained radiological changes such as bone erosion in the region of the sella turcia. Such a procedure might be described as an 'exploratory sellotomy' and provides a relatively simple way of obtaining biopsy material. Miscellaneous conditions encountered by the author are: primary carcinoma of the pituitary; secondary carcinoma—it has been found that 18 per cent of pituitary glands removed for advanced breast cancer contain histological evidence of secondary deposits (Roberts, 1970); cysts of the pituitary gland; mucocoele of the sphenoid sinus.

Pre-operative assessment

The clinical and endocrine pre-operative evaluation of patients with acromegaly of Cushing's disease is complicated and the surgeon is well advised to work in close cooperation with an expert endocrinologist. The following investigations have a direct bearing on the operation and are therefore of interest to the surgeon.

Hormone assay
It is now possible to assay the circulating blood level of all seven pituitary hormones and some or all of these (according to the clinical condition) should be assayed pre-operatively. These investigations serve to confirm the diagnosis and to endorse the clinical indications for surgery. They also act as a base line to evaluate post-operative progress.

Skull radiographs
These are indicated to delineate the shape and size of the pituitary fossa.

Sinus radiographs
They should be taken in order to exclude the existence of a sinus infection. Such an infection would obviously increase the risk of meningitis and should be dealt with before trans-sphenoidal hypophysectomy is contemplated. Sinus radiographs are also useful to the surgeon in that they delineate the anatomy of the ethmoid and the sphenoid sinuses and alert the operator to aberrations of the normal anatomy in this region.

Pneumoencephalography
This should be undertaken in those cases where a supra-sellar extension of the pituitary tumour is suspected. In practice this means that most patients with acromegaly or who have a chromophobe adenoma require this investigation but that patients such as those with breast cancer or in Cushing's disease, where the gland is usually of normal size, do not. This investigation also gives useful information concerning the position of the optic chiasma (whether it is pre- or post-fixed), the position of the diaphragma sellae and the precise shape of the pituitary fossa and of the sphenoid sinus.

Photography
Pre-operative photographs in cases of Cushing's disease and acromegaly provide a useful record to which reference can be made when post-operative evaluation is undertaken. The same applies to visible neoplastic lesions when hypophysectomy is undertaken for advanced breast cancer.

The operation

The operation to be described is the trans-sphenoidal–trans-ethmoidal approach as practised by the author.

Preparation

In order to maintain the patient's circulating cortisone level over the period of the operation, 100 mg of hydrocortisone are injected 1 h before the patient comes to the operating theatre. At the same time the nose is painted with 25 per cent cocaine paste containing supra-renal extract (Mosher's Paste). This serves to shrink the nasal mucosa and decrease the vascularity of this region during surgery. A further application of the same paste is made when anaesthesia has been induced. Haemorrhage during the operation may be sudden and severe and it is important that provision for at least two units of cross-matched blood should be readily available.

Anaesthesia

To give a detailed description of anaesthesia for hypophsectomy is outside the scope of this article but some factors having a direct bearing on the quality of the operation need to be mentioned. Firstly, the technical problems are such that the services of a skilled and experienced anaesthetist should be sought. Secondly, airway problems during surgery are the same as those encountered in nasal surgery and require the use of a cuffed endotracheal tube and of a pharyngeal pack. The tube should be placed in the left side of the mouth so as to interfere as little as possible with the surgeon's instrumentation. Thirdly, profound hypotension during the intra-sellar part of the operation is highly desirable and contributes materially towards the precision of the dissection and to the completeness of the hypophysectomy. In order to monitor the circulatory pressures during this extreme hypotensive period it is desirable that a venous catheter and an arterial line should be installed in order to record central venous pressure and arterial pressure respectively.

The patient is placed in the supine position and the operating table is tilted some 15 degrees into the reverse Trendelenburg position. In order to protect the cornea of the right eye from damage, the upper and lower lids are apposed using one silk suture. While surgery for approach to the pituitary is in progress an assistant proceeds simultaneously to remove muscle and fascia lata from the outer aspect of the right thigh for use later as an autograft in the pituitary fossa.

Incision

A right external ethmoidectomy incision is made and this is extended downwards for approximately 1 cm beyond the point where the usual classic incision ends. This extension allows a more liberal removal of bone in the region of the naso–lacrimal duct and this in turn allows the surgeon to align his visual axis so that he can look more directly into the hypophyseal fossa from below. Bleeding is considerable and in order to facilitate localization and clipping of the responsible vessels it is advisable to mobilize the periosteum immediately after making the initial incision.

The approach

The lacrimal sac is located and retracted laterally. The periosteum is then separated from the orbital plate of the ethmoid bone and retracted by means of a malleable spatula retractor. During this manoeuvre the anterior ethmoid artery becomes visible and is coagulated. Bone removal is then carried out as for an external ethmoidectomy, the initial entry being made by means of a gouge through the middle of the lacrimal fossa where the bone is thinnest. For reasons previously mentioned the removal of the frontal process of the maxilla is extended downwards to within a few millimetres of the pyriform aperture and care is taken to avoid damage to the naso–lacrimal duct.

The ethmoid air-cells are then removed using Luc's or Henckel's forceps. Great care is taken superiorly to avoid fracturing the floor of the anterior cranial fossa. Using the anterior ethmoidal artery as a guide final bone removal of the superior ethmoid air-cells is effected by Hajek's punch forceps, ensuring that the bite of the forceps is parallel to the plane of the anterior fossa floor. It is of interest that the ethmoidal and sphenoidal air-cells in acromegalic patients show considerable mucosal thickening which has frequently progressed to the point of frank polyposis. After removal of the ethmoidal air-cells, the anterior two-thirds of the middle turbinate are excised using a turbinectomy scissors and Luc's forceps. This improves visual access and does not appear to cause any harmful side effects other than transitory and minimal post-operative crusting.

In order to afford access to the left sphenoidal sinus the posterior part of the bony nasal septum is now removed. A gouge of moderately large size is driven through the bony septum and both layers of mucosa at a position approximately 2 cm in front of the posterior border. The posterior and upper part of the septum is removed and the surgeon is then afforded a good view of the anterior surface of the sphenoid sinus.

This is entered with care to avoid damaging the roof of the sinus which may be considerably expanded or even dehiscent in cases where there is a large pituitary tumour. The intersphenoid septum is removed and its attachment, being usually in the midline posteriorly and above, forms a good guide to the surgeon as to the exact position of the midline. The removal of the anterior wall is extended laterally and upwards to the limits of the sinus and the floor of the sphenoid sinus is then partially removed using a dental drill (with a fine tapered handle) through the right nostril. If the sphenoid sinus is unusually small, surgical access may be improved by enlarging the sinus backwards into the clivus thereby exposing the larger part of the floor of the pituitary fossa. At this stage it is important that the surgeon should check his bearings by a clear identification of the bulge of the pituitary fossa into the roof of the sphenoid sinus and by identifying the position of the midline.

Such anatomical variations as the presence of a large posterior ethmoidal cell, extreme deflection or absence of the intersinus septum, or the presence of an abnormally small sphenoid sinus are relatively common and the surgeon may need to refer to pre-operative radiographs of this region before proceeding further. If all else fails then an image intensifier should be brought into use so that the surgeon can check the position of his instruments by reference to the screen of the intensifier.

Exposure of the gland

At this stage Ferris–Smith's self-retaining retractor is inserted and the operating microscope brought into use (with F 300 mm objective). Using a slim-shafted dental drill through the right nasal cavity the bony floor of the pituitary fossa is gradually burred away so as to expose the dura as far as the cavernous sinuses laterally and to the limits of the sphenoid sinus antero–posteriorly. Great care is required to prevent

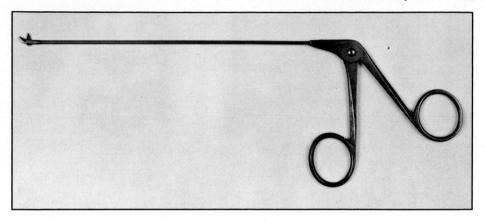

Figure 19.5 Upward cutting alligator micro-scissors used by the author for cutting the dura whilst fashioning the anterior dural flap

trauma to the superior and inferior intercavernous sinuses. Before any piece of bone is removed it should first be carefully separated from the underlying dura by means of a blunt dissector.

To enter the fossa a small transverse incision is made in the dura with a fine sickle knife or micro-scissors at a point slightly behind the centre of the exposed dura and just in front of the inferior (posterior) intercavernous sinus. As soon as glandular or tumour tissue is apparent a fine curved (Angell-James No. 1) dissector is inserted so as to free the anterior and inferior aspects of the gland from the dura. Using a fine alligator scissors (*Figure 19.5*) it is now possible to extend the incision forwards and laterally so as to form a U-shaped dural flap which is hinged antero–superiorly. This is retracted forward by means of a fine silk stay-suture. The use of diathermy for incising the dura is now avoided by the author because coagulation causes partial fusion of the dura and the underlying glandular tissue and makes it more difficult to establish the correct plane for dissection. Also it is possible to attain a greater degree of precision and more easily avoid damage to the cavernous and intercavernous sinuses by using the sickle knife and the alligator scissors.

Removal of gland

Before removal of the hypophysis is attempted, the gland is first mobilized using blunt, suitably curved Angell-James dissectors (*see Figures 19.6* and *19.7*). These are gently inserted in turn between the gland and the dura and moved around the gland taking care that the dissection is performed by the side or heel of the instrument, rather than the tip. This helps to guard against penetration of the cavernous sinuses or inadvertently 'hooking' adjacent structures. After the lateral lobes have been mobilized (and it must be remembered that there is often considerable lateral extension of these where a tumour is present) the gland is dissected away from the diaphragma sellae. In so doing, the subarachnoid space is usually entered resulting in a free flow of cerebrospinal fluid.

At this stage the stalk can be identified and deliberately divided with a sickle knife or upturned scissors in about 50 per cent of cases. Removal of the gland should not be

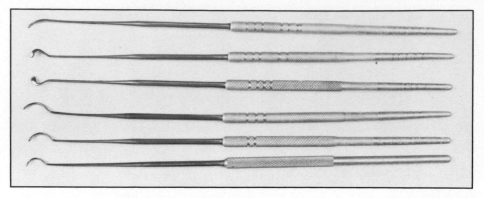

Figure 19.6   Angell-James dissectors for hypophysectomy. Note that the instruments are conveniently labelled by parallel grooves cut into the shaft

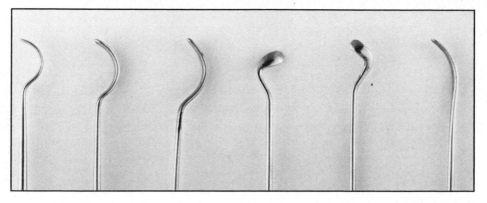

Figure 19.7   Shows an enlarged view of the tips of the Angell-James instruments shown in *Figure 19.6*

attempted until mobilization is as complete as possible because the presence of the hypophysis in the fossa is of great help in the control of bleeding which might otherwise be considerable. In those cases where the gland is of normal size, or is only slightly enlarged it may be 'delivered' complete using the blunt dissectors. Where there is a large tumour present, however, removal is then piecemeal by means of an Angell-James grasping forceps (Angell-James, 1967).

Final stages

When the main mass has been removed, the fossa is inspected for small remnants of glandular tissue. These are most likely to be found in the lateral recesses of the fossa, or attached to the diaphragma sellae immediately behind the hypophyseal stalk. If bleeding is severe this can be controlled by small pieces of lint dipped in 1:1000 adrenaline. When the surgeon is satisfied that all pituitary tissue has been removed the fossa is packed with a piece of muscle which has a volume slightly larger than that of the removed gland. This is held in position by a silk dural suture which apposes the edges of the incision. Since adopting this dural suture technique we have been able to reduce to zero our incidences of post-operative CSF rhinorrhoea and of post-operative meningitis. A piece of fascia lata is now laid over the dural suture line followed by a layer of gelatine foam. The sphenoid sinus and the posterior ethmoidal air-cells are then packed with muscle homograft obtained from the thigh. Subsequently, the right nasal cavity is packed with half-inch ribbon gauze impregnated with an antibiotic ointment. The wound is closed in two layers, the inner layer being that of the periosteum and particular care is taken to get good apposition here in order to ensure that the patient does not have an ugly depressed scar. A single layer of tulle gras is placed over the closed eyelid and a pressure dressing is applied.

Post-operative care

First 24 h
The patient should be carefully observed for signs of intracranial bleeding. State of consciousness, pupil size, movement of the limbs, blood pressure and general state of the patient should be observed and recorded every half hour. Post-operative polyuria is often considerable and it is necessary to keep the intravenous drip in position for one or two days after surgery to ensure adequate fluid replacement. Antibiotic cover is given in the form of ampicillin 500 mg six-hourly for a period of seven days. The level of circulating steroids is maintained by giving hydrocortisone 25 mg eight-hourly intravenously, but the dosage can be quickly reduced so that on leaving hospital the patient is on a maintenance dose of 12.5 mg twice daily.

After 24 h
The pressure dressing can be removed after approximately 48 h and the nasal pack and the skin sutures after three to four days. The skin sutures in the thigh wound should be left in position for 10–14 days. Excessive polyuria is controlled by injections of vasopressin for the first two days and subsequently by nasal insufflation of the same compound. In the immediate post-operative period it is important that sepsis should not be introduced into the nose and nasal manipulation should therefore be kept to a minimum. Visitors and attendants who have a current coryza should be debarred from any contact with the patient.

    After the antibiotic therapy is stopped on the seventh day the patient should be watched carefully for any signs of CSF rhinorrhoea or meningitis for a further three days, and if satisfactory, can then be discharged home.

Maintenance therapy

The following long-term drug therapy is usually necessary:

(1) Cortisone 12.5 mg twice daily by mouth. The first tablet should be taken early in the morning, the second one is taken after lunch, rather than in the evening as the

patient's cortisone requirement at night is minimal. The patient should be given a steroid card and instructed to double the dose should illness or any other type of serious stress occur.

(2) Thyroxine 0.2 mg daily is usually, but not always, necessary. Before such therapy is instituted it is advisable to check the patient's thyroid profile at monthly intervals and thyroxine should be given only when there are indications of developing hypothyroidism.

(3) Antidiuretic hormone is rarely necessary after three months. It is most easily administered in the form of a nasal spray and the patient should be encouraged to use it as little as possible because its too frequent use appears to diminish the rate of natural adaptation.

(4) Testosterone injections should be given to male patients who complain of loss of, or diminished, libido following operation.

Complications

The complications following hypophysectomy may be general or local. In comparison with the trans-frontal operation, trans-ethmoidal hypophysectomy is a relatively minor procedure causing little systemic upset and minimal tissue damge. General complications are therefore uncommon. Deep vein thrombosis of the calf is encountered occasionally and in the author's experience it is most likely to occur in patients who have a severe post-operative polyuria. Adequate intravenous replacement during the post-operative period is essential and frequent and early leg exercises should be encouraged.

The local complications are as follows:

Haemorrhage
Intracranial bleeding is fortunately rare, but may occur and was responsible for one case of mortality in the author's series where the patient suffered a subarachnoid haemorrhage 12 h post-operatively and died after 72 h. Most patients during the immediate post-operative period have a moderate headache but if this is exceptionally severe or of increasing severity or is associated with a diminishing level of consciousness or localizing neurological signs then intracranial bleeding should be suspected. In these circumstances the fossa should be re-explored and bleeding points dealt with by using clips or bipolar diathermy. Troublesome venous oozing can usually be controlled by pressure from a large muscle pack or the local use of gelatin foam. If the bleeding is within the cranial cavity and inaccessible by the trans-sphenoid route then the assistance of a neurosurgeon should be sought.

Visual impairment
This may be due to damage to the optic nerve, the chiasma or to the optic tracts. The complication is avoided by keeping the dissection strictly below the level of the diaphragma sellae. In those cases where the diaphragm is so widely patent as to form a barely recognizable rim, great care is necessary and the surgeon should frequently re-check his bearings by reference to the level of the roof of the ethmoid labyrinth. The plane of the sellar diaphragm coincides with a line projecting backwards from the plane of the roof of the ethmoidal labyrinth and constitutes a useful reference point.

Ophthalmoplegia

Damage to the third, fourth and sixth cranial nerves as they travel in the cavernous sinuses should be avoidable by the use of a careful dissection technique with good haemostasis.

CSF rhinorrhoea

This should be tested for frequently during the post-operative period by getting the patient to bend the head forward and watching for clear fluid dripping from the nose. Sometimes the flow of cerebrospinal fluid is slight only and may be delayed so that the head needs to be held forward in the appropriate position for at least 1 min. In the author's experience this complication has not occurred since adopting the technique of suturing the dura after removal of the gland. In those cases where it previously occurred it usually resolved spontaneously after a few days. In the case of a persistent leak the fossa has to be re-explored and care must be taken to inspect the roof of the ethmoid carefully as the leak may be occurring in this location.

Meningitis

When this complication arises, it is usually in association with CSF rhinorrhoea. Every effort should be made to detect the offending organism by culturing the fluid obtained by lumbar puncture as well as that obtained from the nose. In order to ensure sufficiently high blood levels of the appropriate antibiotic it is advantageous to administer it by the intramuscular or intravenous route.

Diabetes insipidus

This causes troublesome polyuria and polydipsia in approximately one-third of all cases and should be dealt with as described under post-operative care. There is some evidence to indicate that this complication is less likely to occur if the stalk is divided at the lowest possible point. Adaptation occurs rapidly and the symptom is rarely troublesome after six to eight weeks (Jenkins, Ash and Bloom, 1972; Davies, 1972).

Nasal crusting

As with other nasal operations there is always some degree of post-operative nasal crusting. For fear of introducing infection it is best not to attempt to remove these for the first two weeks after operation. Subsequently, in the interest of the patient's comfort the nose should be inspected and any large crusts removed.

Alternative methods of ablation

The principal methods which have been used for pituitary ablation are shown in *Table 19.4.*

Surgical removal by the transcranial and trans-sphenoidal routes have already been discussed and the alternative methods will now be considered.

Conventional tele-radiation

Gramegna in 1909 was the first to employ radiation for the management of pituitary diseases. The normal pituitary gland is extremely resistant to radiation and it has been estimated that a dose of 300 000 rad is required to achieve total destruction (Angell-James, 1967). Emmanuel (1966) reported his results in 34 acromegalics after irradiation with a two-million volt Van der Graff generator. Visual fields and headaches responded dramatically but improvement of the acromegaly *per se* was seen in only approximately 18 per cent. Jenkins, Ash and Bloom (1972) achieved similarly disappointing results in the treatment of acromegaly and a satisfactory fall in growth hormone level was achieved in only one out of ten patients. Orth and Liddle (1971) treated 51 cases of Cushing's disease with external irradiation giving 4000–5000 rad. Ten patients were judged to be cured and 13 patients showed some improvement.

Table 19.4   Methods of pituitary ablation

Irradiation	Conventional tele-radiation
	Heavy-particle irradiation
	Radioactive implants
Surgical ablation	Transcranial hypophysectomy
	Trans-sphenoidal hypophysectomy
	Cryosurgery
	Ultrasonic

Tele-radiation of the pituitary gland is not without danger. Peck and McGovern (1966) reported four examples of brain necrosis. Haemorrhage was encountered in Ellis' series (1949). The possibility of inducing malignant tumours has been suggested by Goldberg, Sheline and Malamud (1963) who cited four examples of malignant pituitary tumours supervening in 75 irradiated patients. The tumours became apparent between ten and 30 years after the initial treatment.

In view of the relatively poor results and the danger of complications conventional tele-radiation is now rarely employed.

Heavy particle (proton beam) irradiation
Linfoot and Greenwood (1965), Kjellberg *et al.* (1968) and Lawrence *et al.* (1970) have reported satisfactory improvements in acromegalics with heavy particle irradiation and have achieved relatively good depression of circulating growth hormone levels. The equipment is extremely expensive and this type of therapy is available only in very few centres in the world. It is contraindicated in patients with a supra-sellar extension

Interstitial irradiation
This is usually achieved by implanting the fossa with yttrium 90 so as to give a dose of approximately 5000 rad. The implant is 'injected' into the pituitary fossa through the nose and the sphenoid sinus under stereotactic fluoroscopic control. The method appears to work best in those cases where ablation of function in a normal gland is required. In a controlled trial conducted in Cardiff (Roberts, 1970) yttrium implants were found to produce as many remissions in carcinoma of the breast as did trans-ethmoidal hypophysectomy. The incidence of CSF rhinorrhoea, meningitis and of ocular complications was, however, considerably higher in the Y-90 cases.

In the treatment of acromegaly interstitial irradiation has achieved only moderate success. Forrest *et al.* (1970) found that implantation with Y-90 or Au-198 was substantially less effective than surgical hypophysectomy in the treatment of this condition. Fraser in 1970 found that in 80 cases of acromegaly implanted with Y-90, 50 per cent gave a 'satisfactory' fall in growth hormone levels. Reduction of growth hormone level to normal was, however, exceptional and the follow-up period did not exceed one year.

In Cushing's disease a satisfactory response is obtained in about 50 per cent of cases where there is no obvious radiological evidence of tumour (Fraser, 1970; Forrest *et al.*, 1970). The incidence of ocular complications, rhinorrhoea and of meningitis is considerable in both these series.

At the present time it appears that interstitial irradiation gives inferior results as compared with trans-ethmoidal hypophysectomy in the treatment of acromegaly, Cushing's disease and of other pituitary tumours. It is of value in producing pituitary ablation for breast cancer because the degree of operative interference and the length of stay in hospital is less than with surgical hypophysectomy.

Cryosurgery

In recent years this method has been used as an alternative method of achieving pituitary ablation. Arguments used in its favour are that it is possible to achieve accurately placed partial destruction thus minimizing the need for hormonal replacement. Seven acromegalics (of whom five had been previously managed by irradiation) were subjected to cryotherapy by Maddy *et al.* (1969). The facial features and headaches improved in all cases and normal growth hormone levels were achieved in five. Adams *et al.* (1968) in a series of 16 cases reported an excellent clinical response in ten patients and normal growth hormone levels followed treatment in 11 cases. They and Conway *et al.* (1969) have encountered examples of delayed ocular palsies post-operatively.

Ultrasound

In 1968 Arslan gave an account of ultrasonic hypophysectomy in 55 patients. The approach was made through the nasal septum and after removal of the roof of the sphenoid sinus the ultrasonic applicator was placed on the 'capsule' of the hypophysis. Out of 15 cases of Cushing's disease, ten showed marked clinical improvement. Similarly five cases out of six acromegalics improved markedly. Satisfactory results were achieved also in the treatment of breast and prostatic cancer and of diabetic retinopathy. The advantage of this method is that the degree of hospitalization is minimal and the complication rate in Arslan's series was low.

The follow-up period however did not exceed three years and there was inadequate assessment of pre- and post-operative growth hormone levels.

In common with the cryosurgical technique this method carries a serious disadvantage in that it is impossible for the operator to know the exact depth and extent of the destruction imposed. This is in marked contrast to the high degree of precision which is attainable by surgical hypophysectomy through the operating microscope where the instrumentation can achieve an accuracy in the order of 1/100 mm.

For this reason and because a sufficiently well analysed and sufficiently large series of cases treated by these two methods has not yet appeared in the literature, ultrasonic and cryosurgical hypophysectomy have not gained widespread general acceptance.

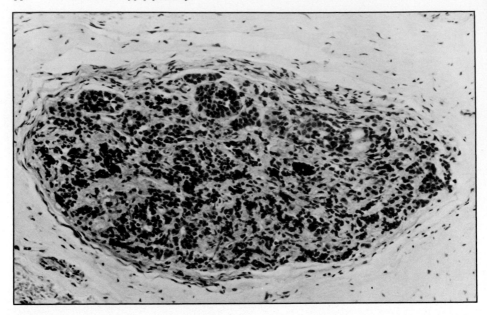

Figure 19.8 Transverse section through pharyngeal pituitary gland removed at trans-ethmoidal hypophysectomy. (Courtesy of Professor E. D. Williams)

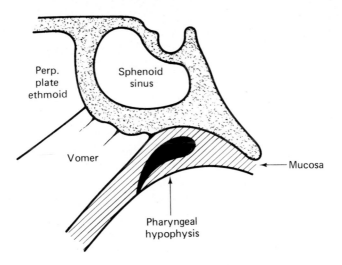

Figure 19.9 Diagrammatic sagittal section through skull showing position of pharyngeal pituitary in roof of nasopharynx

The pharyngeal hypophysis

This consists of a small collection of adeno–hypophyseal cells situated in the mucosa of the roof of the naso–pharynx immediately behind the upper end of the posterior extremity of the nasal septum (*see Figures 19.8* and *19.9*). It represents the proximal

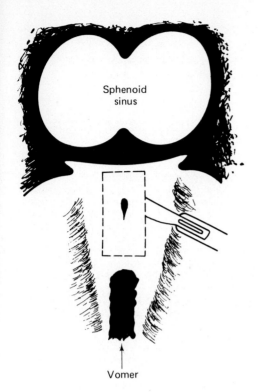

Figure 19.10   Diagram showing removal of a rectangular piece of mucoperiosteum (containing pharyngeal pituitary gland) from roof of sphenoid sinus after the upper part of vomer has been removed

end of the stalk of Rathke's pouch at its junction with the primitive foregut and is invariably present to a greater or lesser degree in human adults and children (McGrath, 1967). Its presence as a functioning entity probably explains the difficulty experienced by various workers in their efforts to produce complete ablation of pituitary function by removing the sellar hypophysis.

When complete ablation of pituitary function is required the pharyngeal hypophysis should be removed by excising an area of mucosa measuring approximately 1 × 2 cm from the vomero–sphenoidal region, as shown in *Figure 19.10* (Richards and Evans, 1974).

When hypophysectomy is performed for acromegaly or Cushing's disease it is better to leave the pharyngeal hypophysis *in situ* as an extra-sellar source of pituitary hormones which will minimize the need for replacement therapy. If, however, the acromegaly or Cushing's disease does not respond to complete sellar hypophysectomy then pharyngeal hypophysectomy may be required in order to eliminate it as a possible source of extra-sellar hormone secretion.

Conclusion

Trans-sphenoidal hypophysectomy is now a well established operation in the treatment of acromegaly and Cushing's disease and in those cases where total ablation of the pituitary gland is required. The procedure is capable of further technical evolution by the use of more precise dissectors, retractors and micro-coagulators etc. Also there is clearly room for considerable development in the operation of partial hypophysectomy. This development, however, must await more accurate localization of the site of production of the various hormones in the adeno-hypophysis.

References

Adams, J. E., Seymour, R. J., Earll, J. M., Tuck, M., Sparks, L. L. and Forsham, P. H. (1968). 'Trans-sphenoidal Cryohypophysectomy in acromegaly: clinical and endocrinological evaluation, *Journal of Neurosurgery*, **28**, 100

Aloia, J. F., Field, R. A. and Kramer, S. (1973). 'Treatment of acromegaly', *Archives of internal Medicine*, **131**, 509

Angell-James J. (1967). 'The Hypophysis', *Journal of Laryngology*, **81**, 1283

Arslan, M. (1968). 'Ultrasonic selective hypophysectomy', *Proceedings of the Royal Society of Medicine*, **61**, 7

Bateman, G. H. (1963). 'Trans-sphenoidal hypophysectomy', *Proceedings of the Royal Society of Medicine*, **56**, 393

Bishop, P. M. F. and Briggs, J. A. (1958). 'Acromegaly: abstract of paper to Study Group on developments in knowledge of anterior pituitary gland', *Lancet* **1**, 735

Cairns, H. (1936). 'The ultimate results of operations for intracranial tumours', *Yale Journal of biological Medicine*, **8**, 421

Chiari, O. (1912). 'Ueber ein Modifikation der Schlofferschen Operation von Tumoren der Hypophyse', *Wiener klinsche Wochenschrift*, **25**, 5

Childs, D. F., Gordon, H., Mashiter, K. and Joplin, G. F. (1975). 'Pregnancy, prolactin and pituitary tumours', *Bristish medical Journal*, **4**, 87

Conway, L. W., O'Foghludha, F. T. and Collins, W. F. (1969). 'Stereotactic treatment of acromegaly', *Journal of Neurology, Neurosurgery and Psychiatry*, **32**, 48

Crooke, A. C. (1935). 'A change in the basophil cells of the pituitary gland common to conditions which exhibit the syndrome attributed to basophil adenoma', *Journal of Pathology and Bacteriology*, **41**, 339

Cushing, H. (1909). 'The hypophysis cerebri: clinical aspects of hyperpituitarism and of hypopituitarism', *Journal of the American medical Association*, **53**, 249

Cushing, H. (1909). 'Partial hypophysectomy for acromegaly', *Annals of Surgery*, **50**, 1002

Cushing, H. (1912). *The pituitary body and its disorders*. J. B. Lippincott; Philadelphia

Dalton, G. (1974). Trans-sphenoidal hypophysectomy for pituitary tumours', *Proceedings of the Royal Society of Medicine*, **67**, 885

Davies, A. G. (1972). 'Antidiuretic and growth hormones', *British medical Journal*, **2**, 282

Decker, K. and Lauter, H. (1960). 'The results of treatment of hypophyseal tumours', *German medical Monthly*, **5**, 265

Dolman, L. I., Roberts, T. S., Poulson, A. M. and Tyler, F. H. (1977). 'Infertility in patients with hyperprolactinemia from a pituitary adenoma', *Archives of internal Medicine*, **137**, 116

Ellis, F. (1949). 'Radiotherapy in the treatment of pituitary basophilism and eosinophilism', *Proceedings of the Royal Society of Medicine*, **42**, 853

Emmanuel, I. G. (1966). 'Symposium on pituitary tumours (3). Historical aspects of radiotherapy, present treatment, technique and results', *Clinical Radiology*, **17**, 154

Falconer, M. A. and Stafford-Bell, M. A. (1975). 'Visual failure from pituitary and parasellar tumours occurring with favourable outcome in pregnant women', *Journal of Neurology, Neurosurgery & Psychiatry*, **38**, 919

Forrest, A. P. M., Thomas, J. P., Richards, S. H., Wood, R. G., Stewart, H. J., Cleave, E. N. and Greenwood, F. C. (1970). 'Radioactive implants of the pituitary for endocrine disease', *Proceedings of the Royal Society of Medicine*, **63**, 616

Fraser, R. (1970). 'Human pituitary disease', *British medical Journal*, **4**, 449

Glick, S. M., Roth, J., Yalow, R. S. and Berson, S. A. (1963). 'Immunoassay of human growth hormone in plasma', *Nature (London)*, **199**, 784

Goldberg, M. B., Sheline, E. G. and Malamud, N. (1963). 'Malignant intracranial neoplasms following radiation therapy for acromegaly', *Radiology*, **80**, 465

Gramegna, A. (1909). Un cas d'acromegalie traité par la radiothérapié, *Revue neurologie*, **17**, 15

Hamberger, C. A., Hammer, G., Norlen, G. and Sjögren, B. (1960). 'Surgical Treatment of Acromegaly', *Acta oto-laryngologica* Suppl. 158, 168

Hardy, J. 'Transsphenoidal microsurgery of the normal and pathological pituitary', *Clinical neurosurgery*, **16**, 185

Hartog, M., Doyle, F., Fraser, R. and Joplin, G. F. (1965). 'Partial pituitary ablation with implants of gold-198 and yttrium-90 for acromegaly', *British medical Journal*, **2**, 396

Henderson, W. R. (1939). 'The anterior basal meningiomas', *British medical Journal*, **26**, 124

Hirsch, O. (1911). 'Ueber Methoden der operativen Behandlung von Hypophysistumoren auf endo-nasalem Wege', *Archives of Laryngology and Rhinology*, **24**, 129

Hirsch, O. (1959). 'Life-long cures and improvements after transsphenoidal operation of pituitary tumours', *Acta ophthalmologica*, Suppl. 56, 60

Hunter, W. M. and Greenwood, F. C. (1964) 'A radio-immunoelectrophoretic assay for human growth hormone', *Biochemical Journal*, **91**, 43

Jenkins, J. S., Ash, S. and Bloom, H. J. G. (1972). 'Endocrine function after external pituitary irradiation in patients with secreting and non-secreting pituitary tumours, *Quarterly Journal of Medicine*, **161**, 57

Joplin, C. F., Fraser, R., Steiner, R., Laws, J. and Jones, E. (1961). 'Partial pituitary ablation by needle implantation of gold-198 seeds for acromegaly and Cushing's disease', *Lancet* **2**, 1277

Kaufman, B., Pearson, C. H., Shealy, C. N., Chernak, E. S., Samaan, N. and Storaasli, J. P. (1966). 'Transnasal-transsphenoidal yttrium-90 pituitary implantation in the therapy of acromegaly', *Radiology*, **86**, 915

Kjellberg, R. N., Shintani, A., Frantz, A. G. and Kliman, B. (1968). 'Proton-beam therapy in acromegaly', *New England Journal of Medicine*, **278**, 689

Kocher, T. (1909) 'Ein Fall von Hypophysis-Tumor mit operativer Heilung', *Deutsche Zeitschrift für Chirurgie*, **100**, 13

Lawrence, A. M., Pinsky, S. M. and Goldfine, I. D. (1971). 'Conventional radiation therapy in acromegaly', *Archives of internal Medicine*, **128**, 369

Lawrence, J. H., Tobias, G. A., Linfoot, J. A., Born, J. L., Lyman, J. T., Chong, C. Y., Manougian, E. and Wei, W. C. (1970). 'Successful treatment of acromegaly: metabolic and clinical studies in 145 patients', *Journal of clinical Endocrinology*, **31**, 180

Linfoot, J. A. and Greenwood, F. R. (1965). 'Growth hormone in acromegaly: effect of heavy particle pituitary irradiation', *Journal of clinical Endocrinology*, **25**, 1515

Macbeth, R. G. (1961). 'An approach to the pituitary via a nasal osteoplastic flap', *Journal of Laryngology and Otology*, **75**, 70

McGrath, P. (1967). 'Volume and histology of the human pharyngeal hypophysis', *Australian & New Zealand Journal of Surgery*, **37**, 16

Maddy, J. A., Winternitz, W. W., Norrel, H., Quillen, D. and Wilson, C. B. (1969). 'Acromegaly: treatment by cryoablation', *Annals of internal Medicine*, **71**, 497

Marie, P. (1886). 'Sur deux cas d'acromégalie: hypertrophie singulière non congénitale des extrémetiés supérieures, inférieures et céphaliques', *Revue medicine* (Paris), **6**, 297

Minkowski, O. (1887) 'Ueber einen Fall von Akromegalie', *Klinischer Wochenschrift*, **24**, 371

Nager, F. R. (1940). 'The paranasal approach to intrasellar tumours', *Journal of Laryngology and Otology*, **55**, 361

Orth, D. N. and Liddle, G. W. (1971). 'Results of treatment in 108 patients with Cushing's syndrome', *New England Journal of Medicine*, **285**, 243

Peck, F. C. and McGovern, E. R. (1966). 'Radiation necrosis of the brain in acromegaly', *Journal of Neurosurgery*, **25**, 536

Rand, R. W. (1966). 'Cryosurgery of the pituitary in acromegaly: reduced growth hormone levels following hypophysectomy in 13 cases', *Annals of Surgery*, **164**, 587

Ray, B. S. (1960). 'The neurosurgeon's new interest in the pituitary', *Journal of Neurosurgery*, **17**, 1

Richards, S. H. and Evans, I. T. G. (1974). 'The pharyngeal hypophysis and its surgical significance', *Journal of Laryngology and Otology*, **88**, 937

Richards, S. H., Thomas, J. P. and Kilby D. (1974). 'Transethmoidal hypophysectomy for pituitary tumours', *Proceedings of the Royal Society of Medicine*, **67**, 889

Roberts, M. M. (1970), 'A comparison of transethmoidal hypophysectomy, yttrium 90 implant and adrenalectomy'. In *The clinical management of advanced breast cancer: proceedings of the Second Tenovus Workshop*, pp. 54–64. Ed. by Joslin, C. A. F. and Gleave, E. N.

Roth, J., Gorden, P. and Bates, R. W. (1968). 'Studies of growth hormone and prolactin in acromegaly'. In *Growth hormone* (*Excerpta Medica International Congress Series 158*), pp. 124–128. Ed. by Pecile, A. and Muller, E. E.

Salassa R. M., Kearns, T. P., Kernohan, J. W., Sprague, R. W., MacCarthy, C. S. (1959). 'Pituitary tumours in patients with Cushing's syndrome', *Journal of clinical Endocrinology*, **19**, 1523

Schloffer, H. (1907) 'Erfolgreiche Operation eines Hypophysentumors auf nasalem Wege', *Wiener Klinischer Wochenschrift*, **20**, 621

Williams, R. A. (1974). 'Trans-sphenoidal hypophysectomy for acromegaly', *Proceedings of the Royal Society of Medicine*, **67**, 881

Wright, A. D., Hartog, M., Palter, H., Tevaarwerk, G., Doyle, F. H., Arnot, R., Joplin, C. F. and Russell-Fraser, T. (1970) 'The Use of yttrium 90 implantation in the treatment of acromegaly', *Proceedings of the Royal Society of Medicine*, **63**, 221

Wright, A. D., Hill, D. M., Lowy, C. and Fraser, T. R. (1970). 'Mortality in acromegaly', *Quarterly Journal of Medicine*, **39**, 1

20 Surgery of the pterygo–palatine fossa
Philip H Golding-Wood

The pterygo–palatine fossa serves as a distribution channel for the nerves and vessels to the face, nose and palate. It contains the third part of the maxillary artery and its terminal branches, the maxillary nerve, and the spheno–palatine ganglion with its branches. It thus becomes the focal point of several surgical procedures that aim at the resection of one or more of these contained structures in the control of severe epitaxis, some aspects of facial pain or the secreto–motor supply to the nasal mucosa or lacrimal gland.

Surgical anatomy of the pterygo–palatine fossa

Knowledge of the anatomy of this area, so vital to safe and effective surgery, cannot be gained from the usual textbooks. These, not being orientated from the surgeon's point of view, give impressions that are frequently misleading and totally unsuitable as a surgical guide (*Figure 20.1*).

The basic essentials are best visualized on a dry skull where the pterygo–palatine fossa can be explored across the maxillary sinus. The anterior wall of the sinus is removed as in a Caldwell–Luc operation and a similar elliptic area of the posterior wall of the sinus is also removed. Simple observations made on such a specimen will teach the neophyte more than a score of articles.

The pterygo–palatine fossa is a cul-de-sac that extends inwards towards the nose from the infratemporal fossa. It lies between the maxillary antrum in front and the pterygoid extension of the greater wing of the sphenoid behind. Above, it opens into the apex of the orbit through the inferior orbital fissure; below, it is closed by the fusion of its own anterior and posterior walls with the lateral projection of the pyramidal process of the palatine bone (*Figure 20.2*).

Medially the fossa is shut off from the nasal cavity by the vertical plate of the palatine bone. Superiorly this bifurcates into a short sphenoidal process posteriorly and a larger orbital process anteriorly. This fuses with the maxilla to form a stout, bony buttress. Between these processes is a deeply rounded notch and, being roofed, the body of the sphenoid forms the spheno–palatine foramen which opens into the

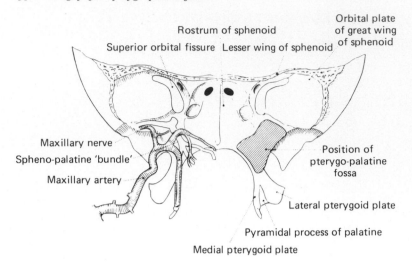

Rostrum of sphenoid

Orbital plate
of great wing
of sphenoid

Superior orbital fissure   Lesser wing of sphenoid

Maxillary nerve

Spheno-palatine 'bundle'

Maxillary artery

Position of
pterygo-palatine
fossa

Lateral pterygoid plate

Pyramidal process of palatine

Medial pterygoid plate

Figure 20.1   Pterygo–palatine fossa and the sphenoid. (From *Operative Surgery*, 3rd edn. Ed. by C. Rob and R. Smith. *Nose and Throat*. London; Butterworths)

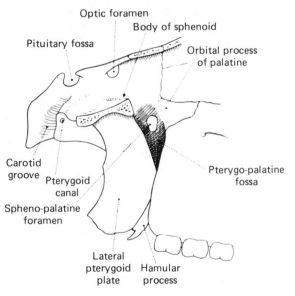

Optic foramen

Body of sphenoid

Pituitary fossa

Orbital process
of palatine

Carotid
groove   Pterygoid
canal

Pterygo-palatine
fossa

Spheno-palatine
foramen

Lateral
pterygoid
plate

Hamular
process

Figure 20.2   Lateral aspect of pterygo–palatine fossa. (From *Operative Surgery*, 3rd edn. Ed. by C. Rob and R. Smith. *Nose and Throat*. London; Butterworths)

nose just behind the posterior end of the middle turbinate. It transmits arteries and nerves from the pterygo–palatine fossa into the nose.

Two foramina in the posterior wall of the fossa provide the basic landmarks. Just below the superior orbital fissure is the foramen rotundum that transmits the maxillary nerve. Surgically, the foramen rotundum marks the upper limit of safety in dissection; any excursion above it endangers structures in the apex of the orbit (*Figure 20.3*).

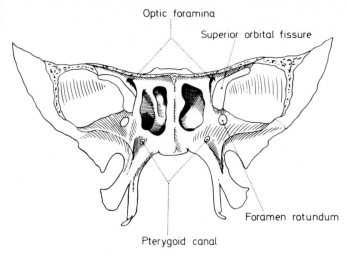

Optic foramina

Superior orbital fissure

Foramen rotundum

Pterygoid canal

Figure 20.3 The sphenoidal foramina. (From *Operative Surgery*, 3rd edn. Ed. by C. Rob and R. Smith. *Nose and Throat*. London; Butterworths)

The Vidian nerve runs forward in the pterygoid canal to enter the fossa. This canal, 1 cm long and ordinarily narrow, widens anteriorly to a funnel-like mouth approximating almost to the size of foramen rotundum. The mouth of the pterygoid canal lies 8–9 mm below and medial to foramen rotundum but it is on a posterior plane and thus a distinct vertical bony ridge generally intrudes between the two foramina.

Ordinarily, the pterygoid canal runs along the infero–lateral aspect of the sphenoidal sinus. Extensions of the sphenoidal sinus, however, may encroach into the pterygoid wings and thus perhaps completely engulf the pterygoid canal. The supero–medial wall of the canal is frequently dehiscent and the Vidian nerve runs beneath the membrane lining the sphenoidal sinus. Similar extension of the supero–lateral aspects of the sphenoidal sinus can similarly surround the optic foramen and these walls may be dehiscent also.

It is important to note that the mouth of the pterygoid canal lies almost in the antero–posterior plane of the medial wall of the maxillary antrum. Thus, its trans-antral exposure requires appropriate lowering of the thickened medial buttress at the posterior window, flush with the medial wall.

Transverse plane of the nerves

Further observation of the bone shows that the line of the infra-orbital canal lies well lateral to foramen rotundum (*Figure 20.4*). Thus, the maxillary nerve on entering the pterygo–palatine fossa, first runs laterally and slightly upwards before it turns forward through the inferior orbital fissure to continue as the infra–orbital nerve within its canal. The surgeon approaching from the front thus finds the maxillary nerve running transversely laterally and slightly upwards immediately after it has left foramen rotundum.

The spheno–palatine ganglion which lies directly in front of the funnelled mouth

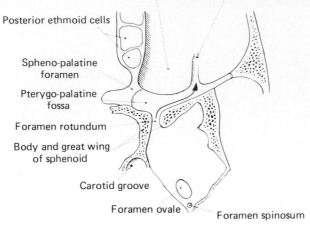

Figure 20.4 Schematic horizontal section through right foramen rotundum. (Arrow shows course of maxillary nerve.) (From *Operative Surgery*, 3rd edn. Ed. by C. Rob and R. Smith. *Nose and Throat.* London; Butterworths)

of the pterygoid canal is laterally compressed into a flattened disc. Just after it has entered the pterygo–palatine fossa, the maxillary nerve gives fibres to the spheno–palatine ganglion and receives others from it. These fibres, usually depicted in textbooks as separate nerve filaments, will almost invariably be found bound together to form a stout bundle, here referred to as the spheno–palatine bundle. Necessarily this bundle passes medially and downwards at approximately 45 degrees from the maxillary nerve. It lies close to the sphenoid and is thus often stretched across the bony ridge separating the foramen rotundum and pterygoid canal (*Figure 20.5*).

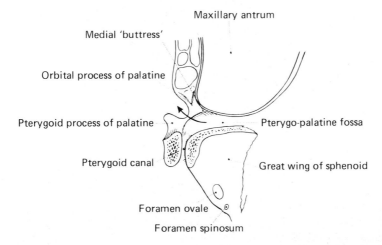

Figure 20.5 Schematic horizontal section through left pterygoid canal. (From *Operative Surgery*, 3rd edn. Ed. by C. Rob and R. Smith. *Nose and Throat.* London; Butterworths)

It is important to appreciate that within the pterygo–palatine fossa, the maxillary nerve, the spheno–palatine bundle and ganglion, with its nasal and descending palatine branches, all lie essentially in a single transverse plane.

Because the flattened spheno–palatine ganglion is seen edgewise, the surgeon approaching from the front seldom sees a fusiform swelling. As the spheno–palatine bundle is traced medially, it seems merely to bifurcate into descending palatine and superior nasal branches. This neural junction is tethered posteriorly by the Vidian nerve emerging from the pterygoid canal. It is only after the Vidian nerve, often bound with the Vidian artery in a fibrous envelope, has been severed, that this neural junction can be manipulated to disclose the entire mouth of the pterygoid canal.

It will be appreciated that Vidian neurectomy alone removes secreto–motor impulses from the glands of the nasal mucosa and from the lacrimal gland, but it does not disturb sensation within the nose or the palate. Removal of the spheno–palatine ganglion will similarly remove those secreto–motor impulses and the sensory innervation from the ipsilateral side of the nose and palate.

Maxillary artery and branches

The maxillary artery, which has entered the pterygo–palatine fossa from between the two heads of the lateral pterygoid muscle, appears from the front to come upward from the floor. Within the pterygo–palatine fossa it runs a characteristically tortuous and variable course, but the basic plan is simple. Arching upwards and forwards it passes medially across the fossa and terminates by bifurcating into spheno–palatine and descending palatine arteries. This essentially transverse arterial arch lies anterior to the transverse plane of the nerves and is thus found superficial to them in any surgical approach from the front (*Figure 20.6*).

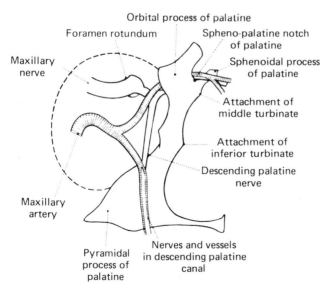

Figure 20.6 Vessels and nerves related to right pterygo palatine fossa. (From *Operative Surgery*, 3rd edn. Ed. by C. Rob and R. Smith. *Nose and Throat.* London; Butterworths)

As it arches upwards, the maxillary artery gives off the large infra-orbital artery which runs laterally and upwards to enter the infra-orbital canal through the inferior orbital fissure. The main trunk continues to run across the fossa lying anteriorly and generally below the line of the maxillary nerve. Its terminal bifurcation is variable. Ordinarily the spheno–palatine and descending palatine arteries continue to run medially in the same transverse plane, diverging upwards and downwards as they do so. The descending palatine arteries turn downwards to join the descending palatine nerve in the pterygo–palatine canal.

The more important spheno–palatine artery runs medially and upwards to enter the nose through the spheno–palatine foramen. In so doing, it passes anterior to the spheno–palatine bundle and/or ganglion and thus skirts the upper rim of the pterygoid canal, separated from it by the superior nasal branches of the spheno–palatine ganglion. Within the nose this artery passes across the sphenoidal roof to reach the septum whence it runs downwards and forwards (as the naso–palatine artery) with the naso–palatine nerve.

Before leaving the lateral wall of the nose, the spheno–palatine artery gives off the posterior nasal branch that supplies the turbinate mucous membrane. This posterior nasal branch generally arises within the spheno–palatine foramen and thus will not be seen in a trans-antral dissection. Not infrequently, however, it arises independently from the maxillary artery, and the spheno–palatine artery thus appears double. Similarly the descending palatine artery divides at a variable point and thus the maxillary artery may be seen to give rise to two descending palatine arteries (*Figure 20.7*).

Pharyngeal and Vidian arteries

Either or both the pharyngeal or Vidian arteries may arise from the spheno–palatine or posterior nasal arteries near the spheno–palatine foramen, and pass backwards to enter the pterygoid or palato–vaginal canals. Either, but particularly the Vidian artery, may be of considerable size and it is of practical importance to recognize that either may frequently pursue an anomalous course. In this event, either vessel arises from the posterior aspect of the maxillary artery immediately after its entry into the pterygo–palatine fossa and then runs medially and upwards over the face of the sphenoid passing deep to the transverse plane of the nerves. Such an anomaly is likely to allow these vessels to escape ligation–resection of the maxillary artery for epistaxis (*Figure 20.8*).

Veins of the pterygo–palatine fossa

Many have feared to invade the pterygo–palatine fossa because they envisaged inordinate difficulties with the venous plexus that they deemed to exist therein. However, whilst the lateral pterygoid muscle outside the fossa is surrounded by a venous plexus, there is no such plexus within the pterygo–palatine fossa itself. Within the periosteum over the posterior wall of the maxillary sinus, one or two fairly prominent veins may be seen running transversely over the fossa. These veins are easily controlled by spot diathermy applied whilst they lie *in situ*. Otherwise there is

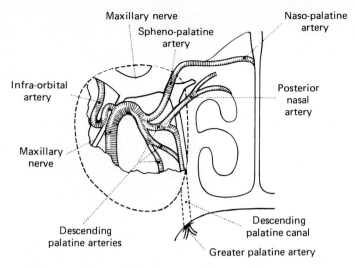

Figure 20.7   Vessels and nerves of right pterygo–palatine fossa. (From *Operative Surgery*, 3rd edn. Ed. by C. Rob and R. Smith. *Nose and Throat*. London; Butterworths)

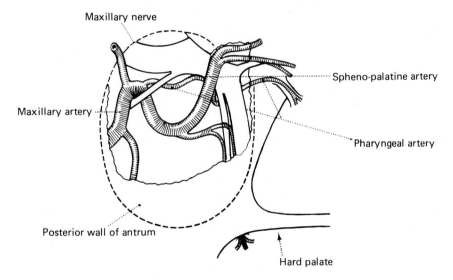

Figure 20.8   Anomalous pharyngeal artery. (From *Operative Surgery*, 3rd edn. Ed. by C. Rob and R. Smith. *Nose and Throat*. London; Butterworths)

only a single small vena comitans in the fat above the maxillary artery and a further minute vein on the maxillary nerve.

Fat

The vessels and nerves within the pterygo–palatine fossa are packed among loosely textured fat that at first seems greatly to hinder dissection, but this difficulty is easily overcome. The fat that lies directly behind the maxillary antrum can be gripped with any suitable cup forceps and pulled away to expose the vessels and nerves; it will come away readily without material bleeding.

Closely applied to the postero–lateral wall of the maxillary antrum, however, is an entirely separate, coarsely lobulated pad of yellow fat (the fat pad of Bichat). This fat pad should be avoided. It will only encroach on the operative field if the posterior antral window is extended too far laterally. This fat, readily recognized by its appearance and consistency, cannot be pulled away. Any attempt to do so will merely drag it into the pterygo–palatine fossa, causing great subsequent difficulty (*Figure 20.9*).

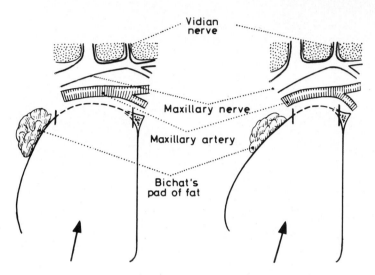

Figure 20.9   Trans-antral approach to pterygo–palatine fossa. (From *Operative Surgery*, 3rd edn. Ed. by C. Rob and R. Smith. *Nose and Throat*. London; Butterworths)

The spheno–palatine ganglion and its branches

The spheno–palatine ganglion, the largest of all the peripheral parasympathetic ganglia, is a distribution centre for sensory fibres from the maxillary nerve reaching it via the spheno–palatine bundle and autonomic fibres from the Vidian nerve.

The sensory fibres pass straight through the ganglion and are distributed by its so-called branches. The nasal branches pass into the nose via the spheno–palatine foramen. Some break up on the lateral wall of the nose, supplying the mucous membrane over the larger posterior part of the superior and middle turbinates. Others cross the sphenoidal roof of the nose to reach the septum and the largest of these (naso–palatine branch) runs downwards and forwards from the septum to reach the incisive canal (*Figure 20.10*).

The descending palatine nerve leaves the spheno–palatine ganglion and passes downwards in the pterygo–palatine canal. Within this canal the nerve divides into two or three branches, the largest of which emerges at the greater palatine foramen

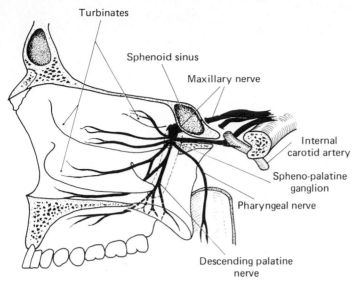

Figure 20.10   The maxillary nerve and spheno-palatine ganglion (From *Operative Surgery*, 3rd edn. Ed. by C. Rob and R. Smith. *Nose and Throat*. London; Butterworths)

and turns forwards to supply the anterior part of the hard palate. The smaller palatine nerves emerge on the palate through the lesser palatine foramen and turn backwards to supply the soft palate. Small nasal branches also arise within the pterygo–palatine canal and pass medially through the vertical plate of the palatine bone to supply the mucosa over the posterior part of the inferior turbinate and the adjacent middle and inferior meati of the nose.

Autonomic supply of the nasal mucosa

The pterygoid canal conveys both parasympathetic and sympathetic fibres to the spheno–palatine ganglion. The nerve of the pterygoid canal (now better known by the earlier name, the Vidian nerve) is of dual origin, its parasympathetic and sympathetic fibres being separately derived.

The small, myelinated parasympathetic fibres arise from a special lacrimatory nucleus in the lower part of the pons and emerge in the nervus intermedius passing with this to join the facial nerve. They leave the facial nerve as a branch from its geniculate ganglion and continue in the greater petrosal nerve. This passes forwards through a hiatus on the anterior surface of the petrous temporal and runs forwards immediately below the dura in a groove on the petrous apex. Here it lies next to the lesser petrosal nerve and receives a twig from it. This minute twig becomes important in the production of 'crocodile' tears.

Further forward, the greater petrosal nerve passes beneath the trigeminal ganglion and thus reaches the foramen lacerum. At the foramen lacerum, the greater petrosal nerve is joined by the deep petrosal nerve that arises from the sympathetic plexus around the internal carotid artery. Both sets of fibres form the Vidian nerve, which passes forwards through the pterygoid canal to the spheno–palatine ganglion (*Figure 20.11*).

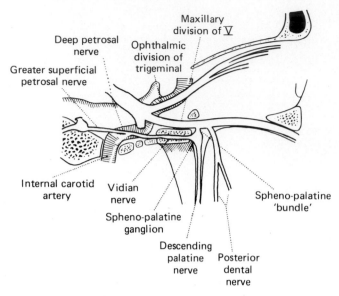

Figure 20.11   Petrosal and Vidian nerves. (From *Operative Surgery*, 3rd edn. Ed. by C. Rob and R. Smith. *Nose and Throat.* London; Butterworths)

The parasympathetic fibres relay in the spheno–palatine ganglion whence the post-ganglionic fibres reach the nasal mucosa via the posterior nasal nerve, the palate via the descending palatine and the lacrimal gland via a communicating twig to the maxillary nerve which passes into the zygomatic branch and thence to the lacrimal gland. These parasympathetic fibres are cholinergic in action and secreto–motor to the nasal mucosa and the lacrimal gland. The unmyelinated sympathetic fibres reaching the spheno–palatine ganglion pass straight through it without relay. They are mostly destined for the nasal mucosa.

Parasympathetic and sympathetic effects

The efferent fibres of the greater petrosal nerve are wholly parasympathetic, vasodilative and secreto–motor to glands of the nasal mucosa. Stimulation of them produces some nasal congestion, lacrimation and marked watery nasal secretion.

Clinically, petrosal neurectomy causes a dramatic change in the nasal mucosa: rapidly this becomes red, glazed, dry and shrunken. Within a few days, however, the colour fades to a normal pink and thereafter the nasal mucosa appears normal though it remains dry; lacrimation can no longer be evoked.

Surprisingly, in view of the sympathetic component, Malcomson (1959) in his experiments on cats, found the Vidian nerve predominantly parasympathetic in effect. This also seems true in humans. Although the mucosal changes are initially less florid with Vidian than with petrosal section, the findings are similar in other respects.

Clinically, however, it had for years been difficult to reconcile the effects of parasympathetic and sympathetic resections on the nasal mucosa. Within days of stellate ganglionectomy or equivalent resection, the nasal mucosa shows considerable congestion and turgescence. This effect, sufficient to occasion clinical discomfort from reduction of the nasal airway in 50 per cent of cases, tends to subside in the ensuing weeks. After two months or so relatively few remark upon it and these can be relieved by submucosal diathermy of the inferior turbinate mucosa. Much attention has been paid to Fowler's report (1943) of a case of unilateral watery rhinorrhoea following ipsilateral stellate ganglionectomy. Such a sequel, however, is certainly unusual. In a long-term follow-up of over 300 patients subjected to bilateral cervico–thoracic sympathectomy (C8–T3), I found a watery rhinorrhoea had developed in only one and this more than one year after operation.

Clinical work had thus established the apparent discrepancy that sympathetic effects seemed limited to the vascular responses of the nasal mucosa, whilst parasympathetic effects were essentially concerned with the secretion of the nasal glands. Recent physiologic advances now explain these clinical observations.

Intramucosal distribution of autonomic fibres

Histochemical investigations have shown that the mucous membrane of the nose has a wealth of autonomic supply that is rivalled only by that of the genitals. As might be expected, there is a rich network of both adrenergic and cholinergic fibres about the nasal blood vessels. This is not merely about the arteries and arterioles, but also about the venous sinusoids. Whereas the veins of other tissues are but sparsely supplied by adrenergic fibres, the venous sinusoids of the erectile tissue in the inferior turbinates have a particularly rich plexus of adrenergic fibres that seem important in regulating blood through the nasal mucosa and thus airflow and heat exchange. Although some cholinergic fibres occur about both arterial and venous vessels, it is the adrenergic innervation that is paramount.

Conversely, the nasal glands are richly surrounded by cholinergic nerve endings but are almost entirely devoid of adrenergic fibres. There are, however, no cholinergic fibres to the ciliated nasal epithelium nor to its goblet cells.

This differing distribution of adrenergic and cholinergic fibres within the nasal mucosa is characteristic of a variety of species and agrees exactly with clinical experience.

Agreement on the intramucosal distribution of adrenergic and cholinergic fibres, however, did not automatically solve the problem of their mode of supply. As Vidian neurectomy became accepted as virtually equivalent to petrosal section in humans, the nature of Vidian fibres came under renewed scrutiny and controversy.

Autonomic efferents of the Vidian nerve

It has long been established that the Vidian nerve contains anatomically sympathetic fibres arising from the periarterial carotid plexus. Animal experiments involving stimulation and section of the Vidian nerve led Jackson and Rooker (1971) to believe that these particular sympathetic fibres, like those to sweat glands, were cholinergic. These authors thus postulated that the adrenergic fibres in the nasal mucosa are derived from the periarterial plexuses of branches of the maxillary and ethmoidal arteries.

This controversy, which had considerable clinical importance, began to be resolved when Malm (1973) demonstrated that the effects of Vidian nerve stimulation varied with the frequency and intensity of the stimulus. High frequency, low intensity stimulation resulting in parasympathetic effects; whereas low frequency and high intensity stimulation gave sympathetic effects. Further experiments by Eccles and Wilson (1973) confirm the duality of Vidian nerve fibres, the cholinergic fibres passing to the nasal glands and the adrenergic supply to the nasal vessels. These last physiological findings are fully in accord with clinical experience.

Nevertheless, the Vidian nerve is not necessarily the only source of cholinergic supply to the nasal mucosa. A few similar cholinergic fibres have been described in both ethmoidal nerves and maxillary nerves.

Periarterial autonomic networks however are almost universal. Although they have generally been regarded as essentially sympathetic in character, the periarterial network about the spheno–palatine artery has been shown by Grote, Juijpers and Huygen (1974) to contain both adrenergic and cholinergic fibres.

These anatomic minutiae may prove to be of great clinical importance. The entire history of autonomic surgery has been bedevilled by the problem of recurrent symptoms traceable to re-innervation. This problem is universal in the sympathetic system, though some forms of sympathectomy remain worthwhile. Recurrence is much less frequent with parasympathectomy, in which the effect is both specific and direct. Furthermore, it is largely amenable to technique as evidenced by recurrence rates after vagotomy, which have varied from 2–30 per cent. It remains mandatory for any autonomic surgery to be as complete as possible for optimal and enduring results.

Autonomic afferents

Although autonomic petrosal fibres were long regarded as purely efferent, the autonomic afferents first demonstrated by Chorobski and Penfield (1932) are now generally accepted. Indeed, central autonomic control would scarcely be feasible without such a feedback mechanism.

Animal experiments show that stimulation of either peripheral or central ends of the Vidian nerve provokes the same sneezing response and leave no reasonable doubt as to the existence of autonomic afferents in the Vidian nerve.

Patients with vasomotor rhinitis commonly find that sharp attacks of rhinorrhoea and sneezing are provoked by exposure to inert dusts. There is much to suggest that this apparent reflex is by autonomic rather than purely somatic sensory pathways. Similarly, clinical experience also suggests that petrosal autonomic afferents also subserve pain.

Central autonomic control

The autonomic system is represented at all levels of the central nervous system, the hypothalamus providing its reflex and integrative centres. There is both motor and sensory autonomic representation in the cerebral cortex, overlapping and integrating with somatic and other cortical areas. This explains the common association of somatic and visceral effects and the undoubted correlation between somatic, autonomic and mental states.

Reactions of the nasal mucosa

It is common in human pathology to find that entirely different aetiological factors can produce the same clinical picture. This is especially so in the upper airways, where various exogenous and endogenous stimuli constantly elicit the same type of reaction. Thus the nasal mucosa constantly responds to almost every form of physiological or pathological stimulus by alteration in vasomotility and secretion. The severe sneezing, serous or mucoserous discharge, hyperaemia and nasal obstruction so long regarded as characteristic of vasomotor rhinitis represent merely an exaggeration of normal responses to simple physical stimuli (such as sunlight or changes of temperature), exposure to irritant although inert dusts, or inhaled antigens.

This defensive activity of shutting out and washing away at the head end of the organism is an effective biologic mechanism against the local intrusion of noxious agents. Equally, the same shutting out and washing away response can result from emotional conflict or endocrine disturbance as so convincingly shown by Holmes *et al.* (1950).

Autonomic effects induced by emotional states are familiar in everyday life. Thus blushing may be induced by shame or embarrassment, whilst blanching may be induced by fear. Tears are usually provoked by emotion, however varied this may be. The lacrimation that ensues is generally associated with some nasal congestion and hypersecretion. This commonplace example of emotional stress indicating localized secreto–motor activity, agrees with the observations of Wolff (1950) that an emotional stimulus causes autonomic effects in a specific part of the body. Thus Wolff speaks of 'stomach reactors' and 'pulse reactors'. Various emotional tensions are apt to find their expression in characteristic autonomic patterns. Witness the coughing and nose blowing by a theatre audience after an emotional scene.

Such localized parasympathetic effects need not occasion surprise, for the so-called balance and antagonism of the sympathetic and parasympathetic may not exist. Whereas the sympathetic–adrenal system acts diffusely and, as a whole, it is characteristic for the parasympathetic system to fire as an isolated unit and thus evoke purely local effects.

My use of first petrosal and then Vidian neurectomy to abolish hitherto continued and in tractable non-specific secreto–motor events in the nose, proved almost uniformly successful in well selected cases (Golding-Wood, 1961, 1962). As these results became amply confirmed, interest in relevant physiological fields quickened. This greatly enhanced our knowledge of the rich autonomic supply of the nasal mucosa and defined the different distributions of adrenergic and cholinergic fibres within it.

Correlation of clinical experience with these physiological advances now permits us rationally to classify the wide variety of dissimilar conditions hitherto lumped together as 'vasomotor rhinitis'. Simultaneously, the indications for Vidian neurectomy have broadened and alternative techniques by which it may be accomplished have been proposed.

A classification of 'vasomotor rhinitis'

It had long been recognized that cases characterized by sneezing, watery rhinorrhoea and obstruction by a swollen mucosa fell into two fairly distinct groups. Prior to 1960 most regarded both groups as allergic and subdivided them as specific and non-specific, atopic and non-atopic, etc.

Irrespective of the terms preferred, the first implies a definable IgE-mediated allergen–antibody reaction with the release of histamine and other chemical mediators. The second group excluded this without implying specific aetiological cause.

The success of Vidian neurectomy in relieving non-atopic sneezing and rhinorrhoea suggested that the symptoms had been produced by localized parasympathetic overactivity and excessive release of acetylcholine. The clinical similarity with atopic cases is inevitable for the chief chemical mediators, histamine and acetylcholine, are pharmacological twins.

Equally it has long been obvious that the great majority of non-specific cases divide themselves into the 'drippers' and the 'blockers'. With the 'drippers' rhinorrhoea and sneezing dominate the picture and obstruction may be completely absent. If present it is seldom more than partial and is then due to a pallid, oedematous mucosa. Conversely, the 'blockers' are characterized by constant or frequent nasal obstruction produced by a red, turgescent mucosa. Frequently these changes alternate from side to side because of the underlying rhythmic changes of the turbinate cycle.

The varied syndromes that can thus be present in these groups cannot be properly considered as a 'rhinitis'. They can all however be classified together as a rhinopathy. Such a rhinopathy is principally manifest either by overaction of the nasal glands, a secreto–motor phenomenon, or by vascular distension within the nasal mucosa, a vasomotor phenomenon.

The rhinopathy may thus be either secreto–motor or vasomotor. Each type can be subdivided according to the dominant aetiological factor:

(1) *Secreto–motor rhinopathy*
   (a) Allergic (atopic)
   (b) Cholinergic
   (c) Reflex
(2) *Vasomotor rhinopathy*
   (a) Chemical (rhinitis medicamentosa)
   (b) Endocrine
   (c) Synadrenergic (post-sympathectomy)
   (d) Idiopathic

Although most cases fall easily into one or other of these groups, it is important to note that mixed cases undoubtedly occur and that infective changes may commonly supervene. The great bulk of the vasomotor rhinopathies will not concern us further in this chapter, for, in pure form at least, they are not provoked by cholinergic impulses and their treatment is that of the causal factor or submucosal diathermy.

Occasionally, gross mucosal congestion and turgescence are accompanied by the sneezing and watery rhinorrhoea typical of the secreto–motor rhinopathy that will be considered further. Such cases seem best treated according to the dominant symptom. Often this involves appropriate treatment of the obstructive factors and when optimal relief of these has been obtained, the secreto–motor aspect can be further assessed.

Secreto–motor rhinopathies

These patients complain of constant or continually recurring 'colds' or 'hay fever'. Profuse, watery nasal discharge is either perpetual or recurs in frequent attacks that last minutes or hours. Often these attacks are preceded by a feeling of irritation in the nose followed by a prolonged bout of sneezing, lacrimation and a streaming nose. Characteristically these attacks occur shortly after waking when they are possibly precipitated by changes of body temperature induced by getting up or by placing the feet on a cold floor. At other times they are induced by dust inhalation or by emotional stress.

The nasal mucosa may appear normal, or pallid, soggy and swollen. In the latter event, there will be some degree of nasal obstruction, not infrequently intermittent but it is the watery nasal discharge that is the predominant symptom. This may be so severe that the nose literally runs like a tap and some patients are driven to the expedient of packing the nostrils before they can attend to ordinary daily tasks.

Symptoms such as these may be purely atopic or purely cholinergic. In most cases the distinction is not difficult, but mixed cases undoubtedly occur and in these it can be extremely difficult to assess the relevant importance of the two factors concerned. The clinical features of these types are shown in *Table 20.1*.

Table 20.1 Clinical features of secreto–motor rhinopathy

Clinical features	Allergic (atopic)	Cholinergic
Sneezing and rhinorrhoea	Seasonal due to pollens; perennial due to occupational dusts	Frequent paroxysms over many years; occasionally unilateral
Lacrimation	Usual	Frequent
Changes in nasal mucosa	Typically bluish, swollen and soggy	Variable; often normal
Nasal eosinophilia	Marked	Frequent but less intense
Response to skin sensitivity tests	Positive reactions related to history	Negative or non-specific
Response to antihistamines	Good	Variable
Polyps	Frequent and large	Occasional and small
Associated asthma	Frequent (40%)	Occasional (15%)

The clinician's first requirement is to differentiate the atopic from the cholinergic group. The history is of particular importance. Enquiry is made as to whether the symptoms can be related to either season or environment. This may give a clue to possible allergens. Equally, it is important to ascertain whether the symptoms began following some period of emotional stress or whether they are greatly aggravated thereby. Such psychosomatic events are usual in the cholinergic variety and such history is not difficult to obtain. Sometimes, however, it may be lacking but its absence does not rule out the cholinergic aetiology. Emotional stimuli are of paramount importance even in stable personalities. Some patients betray an associated anxiety state. The provocative effects of bereavement, separation, domestic unhappiness and marital infidelity are familiar to all. Although time usually brings adjustment to such emotional stress, the rhinitis is apt to continue; once set in motion, it may follow a path independent of the psychic trauma that provoked it.

Endocrine changes such as those that occur in sexual excitement, menstruation or pregnancy may occasion hypersecretion in the nose, although usually hyperaemia and obstruction predominate. When such endocrine events are accompanied by feelings of frustration, resentment, or guilt, the nasal effect is magnified and troublesome symptoms readily recur.

In patients with the cholinergic type, physical agents (e.g. cold, heat, ultraviolet light, or local irritants) are liable to provoke attacks. These stimuli are neutral in the immuno–biological sense and do not provoke antibody reaction. Such patients frequently find aerosol sprays markedly irritant in the nose.

Skin sensitivity tests usually serve to identify the atopic cases, provided they are reasonably interpreted. In themselves, positive skin tests are never proof of allergy for they are often encountered in normal control subjects. Patients are all checked by a full range of intradermal skin tests against possible allergens. The positive responses, if any, are checked against the patient's history and the results of the control test. In general, such intradermal skin tests suffice for the recognition of the atopic cases; if such patients show a raised IgE level, that matter may be regarded as proven. Nasal provocation tests are more accurate than straightforward intradermal skin tests but they are too time-consuming for ordinary clinical practice. Patients in the cholinergic group have uniformly negative skin tests or may show scattered positive responses unrelated to the patient's history.

Eosinophilia in nasal secretions has too often been regarded as pathognomonic of an allergic condition. This is fallacious. Whilst eosinophilia typically occurs in nasal and bronchial tissues after allergen–antibody reaction, it can equally well occur with shifts in autonomic balance. Thus, nasal eosinophilia in secreto–motor rhinopathy may disappear promptly following Vidian neurectomy.

A satisfactory response to antihistamines gives no more than a vague presumption of histaminic pathogenesis. Most synthetic antihistamines also have an anticholinergic effect.

Reflex activity is clearly important in secreto–motor rhinopathy, as evidenced by the attacks which are so often evoked by simple noxious nasal stimuli. Occasionally such symptoms seem to be evoked purely by marked septal deformity or by an impacting spur that irritates the lateral nasal wall. In such patients, appropriate septal surgery is the first requirement. Patients whose symptoms are relieved by such attention can be classified in the reflex group.

Racial influences
There is a marked difference in the incidence of vasomotor and secreto–motor rhinopathies in different races. At least in Britain, Arabs and Indians seem to be prone

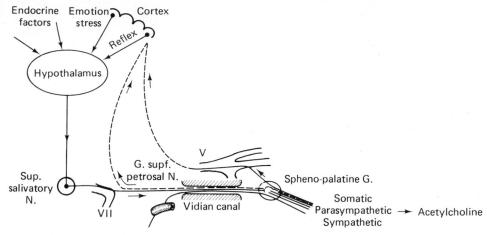

Figure 20.12 The neural mechanism of secreto–motor rhinopathy. (Reproduced by permission of the Editor of *Journal of Laryngology and Otology*)

to severe vasomotor and secreto–motor rhinopathy and the two are not infrequently seen in association. Jamaicans, however, seem relatively immune.

Neural mechanism of non-atopic secreto–motor rhinopathy

The author's initial concept (Golding-Wood, 1962) that all the factors involved in non-atopic secreto–motor rhinopathy can be welded into a single unifying hypothesis, i.e. that it is due to localized parasympathetic over-activity, is generally accepted. This mechanism can be presented diagrammatically (*Figure 20.12*).

The hypothalamus, as the chief reflex and integrative centre of the autonomic system, responds to emotional stimuli, endocrine changes, and perhaps, other factors as yet unknown. Similarly it initiates reflex activity in response to afferent stimuli from the nasal mucosa. These afferent fibres may be somatic trigeminal fibres or purely autonomic fibres within the Vidian nerve.

In response to hypothalamic stimuli, the superior salivatory and lacrimal nuclei fire parasympathetic impulses that travel over the greater petrosal nerve to the spheno–palatine ganglion. Here the parasympathetic fibres relay before being distributed through the nasal mucosa and the lacrimal gland, where their secreto–motor and vasodilator effects are exerted by the release of acetylcholine. Racial, constitutional, and other genetic factors set the trigger pressure; they do not alter the mechanism.

Cholinergic effects can thus be abolished by surgical section of the final effect or pathway. The chief possibilities are as follows:

(1) Greater petrosal neurectomy in the middle cranial fossa, a purely parasympathetic section.
(2) Vidian neurectomy in the pterygoid canal. This is predominantly para-sympathetic.
(3) Spheno–palatine ganglionectomy. Whilst technically simpler, this is unnecessarily destructive of somatic afferent fibres important to the integrity of the nasal mucosa. These, of course, are preserved in Vidian neurectomy which is the preferred technique.

Rationale of Vidian neurectomy in atopic patients

The secreto–motor effects induced by histamine release in IgE-mediated atopy would seem quite distinct from those cholinergically determined, despite the understandable clinical similarity. Although the general management of atopic patients requires no comment here, it is apparent that an allergic constitution is not the only factor involved. Even in seasonal pollenosis, symptoms are not consistently related to the pollen concentration of inspired air. It is no new idea that autonomic tone can influence a truly allergic manifestation. Almost 70 years ago, Eppinger and Hess (1910) classified allergic states as vagotonic disease. Although this went too far, there is no doubt that allergic attacks are partly conditioned by variation in autonomic balance. Van Dishoeck (1961) found that in atopic patients unilateral stellate block markedly increased the local response to a small stimulus. More recently Nomura and Matsuura (1972) satisfactorily relieved house-dust atopy by Vidian neurectomy. They showed that, after operation, provocative tests on the nasal mucosa were negative on the operated side but remained positive on the unoperated side. These authors believed that an allergic reaction may also be a triggering response for cholinergic activity and that, when specific desensitization fails, Vidian neurectomy is indicated. This suggestion that atopy may be one of the factors influencing hypothalamic activity and that it may thus have a common cholinergic pathway, is interesting but further work is necessary before this position becomes clear. Surgery should not diminish circulating or interstitial IgE but the clinical response of atopic patients in whom desensitization has failed is certainly encouraging enough to be considered an indication. Nevertheless the results do not appear as good or as well maintained as in the strictly cholinergic cases.

Practical considerations of pterygo–palatine fossa surgery

Within the pterygo–palatine fossa, the surgeon may be concerned with one of several different procedures:

(1) Maxillary artery ligation
(2) Maxillary neurectomy
(3) Spheno-palatine ganglionectomy
(4) Vidian neurectomy

Only the now classic trans-antral route allows a flexible approach for any or all of these procedures, each of which has a distinct place in our armamentarium. Each requires the same instruments, anaesthesia, and operating microscope and the first three can only be carried out by the trans-antral route. Details of these techniques are given in the author's appropriate chapters in *Operative Surgery (Nose and Throat)* (Butterworths). Here it is principles rather than operative details that concern us, but the essentials of these techniques require to be stated here, before the clinical use, indications, complications and the possible alternative methods for Vidian neurectomy are considered.

The classic trans-antral technique

Preliminary considerations

Any sinus infection will have been eliminated or resolved. The configuration of the maxillary antrum can be judged in standard x-ray views and a submento–vertical view. This latter is invaluable in judging the working room available and the relative thickness of bony walls.

Anaesthesia and position

General endotracheal anaesthetic with hypotension is employed. A systolic blood pressure of approximately 60 mmHg is often critical in giving the relatively bloodless field required for all but emergency ligations of the maxillary artery. The patient is positioned as for a Caldwell–Luc operation. Local anaesthesia with heavy basal sedation has been employed successfully by others.

Instruments

A Zeiss microscope with 10 × magnification and a 300 mm objective, is used. A few special instruments designed by the author are invaluable. Shouldered probes for diathermy within the pterygoid canal are essential for safety.

The trans-antral tunnel

The anterior wall of the maxillary antrum is removed as for a Caldwell–Luc operation. Ordinarily the antral mucosa is virtually normal and access to the posterior antral wall is unimpeded. Should the medial antral wall bulge laterally and impede vision, it may be mobilized and pushed medially towards the nose to give adequate access and replaced subsequently. The mucosa over the posterior antral wall is removed and a posterior antral window outlined by chisel cuts through the thin postero–lateral bony wall. The inexperienced are apt to cut this posterior window too high. It should be remembered that the level of foramen rotundum will be below the level of the antral roof. Orientation is easier if this window is cut before turning to the microscope. Only the bone is cut through; the underlying periostial layer is to be preserved. Once the bone is removed any prominent veins running across the periosteum can be lightly coagulated.

Ligation of the maxillary artery

Practical experience of this procedure should be mandatory for any surgeon contemplating Vidian neurectomy by the trans-antral route. Ligation in continuity is unsatisfactory and ligation–resection is required. Scissors are thrust directly backwards through the periosteum and opened widely in both horizontal and vertical planes. Any attempt to dissect and portray the maxillary artery and its branches as they lie *in situ*, is likely to prove both difficult and frustrating. A simple trick ensures success. An appropriate hook is slipped behind any presenting loop of the maxillary artery. This is drawn gently towards the operator and so the vessel is held under tension. Thus held, scissor dissection will quickly display the entire arterial pattern and permit the ready identification of any breach. Whilst the artery is held similarly on a hook, clips are applied for its occlusion. Practically all surgeons with pioneering experience in this procedure can recall cases where apparently appropriate ligation–division of the maxillary artery has failed to stop epistaxis arising within the territory of this vessel and subsequently stopped by ligation of the external carotid. This continued bleeding is due to one of three possible errors in this technique:

(1) The infra-orbital branch may be mistaken for the main trunk which is allowed to remain intact.
(2) The maxillary artery is divided lateral to its bifurcation into ascending spheno–palatine and descending palatine arteries. If this terminal bifurcation remains intact, anastomotic backflow can lead to continued bleeding from the spheno–palatine artery or its branches (*Figure 20.13*).
(3) An anomalous pharyngeal and/or Vidian artery has been overlooked and allows bleeding to continue. Such a vessel can easily be found by dissection backwards through the fat to the face of the sphenoid along a curved line extending downwards and inwards from foramen rotundum (*Figure 20.14*).

Resection of the maxillary nerve
By steps similar to the above, the maxillary artery is defined and the main trunk clipped for safety and the vessel is otherwise left intact and pushed inferiorily whilst the maxillary nerve is sought in the fat above it. This nerve can also be steadied on a hook and traced backwards to the foramen rotundum, the lower edge of which can be defined by a small rugine. Remembering that the foramen rotundum is the upper limit of safe dissection, the operator should approach both nerve and foramen from

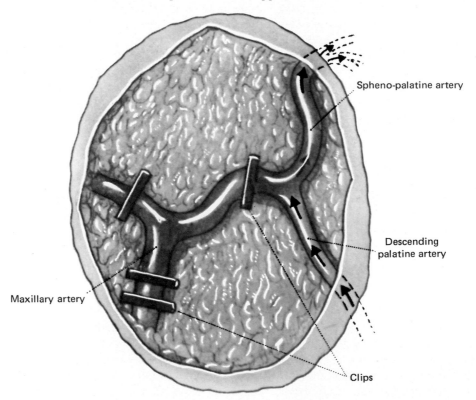

Figure 20.13   Anastomotic backflow in faulty ligation of maxillary artery. (From *Operative Surgery*, 3rd edn. Ed. by C. Rob and R. Smith. *Nose and Throat*. London; Butterworths)

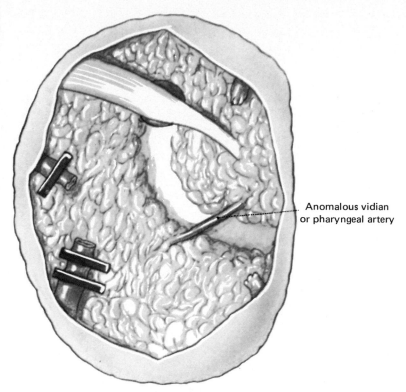

Anomalous vidian
or pharyngeal artery

Figure 20.14 Seeking an anomolous vessel in maxillary ligation. (From *Operative Surgery*, 3rd edn. Ed. by C. Rob and R. Smith. *Nose and Throat.* London; Butterworths)

below and work upwards towards it. The maxillary nerve is resected flush with foramen rotundum with a sickle knife. The distal part of the nerve can then be drawn into the wound and at least 1 cm of the nerve resected.

Spheno–palatine ganglionectomy

Once the maxillary nerve and the edge of the foramen rotundum have been exposed, it is easy to locate the spheno–palatine bundle that arises from the maxillary nerve immediately after it emerges from the foramen. This bundle is traced downwards and medially towards the mouth of the pterygoid canal. This area may still be hidden under cover of the medial buttress of the posterior antral window (*Figure 20.15*). An appropriate segment of this buttress is now lowered flush with the medial wall of the antrum by appropriate chisel cuts. A small chisel is safer and quicker than any burr and the latter should not be used once the periosteum has been opened. Once the medial bony buttress has been lowered, the terminal bifurcation of the maxillary artery is held on a hook and the spheno–palatine branch resected. This allows the spheno–palatine bundle to be traced dowards and medially under full vision. About 8 mm medial to and below the foramen rotundum the position of the spheno–palatine ganglion will be clear from the divergence of its descending palatine and nasal branches. Whilst these are elevated on a hook, a sickle knife is swept beneath them to cut the Vidian nerve as it emerges from the pterygoid canal. A sickle-knife is now used

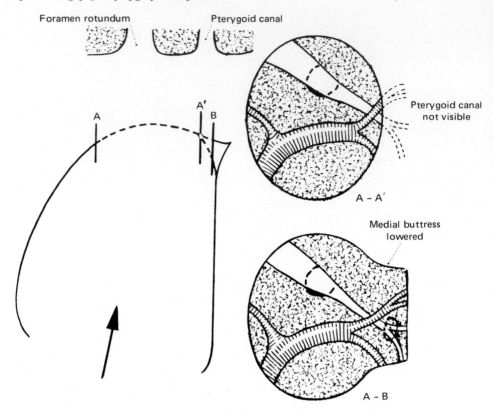

Figure 20.15 Influence of medial buttress in trans-antral approach. (From *Operative Surgery*, 3rd edn. Ed. by C. Rob and R. Smith. *Nose and Throat.* London; Butterworths)

to cut the spheno–palatine bundle and its terminal branches. The spheno–palatine ganglion will thus lie free to be removed.

Vidian neurectomy

The Vidian nerve is exposed by following the essential steps enumerated above. The trans-antral tunnel is used to enter the pterygo–palatine fossa. The maxillary artery is secured and clipped and then pushed downwards whilst the maxillary nerve is sought and used as a guide to expose the lower border of the foramen rotundum. The spheno–palatine bundle is now traced downwards and medially, the overlying bony buttress being lowered to facilitate this and the spheno–palatine artery resected for better exposure. The point of divergence of terminal branches of the spheno–palatine bundle is determined and whilst these are elevated on a hook, the sickle knife is swept beneath them to cut the Vidian nerve as it emerges from the pterygoid canal (*Figure 20.16*). Once the Vidian nerve is divided, the spheno–palatine bundle can be swung upwards or downwards like a bucket handle to better expose the mouth of the pterygoid canal. The mouth of this canal is now fully exposed with a small rugine from either the medial or the lateral side of the descending palatine nerve, whichever seems the more appropriate.

Simple surgical section of the Vidian nerve leaving the ends in relative apposition would invite recurrence. Diathermy of the pterygoid canal is now used to complete

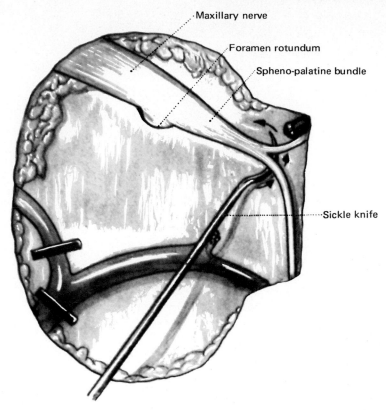

Figure 20.16   Vidian neurectomy. (From *Operative Surgery*, 3rd edn. Ed. by
C. Rob and R. Smith. *Nose and Throat.* London; Butterworths)

the destruction of the Vidian nerve over an area and to secure haemastasis (*Figure 20.17*). A blunt-headed and shouldered probe is inserted to fit snugly into the mouth of the pterygoid canal. The probe most often required is 3 mm in diameter across the shoulder. Diathermy with a coagulating current is applied via the probe intermittently for approximately 5 s. Proper use of the author's probes appears to have eliminated the possible risks of external ophthalmoplegia that can be provoked by over-penetration of the pterygoid canal with a faulty probe.

The indications for pterygo–palatine fossa procedures

Indications for maxillary artery ligation

Acute massive epistaxis
Whilst vascular ligation is required in only 1–2 per cent of severe acute epistaxes, it should be considered when the usual conservative procedures fail to control bleeding within two to three days. The appropriate artery must be properly selected but this is seldom difficult. Bleeding from the anterior ethmoid artery (internal carotid system)

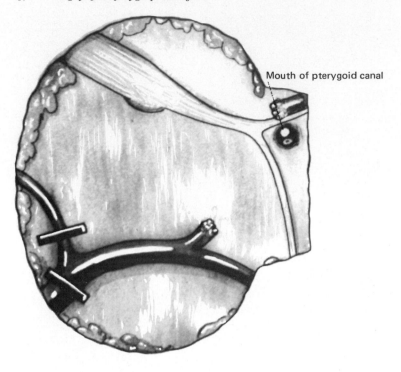

Mouth of pterygoid canal

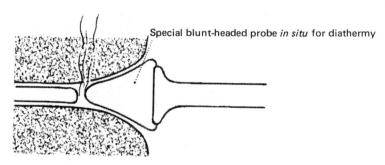

Special blunt-headed probe *in situ* for diathermy

Figure 20.17 Diathermy of pterygoid canal. (From *Operative Surgery*, 3rd edn. Ed. by C. Rob and R. Smith. *Nose and Throat*. London; Butterworths)

is uncommon for the vessel supplies only about 7 per cent of the nasal mucosa, all above the middle turbinate on the lateral wall of the nose. Such ethmoidal bleeding is usually traumatic in origin and evidence of ethmoidal fracture is frequent.

The vast majority of severe bleeds arise from the area of maxillary supply (external carotid system). This is generally evident from bleeding below the middle turbinate on the lateral wall or from the septum. If such location cannot be determined, a maxillary source can almost certainly be presumed in the absence of clear evidence of ethmoidal bleeding. In the circumstances of severe bleeding from the maxillary supply, a trans-antral maxillary ligation is ideal but circumstances in an elderly enfeebled patient exhausted by blood loss, may suggest external carotid ligation under a local anaesthetic as preferable. Even although the distal anastomosis may open within a week, external carotid ligation can be depended upon to arrest bleeding from this source. Such external carotid ligation will however cause blindness in the exceptional circumstance that the ophthalmic artery on the operated side arises anomalously from the middle meningeal branch of the maxillary artery *before* the latter enters the pterygo–palatine fossa. Such risks approximate to 1 in 3000. With other indications for vascular ligation, external carotid ligation is inappropriate and any vascular ligation must be maxillary.

Recurrent epistaxis

Here the problem is not control of the individual bleed but the elimination of frequent recurrence. Such cases are often due to hypertension but hypotensive therapy, which will generally suffice, may be contraindicated or ineffective. In these, as in other recurrent cases, maxillary ligation is generally highly effective in preventing further recurrences. Several years later, however, further ligations may be required to control the established anastomotic circulation.

Hereditary telangiectasia

The control of severe frequently recurrent epistaxis from this cause is proverbially difficult. Vascular ligation all too often proves diappointing but seems to provide effective help for possibly 30 per cent of patients, at all events for two years or so. Maxillary ligation alone will seldom suffice. It should be combined with ethmoidal ligation and division of the labial supply to the lower part of the septum. At times, at least, subsequent recurrence can be shown by angiography to have followed the opening of new vessels generally derived from the ophthalmic artery. Septal dermatoplasty is an alternative to vascular ligation but, in my experience, with revascularization of the graft epistaxis again becomes recurrent after two to three years.

Nasopharyngeal angiofibroma

The extirpation of these vascular tumours, ordinarily attended by massive bleeding, is difficult to control. Almost always, however, these tumours are supplied by the spheno–palatine artery of one or other side. This can be demonstrated by angiography. Preliminary trans-antral ligation of the feeding vessels removes the hazard of bleeding from the next step of tumour extirpation, which is thus greatly simplified. These naso-pharyngeal tumours also not infrequently extend into the medial part of the pterygo–palatine fossa and in such a case the trans-antral exposure with appropriate vascular ligation is almost essential to complete removal of the tumour.

Indications for maxillary neurectomy

Tic douloureux

The diagnosis and treatment of this condition have been fully considered in Chapter 18. Although all forms of peripheral neurectomy have so far proved temporary and followed by recurrence within 1–1½ years, they retain a place prior to any sensory root section and may prevent the anaesthesia dolorosa that can otherwise prove such a permanent handicap. The pain that recurs 9–12 months after infra-orbital or supra-orbital neurectomy, appears to have been due to nerve regeneration.

The resection of at least 1 cm from the maxillary nerve flush with the foramen rotundum, seemed to me sufficient to prevent such regeneration in a somatic nerve across such a gap. Nevertheless, my experience of 35 such cases has been that without other measures local tic douloureux has inevitably been followed by recurrence in 14–18 months.

Later I was to observe in a revision operation that an almost normal looking maxillary nerve had been regenerated across a gap of 1.5 cm and the further resection of it gave gratifying relief. Since then, in any case of maxillary neurectomy, I have plugged the foramen rotundum with a silastic or acrylic implant together with an x-ray marker.

Such patients are yet too few and follow-up too short to permit dogmatic assertion that it will avert recurrence and give relief as long-lasting as sensory root section. Nevertheless, I now have several patients who have passed two years without recurrence, an event hitherto unknown in my experience. It appears that such plugging of foramen rotundum is a well worthwhile and safe extension of ordinary maxillary neurectomy and may give a successful long-term result.

Where tic douloureux is limited to the second division of the trigeminal and cannot be controlled by conservative means, then maxillary neurectomy with an appropriate plug to the foramen rotundum is well justified and may suffice to allow the elderly patient to live out his life in comfort with the minimal degree of sensory loss or other inconvenience.

Persistent maxillary neuralgia

One occasionally sees patients with persistent pain strictly confined to the territory of the maxillary nerve or within this. Such pain is seldom severe but the constancy of it through weeks, months or even years can prove wearing in the extreme. Careful examination fails to reveal any still existing pathology but the history will often show that the pain started following some surgical intervention, such as an upper dental extraction or a Caldwell–Luc operation. It may however have preceded the latter, having started with an acute maxillary sinusitis. At other times no precipitating lesion or injury can be recalled.

The nature of this type of neuralgic pain remains obscure and it needs to be carefully distinguished from conversion hysteria or other psychic states or atypical facial neuralgia (*see* Chapter 18). Provided that this can be done, and the author has met 37 cases over the past 25 years, it can be relieved by maxillary neurectomy at the foramen rotundum. Such relief has been found on follow-up to endure for years but from earlier remarks it would seem wise to plug foramen rotundum to hinder nerve regeneration. Such maxillary neurectomies have invariably shown that the resultant anaesthesia is much less extensive over the skin than would be expected from the generally accepted trigeminal dermatomes. The area of skin subserved by the zygomatic–temporal and zygomatic–facial branches, still carry apparently unimpaired sensation following maxillary neurectomy and pain within this area will not be affected by it. The explanation appears to be in the communicating twig to the zygomatic branches from the ophthalmic division and pain that resides or persists in the zygomatic area can be relieved by a limited lateral orbitotomy to resect this communication (Golding-Wood, 1970).

Indication for spheno-palatine ganglionectomy

Periodic migrainous neuralgia

The distinctive characteristics of this syndrome have been described in Chapter 18. Ordinarily these patients can be relieved by ergotamine in adequate dosage and surgery is to be considered only where medical therapy has failed. Although the pain appears largely vascular in character, the role of autonomic influences remains uncertain. Both petrosal neurectomy and spheno–palatine ganglionectomy have been used, but the long periods of spontaneous remission so characteristic in this condition render the assessment of operative results difficult.

Petrosal neurectomy was found by Gardner (1955) to give effective relief but he found subsequent recurrence of pain that he deemed due to nerve regeneration. More recently Fisch (1975) has claimed much improved results from petrosal neurectomy that he attributes to his micro-surgical technique and use of a Silastic screen between the nerve ends to hamper regeneration. The author has attained apparently comparable results from spheno–palatine ganglionectomy together with resection of the maxillary artery within the pterygo–palatine fossa. The patient has ordinarily been admitted near the start of a cluster of attacks and in virtually every case operation has secured prompt cessation of the attacks. This has characteristically endured far beyond the ordinary periods of remission that the patient had hitherto known. After two or three years, however, there is a tendency for pain to recur, although frequently such recurrence has been notably less severe and the clusters less prolonged. On two occasions, the recurrence of pain has been on the other side of the face. On several occasions it has been found that such recurrent pain has strangely proved amenable to ergotamine whereas prior to operation, it had not been so. Further experience and longer follow-up is required before these surgical measures can be properly assessed. Nevertheless, the results at present seem well worthwhile.

Indications for Vidian neurectomy

Intractable secreto–motor rhinopathy
   (a) Cholinergic
   (b) Allergic

The cholinergic group   In many such patients, the symptoms are insufficient to require surgery; adequate relief can be obtained by use of antihistamines (which have an anticholinergic action), oral decongestants or simple alterations of the patient's way of life. Only those whose symptoms are completely intractable are considered for surgery. Those patients who elect surgery without hesitation rather than put up with the symptoms, may with confidence be offered Vidian neurectomy, provided the operator is confident of his technique

The allergic group   These atopic patients are not ordinarily regarded as candidates for surgery. Where customary anti-allergic measures including full specific desensitization and 'Rynacrom' have failed and symptoms remain severe, Vidian neurectomy offers good prospects of marked improvement.

The mixed group   This group includes at least some of those patients whose atopic symptoms are not relieved by appropriate anti-allergic treatment. Sometimes cholinergic influences are clearly apparent but this is not always so. In practice, the atopy should be treated and Vidian neurectomy considered only if the residual symptoms remain severe.

Senile rhinorrhoea   The ordinary dewdrop of the aged does not require surgery. Occasionally, however, this senile type of rhinorrhoea is unquestionably severe and extremely distressing, although the nasal mucosa shows no apparent change and sneezing is not much in evidence. These aged patients are often in poor cardiovascular condition but their symptoms distress them to the extent that they beg for operative relief, seemingly undeterred by mention of appreciable risk. The few so operated were incredibly happy from the maintained relief from this source of distress.

Chronic epiphora   Where, as is usually the case, there is demonstrable disorder of the naso–lacrimal ducts, this pathology is to be attacked directly. Where symptoms of epiphora cannot otherwise be relieved, either lacrimal adenectomy or Vidian neurectomy are likely to be equally affective.

Occasionally, epiphora persists after lacrimal adenectomy. Such cases are difficult to relieve since accessory glands and goblet cells of the conjunctiva contribute markedly to the epiphora. These glands do not appear to be under any neural control, and although Vidian neurectomy may give a little improvement, it is not to be recommended lightly.

Crocodile tears   Severe lesions of the facial nerve at or proximal to geniculate ganglion tend to be followed 6–12 months later by the development of crocodile tears. This purely gustatory lacrimation is one of several bizarre phenomena that result from the collateral nerve sprouting that is so enormously effective in the autonomic system. When an autonomic nerve degenerates, any adjacent normal autonomic fibres give off sprouts which can connect with appropriate cholinergic or adrenergic endings. Either useful function or bizarre sequelae result. A facial palsy with a dry eye due to involvement of the petrosal nerve provides just the conditions for an abnormal gustatory reflex, for secreto–motor salivary fibres pass in the tympanic nerve and lesser petrosal nerve to reach the lacrimal gland by a process of collateral sprouting. The communicating twig between lesser and greater petrosal nerves facilitates the passage of these sprouts.

The patient's embarrassment when, with every meal, tears roll down the affected cheek, is easily understood. In treatment I prefer tympanic neurectomy because it preserves emotional tearing (Golding-Wood, 1963). Where, however, a local ear condition contraindicates this, or symptoms have recurred, then Vidian neurectomy can be depended upon to give complete relief from this nuisance, though emotional tearing is, of course, lost on that side.

Recurrent nasal polyposis   Nasal polypi may occur in any case of secreto–motor rhinopathy but seem considerably more common where there is evidence of atopy. Infective changes in the nose and/or sinuses seem to provide the essential stimulus for the production of polyps. The other factors merely provide the relatively swollen, oedematous mucosa that is likely to lead to the obstruction of sinus ostia and infection. Every rhinologist is only too aware of the problems posed by patients with severe, recurrent polyposis. A growing number of rhinologists have recorded their results in such cases of bilateral polypectomy with unilateral Vidian neurectomy. There appears to be general agreement that if patients so treated are followed up for periods of at least two years, the polyps rarely recur on the side of the Vidian neurectomy though they frequently do so on the non-neurectomized side. This characteristic finding appears independent of the type of polypectomy elected and of the technique of Vidian neurectomy.

There is much to suggest that the initial tissue changes in nasal polyposis are oedema and cellular infiltration of the nasal mucosa produced by secreto–motor rhinopathy, whether atopic or cholinergic. These changes (and perhaps the viral agents postulated by Weille, 1966) favour bacterial invasion and chronic infection, which in turn produces the hyperplastic tissue. Surgical measures must clearly aim at the removal of obstructing polyps and adequate drainage of involved sinuses. This generally seems best accomplished by some form of ethmoidectomy. Vidian neurectomy may do much to correct the underlying mucosal factors.

My own preference is to carry out a trans-antral Vidian neurectomy proceeding with the ethmoidectomy afterwards in the superbly bloodless field given by the associated resection of the spheno–palatine artery.

Follow-up examinations, however, as yet have been too few to claim an established place for this indication. In severe nasal polyposis at present it appears a worthwhile measure but it most certainly does not eliminate further recurrence at a later date.

Alternative methods of Vidian neurectomy

Vidian neurectomy can be accomplished by several routes as follows:

(1) Trans-antral a) Classic (Golding-Wood, 1961)
              b) Subperiosteal (Nomura, 1974)
(2) Trans-nasal a) Trans-septal (Minnis and Morrison, 1971)
              b) Direct (Patel and Gaikwad, 1975)
(3) Trans-palatal (Chandra, 1969; Mostafa, Abdel-Latif and el-Din, 1973)

Soon after the success of Vidian neurectomy by the original trans-antral technique had been widely confirmed, other operative approaches were described. The main purpose of their protagonists was to avoid the 'difficulties and dangers of the trans-antral route'. However, these so-called difficulties and dangers are mainly illusory, provided the surgical anatomy of the pterygo–palatine fossa is properly appreciated, and the surgeon has basic experience of maxillary ligation and other pertinent procedures. Only the classic trans-antral route will ordinarily permit any manoeuvre desired in the pterygo–palatine fossa to be carried out under direct vision. Any successful method of Vidian neurectomy should give equivalent immediate results. The route chosen, however, may influence not only the possible complications but also the likelihood of complete neurectomy and the possibility of later recurrent symptoms. Although most authors can record initial result rates of about 90 per cent, the only long-term follow-up figures available are my own. It should be noted that these figures relate to a procedure in which the spheno–palatine artery is deliberately resected. All other methods seek to avoid the vessels. Thus they leave an intact periarterial plexus that may contribute collateral sprouts that could well re-innervate the nasal glands; this is certainly a considerable theoretic disadvantage. Whether it matters in practice, however, only long-term follow-up studies can show.

The trans-antral subperiostial route

Nomura's method follows my own until the posterior antral window is cut. The medial buttress and posterior part of the medial antral wall are removed immediately. A periosteal elevator is inserted between the periosteum of the pterygo–palatine fossa and the vertical plate of the palatine bone until it meets the pterygoid process of the sphenoid bone. The periosteal envelope that encloses the contents of the pterygo–palatine fossa is now stripped laterally and upward until the elevator locates the mouth of the pterygoid canal. This is felt rather than seen because the periosteum descends into the canal enclosing the Vidian nerve and vessels in a fibrous funnel. To minimize bleeding, this entire funnel is coagulated before being sectioned. Subsequently it is imperative that the entire circumference of the pterygoid foramen be cleared and the tissues deeply resected within it.

I believe that this method is generally excellent and the relatively inexperienced may prefer it to the more difficult dissection across the soft tissue of the pterygo–palatine fossa. Should bleeding give difficulty, however, or the pterygoid canal be so enclosed by the sphenoid sinus that the walls crumble away on the pressure of the coagulating probe, then the surgeon is far less able to correct the situation.

Trans-nasal approaches

These approaches depend upon the fact that the spheno–palatine foramen, which is 5 mm in diameter, has a fairly prominent posterior lip and lies relatively open from the front for the anterior lip diverges laterally. In a dry skull one can see the open mouth of the pterygoid canal immediately lateral and slightly behind the spheno–palatine foramen. Thus, a coagulating probe can be passed through the spheno–palatine foramen and into the pterygoid canal but in operating conditions this procedure is necessarily blind and the diameter of the probe is greatly restricted.

The original papers must be consulted for details of the technique but in either case the pterygoid canal is entered, necessarily blindly, with a narrow probe. An Angell-James pituitary diathermy probe approximately 1.5 mm in diameter is generally used. Ordinarily this probe will feel as though it is gripped within a canal and will be arrested about half way along the 1 cm length. Diathermy coagulation is then applied.

In small series, both these two teams of authors had excellent results without material complication. In ordinary circumstances the approach should be safe enough but in the not infrequent cases in which the pterygoid canal is widely dehiscent into the sphenoid sinus, there are clearly risks of being lost. I believe, however, that there is a more serious inherent risk in this technique. Originally I had used an ordinary theatre probe 2 mm in diameter for coagulation within the pterygoid canal. Over 50 patients were treated without incident before three developed a gross ophthalmoplegia with severe palsy of the third, fourth and sixth cranial nerves immediately following operation. After six months these improved, but one required muscle balance surgery. The same serious complication was later reported by others (Martin, 1967; Hilger, 1969). Later I was to find that whilst the pterygoid canal typically narrows to obstruct the passage of such a probe, in 2 per cent of skulls it will admit a probe of 2.5 mm in diameter throughout its entire length. This was a striking parallel to the incidence of this complication, which seemed due to over-penetration of the probe and diathermy coagulation damaging these nerves in the middle cranial fossa. The blunt headed and shouldered probes subsequently designed to avert this risk of over-penetration, appear to have eliminated this risk of ophthalmoplegia for certain. Since using these probes, I have had no further ophthalmoplegia in over 15 years and 300 patients. Probes of this design are, I believe, imperative for the safe conduct of this operation. The risk would seem to remain inherent in either form of trans-antral technique, since room to manipulate a similarly headed probe is lacking. The report by Sood, Krishnamurthy and Kapoor (1976) of unilateral blindness following a trans-septal Vidian neurectomy is sufficient to show that these risks are not merely theoretical.

The trans-palatal technique

This technique, introduced by Chandra (1969), and improved by Mostafa, Abdel-Latif and el-Din (1973) will appeal to surgeons who wish to avoid the pterygo–palatine fossa.

It requires general anaesthesia with an oral cuffed tube and a pharyngeal pack. The patient is placed in a semi-reclining position with the head thrown well back. A Boyle–Davis gag is useful to keep the mouth open and this position permits easy displacement of the soft palate and allows blood to drain away from the operative field.

A curved incision is made over the hard palate curving backwards on either side from a point in the midline at least 1 cm anterior to the posterior edge of the hard palate. The soft palate is freed and displaced downwards and 5 mm of bone removed from the posterior edge of the hard palate to give a better exposure. The orifices and cushions of the eustachian tubes are important landmarks. A Zeiss microscope is used and a 300 mm focal length objective is required for sufficient working room. An incision is made through the mucosa to expose the medial pterygoid plate at its junction with the basi-occiput. This landmark is vital, because the foramen lacerum and the internal carotid artery it contains, lie immediately postero–lateral to it. The base of the medial pterygoid plate is removed over the line of the pterygoid canal with a cutting burr. Posteriorly, a bar of bone must be left intact across this to avoid opening the foramen lacerum. Usually the pterygoid canal is only 2–3 mm deep and is readily opened. The Vidian nerve is cut and cauterized and its fellow similarly dealt with on the other side. The palate is then closed in two layers.

Ordinarily, the trans-palatal technique should be dependable for a pure resection of the Vidian nerve, but in patients in whom extensions of the sphenoid sinus engulf the pterygoid canal, real difficulty could ensue. Much has been made of the fact that a trans-palatal approach gives access to both pterygoid canals, whereas the trans-antral route requires bilateral operation. With proper technique, however, this is of no great moment, because the bilateral trans-antral operation ordinarily requires only 50 min. The trans-palatal route is not an automatic guarantee of safety. It seems ironic that a method designed to avoid the maxillary artery and a non-existing venous plexus, should lead one to take a cutting burr so close to the internal carotid artery. Nevertheless, the trans-palatal approach has great merit when the trans-antral route is contraindicated by lack of room or other reason.

Possible complications

The complications of any form of pterygo–palatine fossa surgery, by the trans-antral route, have been remarkably few and the procedure usually gives but little more reaction than a simple Caldwell–Luc. The possible sequelae may be enumerated as follows:

(1) Marked swelling of the cheeks may occur but it subsides within a few days. Although this was common in the author's early experience, it has been almost eliminated by the anaesthetist's care to avoid rapid oscillations of blood pressure and too early resumption of normal pressure post-operatively.

(2) Some numbness of the infra-orbital area and especially the upper lip is common and may last several weeks. Patients are warned of this effect and they have not been unduly troubled by it.

(3) Rarely, a continuous and troublesome neuralgic pain over the infra-orbital area has been present. The occurrence of this has been limited to one side in each of two patients (of a total of over 400). In each case this pain resisted even maxillary neurectomy and appeared to have been in an hysterical conversion syndrome.

(4) External ophthalmoplegia due to over-penetration of the pterygoid canal occurred in three patients in my earlier series (Golding-Wood, 1973) and it has been recorded by others. It appears to be eliminated by proper use of shouldered probes. However, a similar risk of over-penetration of the pterygoid canal would seem an inherent risk of trans-nasal techniques.

(5) There is some risk of post-operative maxillary sinusitis, but it is greatly reduced by post-operative use of a broad spectrum antibiotic. Should it occur, such infection responds to antral washouts which can be carried out as usual and as early as required together with appropriate antibiotics. In no case has there been any evidence of wider spread of infection.

Results of Vidian neurectomy

As is apparent, the prime indication for Vidian neurectomy is in secreto–motor rhinopathy and only its results on such indication now remain for consideration.

Cholinergic type

Given proper diagnosis and meticulous technique, prompt and complete cessation of the rhinorrhoea uniformly occurs. Former severe paroxysms of sneezing are vastly reduced, but the reflex is not lost and local irritation can evoke the response. Rarely however do patients complain of this.

Perhaps because many earlier episodes were confused with colds, on post-operative follow-up it is common to hear the patient remark 'I never get even a cold these days, either'. When previously mucosal oedema had produced some nasal obstruction, patients almost invariable comment on their newly acquired ease of breathing.

Significant symptomatic relapse is unusual, and practically limited to 2–3 per cent of patients who experience partial return of symptoms 1–2 years after operation. These patients, who still remain grateful for operation, have seldom relapsed further, even in another decade.

In the author's entire series of 280 patients in this group, there were but four complete failures, all within the first 20 and apparently due to technical inadequacy. The patients relapsed completely a few months after apparently successful operation but the reason remains obscure. Occasionally a patient presents with an apparent relapse that proves to be due to a subsequent development of allergy. This however can be relieved by appropriate treatment.

A bilateral response can follow unilateral operation, the unoperated side responding almost as well as the operated side after a lag of 1–3 weeks. This strange and wholly unexpected result has been repeatedly confirmed by others, but an entirely satisfying explanation is still lacking. In my experience it occurred in 30 per cent of patients, but the second side relapsed in half of these after about a year. Hence for many years I have operated on both sides in the initial session.

Confirmatory results have been widely recorded by many authors and from most countries. Properly used, Vidian neurectomy will give virtually complete relief in over 90 per cent of cholinergic cases and this appears to be indefinitely maintained in the vast majority.

Allergic and mixed types

My rule has been to first treat any evidence of atopy and consider operation when no other reasonable measure remained.

Some 80 per cent of patients derive distinct improvement from operation, though sneezing has remained more prevalent and the airways less clear than in the cholinergic group. More than 50 per cent of these patients respond as well as those in the cholinergic group but it is not yet certain whether or not there is some increased liability to relapse.

The nasal effects of Vidian neurectomy

No adverse effects are normally found in the nasal cavity. The secretions are somewhat sticky, but crusting or other troubles are conspicuous by their absence. The ciliary transport of a drop of Indian ink through the nose, remains within normal limits and equal on operated and unoperated sides. Any subsequent acute coryza runs the normal course.

A purely postural engorgement of the nasal mucosa has been seen but in only three patients. Whilst their turbinate mucosa was entirely normal when they were sitting, it would become engorged and swollen within a few minutes of lying down. Simple submucosal diathermy of the affected turbinates sufficed for complete relief in each case.

Histologic changes

In cholinergic cases, Vidian neurectomy sharply reduces the number of mucus glands in the nasal mucosa. Those that were formerly markedly hyperactive, quickly revert to normality. Eosinophils in the mucosa also reduce to normal.

Mostafa, Abdel-Latif and el-Din (1973) found Vidian neurectomy to give analogous changes even in atopic rhinitis. The previous oedema of basement membrane propria, quickly disappeared. Simultaneously, the vascularity improved as the vessels were allowed to open when the compressive effects of oedema had subsided. The epithelium that formerly was desquamated, rapidly regenerated to normal. The marked esosinophilia found before operation quickly reduced after it. Pre-operatively, mast-cells were few and showed marked degranulation, indicative of histamine release. Post-operatively, the mast-cells rapidly increased in number and showed minimal degranulation indicating that histamine release is retained within these cells. These same workers confirm the results of others, that polyps shrank post-operatively and that mucinous and oedematous fluids were absorbed, leaving empty spaces. By carrying out biological assays of the histamine content of the nasal mucosa before and after operation in patients with atopic rhinitis, Vidian neurectomy was found to result in a 50 per cent reduction in the histamine content. As the number of cases and the timing of these observations was not stated, however, this work requires further assessment by others.

The ocular effects of Vidian neurectomy

Normal lacrimation ceases because the secreto–motor supply to the lacrimal gland is necessarily lost. The relatively dry eye can be shown by Schirmer's test. Some patients experience temporary ocular discomfort that however is easily relieved by artificial tear drops, 1–3 per cent methylcellulose, that can be discontinued after a few weeks. This suspension of normal lacrimation has not appeared to carry any risk of the kerato–conjunctivitis sicca that attends the dry eye of the Sjogren syndrome, for the conjunctival goblet cells remain active. Whilst these ocular effects might be aggravated in hot, dry or dusty climates, there does not seem any report from other quarters of the globe that significant trouble has ensued from this cause.

Patients must be informed that following the operation they will not be able to cry. At first they will feel deprived of the psychological relief given by weeping in times of emotional stress. Some patients have commented that their feelings remain churned up for several hours when otherwise they might have been speedily relieved by a good cry. Nevertheless, they have adjusted to this within a few months and thereafter have not been perturbed by the loss of emotional tearing. Although the eye remains relatively dry, the use of contact lenses seems seldom to have been made more difficult.

Secreto–motor rhinopathy, severe and intractable enough to justify Vidian neurectomy, is not found in more than ten patients annually/500 000 population. The affected individuals have been utterly miserable for years and their gratitude for operative relief is correspondingly great. The surgeon's responsibility remains great because any technical failure will not only mar the result, but also will cause a rapid build up of scar tissue in the pterygo–palatine fossa, which will render any revision operation extremely difficult.

Patients whose nasal airways are primarily obstructed by chronically congested or hyperplastic turbinates are not ordinarily candidates for this type of surgery.

Collectively the procedures to be undertaken within the pterygo–palatine fossa form a very considerable addition to our armamentarium. Whilst these operations are not for the inexperienced operator, they contain nothing to deter any skilled and adequately equipped ENT surgeon. Initial practice on a dry skull and on cadavers is essential, as is practical familiarity with the landmarks and tissues gained in the simpler procedures such as ligation of the maxillary artery.

References

Chandra, R. (1969) *Archives of Otolaryngology*, **89**, 52

Chorobski, J. and Penfield, W. (1932) *Archives of Neurology and Psychiatry*, **28**, 1257

Eccles, R. and Wilson, H. (1973) *Journal of Physiology*, **230**, 213

Eppinger, H. and Hess, L. (1910) *Die Vagotonie, eine Klinische Studie*, Berlin

Fisch, U. (1975) Personal communication

Fowler, E. P. (1943) *Archives of Otolaryngology*, **37**, 710

Gardner, W. J. (1955) In *Pain*. Ed. by White, J. C. and Sweet, W. H., Springfield, Illinois; Thomas

Golding-Wood, P. H. (1961) *Journal of Laryngology and Otology*, **75**, 232

Golding-Wood. P. H. (1962) *Journal of Laryngology and Otology*, **76**, 969

Golding-Wood, P. H. (1963) *British Medical Journal*, **1**, 1518

Golding-Wood, P. H. (1970) *Laryngoscope*, **80**, 1179

Golding-Wood, P. H. (1973) *Laryngoscope*, **83**, 1673

Grote, J. J., Juijpers, W. and Huygen, P. L. M. (1974) *Acta Otolaryngologica*, **79**, 124

Hilger, H. J. (1969) Personal communication

Holmes, T. H., Goodell, H., Wolff, S. and Wolff, H. G. (1950) *The Nose*, Springfield, Illinois; Thomas

Jackson, R. T. and Rooker, D. W. (1971) *Laryngoscope*, **81**, 565

Krajina, Z. (1973) *Acta Otolaryngologica*, **76**, 366

Malcomson, K. G. (1959) *Journal of Laryngology*, **73**, 73

Malm, L. (1973) *Acta Otolaryngologica*, **76**, 366

Martin, J. C. (1967) Personal communication

Minnis, N. L. and Morrison, A. W. (1971) *Journal of Laryngology and Otology*, **85**, 255

Montgomery, W. W., Katz, R. and Gamble, J. F. (1970) *Annals of Otology, Rhinology and Laryngology*, **79**, 606

Mostafa, H. M., Abdel-Latif, S. M. and el-Din, S. B. (1973) *Journal of Laryngology*, **87**, 773

Nomura, Y. and Matsuura, T. (1972) *Acta Otolaryngologica*, **73**, 493

Nomura, Y. (1974) *Laryngoscope*, **84**, 578

Patel, K. H. and Gaikwad, G. A. (1975) *Journal of Laryngology*, **89**, 1291

Sood, G. S., Krishnamurthy, G. , Kapoor, S. *et al.* (1976) *Journal of Laryngology*, **90**, 311

Toppozarda, H. H. and Talaat, M. A. (1976) *Otology, Rhinology and Laryngology*, **38**, 164

Van Dishoeck, H. A. E. (1961) *Congress of International Otorhinolaryngology*

Weille, F. L. (1966) *Annals of Allergy*, **24**, 549

Wolff, H. G. (1950) In *Feelings and Emotions* p. 284. Ed. by Reymert, M. L. New York

Index

Abnormalities,
  acquired, 59–71
  congenital, 47–59
Acne rosacea, 4, 18
Acoustic neuroma, 404
Acromegaly, treatment of, 426, 427, 431, 440, 441, 443
Actinomycosis, 203
Acupuncture in facial pain, 423
Adenocarcinoma of sinuses, 374
Adenoid cystic carcinoma, 361
Adenoiditis, sinusitis caused by, 245
Adenoma, benign papillary, 358
Agamma-globulinaemia, sinusitis and, 268
Airway,
  examination of, 6
  loss of lining, 64
  patency of, 2
Alar base,
  cleft lip and palate, in, 54, 55
  excision of, 53
  rodent ulcer of, 68
Alar cartilages, exposure of, 120, 123
Alar dome,
  cleft lip and palate, in, 55
  deformity, 61
Alar margin, loss of, 65
Albright's syndrome, 370
Allergy, 210
  perennial, 211
  sinusitis and, 251, 286, 288
  vestibulitis in, 15
Ameloblastoma, 371
Anatomy of nose, 73
Angiofibroma,
  nasopharyngeal, 162
  treatment of, 471
Angioneurotic oedema, 265
Angiosarcoma, 362
Anosmia, 235
  atrophic rhinitis, in, 177
  examination of, 9
  fractures of maxilla, following, 39

Anosmia (*continued*)
  nasal fractures, from, 24, 29
  polypi causing, 228
Anterior ethmoidal nerve syndrome, 89
Anterior ethmoidal syndrome, 412
Anterior rhinoscopy, 281
Anthrax, rhinitis in, 175
Anticholinesterases causing rhinitis, 218
Antral puncture, 290
Antro-choanal polypi, 233
Antrostomy, intranasal, 286, 293, 310
  children, in, 312
  technique, 294
Antrum,
  infection of, facial fractures, following, 45
  pain in, sinusitis, in, 256
  washouts, 310
Arterial ligation in epistaxis, 160
Arterio-arterial anastomoses, 151
Ascaris in nose, 145
Aspergillosis, 202, 269
Asthma,
  polypi and, 228
  sinusitis and, 251
Atopy, 209
Atypical facial neuralgia, 422
Auditory meatus, external, pain in, 390
Autonomic faciocephalgia, 420

Bacterial infection, sinusitis and, 253
Baro-sinusitis, 411
Barotrauma, sinusitis from, 249
Basal-cell carcinoma (*See* Rodent ulcer)
Bernouilli's phenomenon, 89, 225
Bernstein's technique, 103
Birth moulding theory of septal deviation, 85
Blastomycosis, 203
Bleeding diathesis, 162
Blindness, from temporal arteritis, 422
Blood vessels,
  nose, of, 148
  pathology of, 154

Boeck's sarcoid (*See* Sarcoidosis)
Boils (*See* Furuncles)
Bone,
    fibrous dysplasia of, 369
    thickening of, following injury, 30
Bone graft for septal support, 61
Bony deformities, 4
Brain-stem lesions, 264, 414
Breast cancer, 382, 430
Breschet's canals, infection of, 331
Bronchiectasis, sinusitis and, 252, 347
Bronchitis, sinusitis and, 251, 347
Bruxism, 419
Burkitt's lymphoma, 370

Caldwell–Luc operation, 293, 294–297, 308, 320,
        337, 344
    modifications, 297
    pain following, 413, 472
    sublabial fistula following, 345
    technique, 295
Candidiasis (moniliasis), 175, 204
Canfield's operation, 297
Capillary haemangioma, 65
Carcinoma,
    adenoid cystic, 361, 376
    basal-cell (*See* Rodent ulcers)
    nerve compression in, 404
    paranasal sinuses, of, 372
    sinusitis and, 346
    squamous-cell, 19, 359, 372
Caries, dental, 260, 406
Carotid artery ligation in epistaxis, 160
Cartilaginous tumours, 364
Cavernous haemangiomas, 363
Cavernous sinus thrombophlebitis,
    complicating sinusitis, 341
    furuncles, from, 14
Cerebello-pontine angle, tumours of, 264
Cerebrospinal rhinorrhoea, 11
    ethmoid operations, after, 298
    facial injury, in, 24
    fractures of maxilla, in, 38
    location of leak, 11
    nasal fractures, from, 24, 25, 29
    trans-ethmoidal hypophysectomy, following,
        439
Cervical myalgia, 417
Chicken-pox, 173
Choanal atresia,
    bony, 78
    membranous, 78
    posterior, 76
        anatomy, 76
        clinical picture, 77
        complications, 79
        examination for, 78
        management, 77, 78
Cholesteatoma, 181, 326
Christmas disease, 162
Chrome workers, septal perforation in, 135
Chromophobe tumours, trans-ethmoidal hypo-
        physectomy for, 430

Cilia,
    chronic sinusitis, in, 277
    cold and, 250
Ciliary neuralgia, 420
Cleft lip and palate, nose in, 54
Cluster headaches, 420
Colds (*See* Coryza)
Columnar mucosa, metaplasia of, 5
Common cold (*See* Coryza)
Congenital abnormalities, 47, 74–81 (*See also specific
        lesions*)
Congenital diseases of nose, 73–81
Conversion hysteria, facial pain and, 394
Cornea, pain afferent fibres in, 389
Coronary artery disease, facial pain from, 415
Coronary thrombosis, epistaxis and, 160
Coryza, 163–172
    anosmia in, 10
    bacteriology of, 169
    causative agents, 165
    clinical picture of, 169
    complications, 169
    diagnosis of, 170
    duration of infectivity, 166
    herpes simplex vesicles in, 16
    immunity against, 167
    incidence of, 163
    incubation period, 166
    local defences, 166
    mode of infection, 166
    mode of transmission, 166
    nasopharyngitis in, 169
    pathology of, 167
    predisposing factors, 163
    prevention of, 170, 265
    prophylaxis, 171
    recurring, 461
    sinusitis from, 244
    transmission of, 165
    treatment of, 172
    vaccines for, 171
    vestibulitis in, 15
Cosmetic surgery, 47–71
Costen's syndrome, 263, 418
Cottle's maxilla–pre-maxilla approach to septum,
        98, 99
Cough in sinusitis, 281
Cribriform plate,
    fracture of, 29
    lesions causing CSF rhinorrhoea, 11
Cryosurgery for pituitary ablation, 441
Cryptococcosis, 203
Cushing's disease, treatment of, 413, 426, 429, 440,
        441
Cystic fibrosis, 227, 252
Cysts of nose, 4, 75
Cytotoxic drugs in Wegener's granulomatosis, 353

Denker's operation, 297
Dental extraction,
    oro-antral fistula following, 343
    pain following, 407

Dental infection,
  osteomyelitis of maxilla from, 337
  sinusitis caused by, 245
Dental neuralgia, 260, 405
  edentulous jaw, in, 408
Dentigerous cyst, 285
  sinusitis from, 246
Depression, facial pain and, 394
Dermoid cysts, 4, 56, 75
Diabetes insipidus, following trans-ethmoidal
    hypophysectomy, 439
Diabetes mellitus, 15
Diabetic retinopathy, trans-ethomoidal
    hypophysectomy for, 430
Digestive tract symptoms of sinusitis, 281
Diplopia,
  facial fracture, in, 39, 40, 43, 45
  mucocoele, from, 321
Diphtheria, nasal, 174, 264
Diving, sinusitis and, 248
Dog bites of nose, 65
Dry sockets, 337, 407

Ear disease, cavernous sinus thrombophlebitis, in,
    343
Embryology of nose, 73
Emotions, rhinopathy and, 461
Emphysema, surgical, 45
Encephalocoeles, 75
Endochondromas, 364
Endocrine changes, rhinopathy and, 462
Endocrine factors,
  common cold, in, 165
  rhinitis, in, 219
Entomophthoromycosis conidiobolae, 201
Eosinophilia, 275, 462
Eosinophilic granuloma, 65
Epileptiform fits, rhinogenic intracranial suppura-
    tion causing, 327, 328
Epiphora, 10
  chronic, Vidian neurectomy for, 474
  fractures of maxilla, following, 39
Epistaxis, 147–162
  age distribution of, 154
  area of bleeding, 151
  arterial ligation in, 160
  atrophic rhinitis, in, 177
  bleeding diathesis and, 162
  blood pressure and, 157
  blood vessel pathology in, 154, 157, 158
  chronic sinusitis, in, 279
  clinical management of, 155
    arterial ligation, 160
    elderly, 159
    young people, 155, 159
  clinical manifestations, 151
  clotting defects and, 162
  contributory factors, 152
  coronary thrombosis and, 160
  duration of haemorrhage, 155
  ethmoid carcinoma, in, 375
  foreign bodies causing, 142, 143

Epistaxis (*continued*)
  fractures of maxilla, in, 32
  frequency of haemorrhage, 155
  history of, 147
  incidence of, 151
  Little's area, from, 152, 153
  lupus vulgaris, in, 187
  malar–zygomatic complex fracture, from, 40
  maxillary artery ligation for, 469, 471
  myiasis, in, 205
  nasal fractures, from, 20, 29
  nasopharyngeal angiofibroma, from, 162
  oestrogens and, 161
  olfactory neuroblastoma, from, 363
  Osler's disease, in, 161
  osteosarcoma of maxilla causing, 371
  recurrent, management of, 155
  rhinosporidiosis, in, 201
  septal capillary haemangioma, from, 363
  venous, 152
  Wegener's granulomatosis causing, 351
Epithelial tumours, 68, 358
Erysipelas, 15, 174, 264
Espundia, 205
Ethmoid,
  carcinoma of, 376, 378
  cartilaginous tumours of, 364
  pain in, sinusitis and, 256
  polypi in, 228
    treatment of, 232
  squamous carcinoma of, 359
  surgery of, 297–302
  tumours of, 265
Ethmoidal artery ligation in epistaxis, 160, 161
Ethmoidal sinus,
  carcinoma of, 374, 375
  compound fracture of, sinusitis and, 249
  mucococle, 320
  operations on, 297–302, 311
    complications, 298
  osteomas, 369
  pain from, 411
  Patterson's operation, 308
  puncturing, 284
  pyocoele, 322
Ethmoidal sinusitis,
  anterior rhinoscopy in, 257, 281
  children, in, 268, 320
  chronic, 273
  complications of, 315, 318, 339
    intracranial, 326, 340
  mucocoele from, 318
  pain in, 256
  signs of, 257
  treatment, 310
Ethmoidectomy,
    external, 300
    external fronto-, 301
    intranasal, 297
    transantral, 308
Exophthalmos in fractures of facial skeleton, 45
Eye,
  disorders, facial pain from, 415
    removal of, 276

Eye (*continued*)
    sinusitis, in, 280
    trans-ethmoidal hypophysectomy, after, 438
    Vidian neurectomy affecting, 480
Eye lid,
    coloboma of, 56
    fistulae in, 325
    hay fever, in, 211
    swelling from facial fracture, 40

Facial pain, 385–424 (*See also* Neuralgia *and under* Pain)
    acupuncture and, 423
    anxiety and, 396
    atypical, 263, 422
    behaviour of, 394
    brain stem lesions, from, 414
    central lesions causing, 413
    classification of, 397
    conversion hysteria and, 394
    coronary artery disease, in, 415
    depression and, 394
    distribution of afferent fibres, 389
    gate-control theory and, 390
    hypochondriasis and, 395
    masticatory, 418
    motivationally disabled, and, 395
    muscle and joint, 415
    myofascial triggers, 415
    myospasm, 417
    neurophysiology of, 386
    personality patterns and, 394
    psychiatric syndromes and, 394
    psychological aspects of, 392
    temporo-mandibular joint, from, 417
    thalamic lesions causing, 414
    types of, 393
    vascular, 420
Facial palsy, 190
Facial skeleton,
    fractures of, 22
    injuries of, 21–46 (*See also under specific region*)
        associated lesions, 24
        later complications, 30
        mechanism of, 22
Familial haemorrhagic telangiectasia, 177
Fibrous dysplasia of bone, 369
Fistulae, 325–326
    posterior choanal atresia, following, 79
Focal sepsis, sinusitis and, 348
Forehead, fistula to, 325
Forehead, skin flaps, 69
Foreign bodies, 141–146, 265
    aetiology, 141
    animate, 142, 143, 145
    children, in, 141
    diagnosis of, 144
    floor of nose, in, 8
    management of, 145
    mode of entry, 141
    pathology of, 142
    radiography, 8
    rhinitis in, 181
    sinusitis caused by, 245, 248, 249

Foreign bodies (*continued*)
    site and type of, 142
    symptoms and signs, 143
    types of patient, 141
    vestibulitis, causing, 15
Fractures, 5, 19
    frontal, 22
    lateral, 22
    mechanism of injury, 22
    sinus involvement in, 20
Fractures of maxilla (*See under* Maxilla)
Fractures of nose,
    associated injuries, 24
    frontal, 26, 61
    lateral, 22, 24
    laterally displaced inner canthal ligament, 27
    later complications, 30
    loss of septal support following, 63
    radiography of, 24
    symptoms and signs, 24
    treatment of, 25
Framboesia (*see* Yaws)
Frontal bone,
    osteomyelitis of, 317
        sinusitis causing, 329
Frontal pain,
    sinusitis, in, 256
Frontal sinus,
    barotrauma and, 269
    catheterizing, 284
    compound fracture of, sinusitis and, 249
    mucocoele, 320
    operations on, 303–308
    osteoma, 367, 369
    osteoplastic operation, 304,
        unilateral, 305
    pyocoele, 322
    trephination of, 303
Frontal sinusitis,
    anterior rhinoscopy in, 281
    complications of, 315
    intracranial complications, 326
    operations for, 301
    osteomyelitis from, 328
    pain in, 256, 411
    signs of, 257
    spread of infection from, 317
    surgical treatment, 268
    treatment of, 286, 301, 303, 310
Fronto-ethmoidectomy, 301
Fronto-ethmoid operation, 310
Frontonasal glioma, 59
Fungal infection, 200, 269
Furuncles, 4, 6, 13, 15

Galloway operation, 93, 95
Galvanism, pain from, 409
Gangosa, 180
Gangreangosa, 180
Gardener's syndrome, 369
Gasserian ganglion injection, 401
Gastroenteritis complicating common cold, 170
Glabella, encephalocoeles, 75

Glabellar flaps, 69
Glanders,
  chronic, 199
  diagnosis, 184
  rhinitis in, 174
Glaucoma, 415
Gliomas, 75, 365
Glossodynia, 415
Glosso-pharyngeal nerve, 389
  pressure involvement, 404
Glossopharyngeal neuralgia, 402
Glue ears, 312
Gonorrhoea, rhinitis in, 175
Goundou, 198
Granulomas,
  giant-cell, 352
  non-healing, 351–356
Gummata, 18, 183, 184

Haemangioma, 363
  capillary, 65
Haemangiopericytoma, 364
Haemophilus influenzae, sinusitis and, 253
Hair follicles, staphylococcal infection of, 5
Hay fever, 210
  clinical features of, 211
  recurring, 461
  treatment, 215
Headache
  cervical myalgia and, 417
  frontal sinusitis, in, 327
  mucocoele, from, 321
  mucosal congestion, from, 411
  ocular disorders, from, 415
  olfactory neuroblastoma, from, 363
  sinusitis, in, 280, 285, 411
  sphenoidal sinus osteoma causing, 369
  vacuum type of, 412
  whiplash injury of spine and, 413
    (*See also* Neuralgia)
Head injury, anosmia following, 10
Heerfordt's syndrome, 190
Hereditary telangiectasia, maxillary artery ligation
    for, 471
Herpes ophthalmicus, 413
Herpes simplex, 4, 16
Herpes zoster, 16
Histamine cephalgia, 420
Histoplasmosis, 204
Hump nose, 47
Hyoid bone, fracture of, 34
Hypertelorism, 74
Hypochondriasis, 395
Hypophysectomy, trans-ethmoidal (*See* Trans-
    ethmoidal hypophysectomy)
Hyposensitization in allergic rhinitis, 213
Hyposmia, from polypi, 228

Iatrogenic disease, 397
Immunoglobulins, 210
  polyposis and, 225
Impetigo, 15

Infections,
  acute, 13–17
  anosmia in, 10
  external nose, of,
    acute, 13
    chronic, 17–18
  polypi and, 226
  posterior choanal atresia, from, 79
Inflammations of nasal cavities, 163–224 (*See also*
    Rhinitis etc.)
Influenza, 172
  anosmia following, 10, 240
Injuries to nose, 19–20 (*See also* Fractures etc.)
Interferon, 167
Intracranial infections, from sinusitis, 315
Intracranial lesions, abnormalities of smell and,
    236, 241
Intracranial suppuration, rhinogenic, 326
Intranasal antrostomy, 293
  children, in, 312
  technique, 294
Intranasal ethmoidectomy, 297
Investigations, 9
Iritis, acute, 415

Jansen–Horgan operation, 232
Jaw joint pain–dysfunction syndrome, 419

Kaninloma, 181
Kartagener's syndrome, 312, 347
Killian operation, 91, 95, 105, 134

Lacrimal obstruction, from nasal fractures, 29
Lacrimation, Vidian neurectomy and, 480
Laryngitis in sinusitis, 280
Larynx,
  involvement in fracture of maxilla, 33
  leishmaniasis, in, 205
  scleroma, in, 191
Lautenslager's operation, 180
Leiomyosarcoma, 367
Leishmaniasis, 184, 205
Leprosy, 184, 195–197, 270
Liposarcoma, 370
Lipsett operation, 53
Little's area, epistaxis from, 152, 153
Lung, in Wegener's granulomatosis, 352
Lung cancer, 382
Lupus erythematosus, 18
Lupus pernio, 189
Lupus vulgaris, 5, 17, 184, 186, 188
Lymphadenitis complicating common cold, 170
Lymphoma, malignant, 366, 378

Macroglobulinaemia, Waldenstrom's, 162
Malar–zygomatic complex,
  fracture of, 32, 33, 37, 39–45
    post-operative complications, 45
    radiology, 41
    symptoms and signs, 40
    treatment of, 41

Malignant lymphoma, 366, 378
Malignant melanoma, 360
Mandible, ameloblastoma (adamantinoma), 371
Masticatory pain, 418
Mastoiditis complicating common cold, 170
Maxilla,
    ameloblastoma (adamantinoma) of, 371
    Burkitt's lymphoma of, 372
    carcinoma of, 376
    fibro-osseous disease of, 369
    fracture of, 20
        alveolar fragment in, 37
        associated injury in, 32
        classification of, 31
        delayed treatment of, 38
        edentulous patient, in, 38
        fixation of, 34
        mechanism of injury of, 30
        mobilization and reduction of, 34
        post-operative complications of, 39
        post-operative treatment of, 38
        radiology of, 33
        reduction and fixation of non-maxillary
            elements in, 36
        special problems in, 37
        symptoms of, 32
        treatment of, 33
    injuries to, 30–39
    involvement in septal deviation, 86
    osteomyelitis,
        children, in, 339
        complicating sinusitis, 336
        management of, 340
        symptoms and signs of, 338
    osteosarcoma of, 369
    pain in, after Caldwell–Luc operation, 413
    removal of, 379
Maxillary antrum,
    compound fracture of, sinusitis and, 249
    foreign bodies in, sinusitis from, 248
    infected (*See under* Sinusitis)
    tumours of, 265
Maxillary artery,
    anatomy of, 451
    ligation of, 465
        epistaxis, for, 161, 469, 471
        hereditary telangiectasia, for, 471
        indications for, 469
        nasopharyngeal angiofibroma, for, 471
Maxillary nerve,
    anatomy of, 451
    resection of, 466
Maxillary neurectomy, indications for, 471
Maxillary sinus,
    inverted papilloma from, 358
    obliteration of, 297
    operations on, 311
    pain from, 411
    pressure changes in, 410
    puncture of, 284, 290
    squamous carcinoma of, 359
    tuberculosis of, 270
Maxillary sinusitis,
    children, in, 268

Maxillary sinusitis (*continued*)
    chronic, 273
    complications of, 315
    dental causes of, 245, 247
    fluid level in, 259
    irrigation in, 290
    osteomyelitis from, 329, 337
    pain in, 256, 472
    signs of, 257
    surgical treatment of, 267, 293
Maxillectomy,
    partial, 381
    total, 379
Measles, 173, 264
Melanin, 362
Melanoma, malignant, 360
Melanoma of nose, 68
Meningiomas, loss of smell caused by, 241
Meningitis, 143, 203, 264
    ethmoid operations, after, 298
    pyococcal, 328
    sinusitis causing, 328
    trans-ethmoidal hypophysectomy, following, 439
Meningocoeles, 227
Mental illness, sinusitis and, 281
Metzenbaum operation, 92, 93
Migraine, 220, 263, 280, 412
Minimum perceptible odour, 237
Molluscum sebaceum, 66
Mott cells, 192
Mount Vernon box fixation of maxilla, 35, 36
Mouth pain, afferent fibres in, 389
Mucocoeles, 369
    intracranial extension of, 322
    radiology of, 321
    sinusitis, from, 240, 318, 320
Mucormycosis, orbital and central nervous system,
    202
Mucosa,
    autonomic supply of, 455
    reactions of, 459
    vascularization and innervation of, 216
Mucosal changes in septal deviation, 89
Mucosal congestion, 411
Mucoviscidosis, 227, 252, 312
Multiple sclerosis, facial pain from, 403, 414
Myalgia,
    cervical, 417
    masticatory, 419
Myiasis, 141, 142, 145, 205
Myofascial triggers, 415
Myxomas, 371

Naevus, pigmented, 66
Nasal cavities, (*See also* Rhinitis etc.)
    inflammations of, 163–224
    tumours of, 357
Nasal cholesteatoma, 181
Nasal crusting following trans-ethmoidal hypo-
    physectomy, 439
Nasal cycle, 217
Nasal discharge,
    aspergillosis, in, 202

Nasal discharge (*continued*)
  chronic diphtheritic rhinitis, in, 191
  chronic sinusitis, in, 279, 281
  foreign body causing, 142, 143, 144
  infants, in, 2
  leprosy, in, 196
  lupus vulgaris, in, 187
  rhinosporidiosis, in, 201
  sarcoidosis, in, 189
  sinusitis, in, 256
Nasal flora, 13
Nasal fossae, examination of, 1, 6
  radiology, 8
Nasal glioma, 363
Nasal hump,
  reduction of, 124
  removal of, 125–133
    osteotomies, 128
    post-operative care, 132, 133
    sex differences, 125
    technique of, 126
Nasal obstruction,
  acute sinusitis and, 250
  allergic rhinitis, in, 211
  anosmia in, 10
  aspergillosis, in, 202
  atrophic rhinitis, in, 177
  chronic diphtheritic rhinitis, in, 191
  chronic sinusitis, in, 279
  common cold and, 164
  ethmoid carcinoma, in, 375
  infants, in, 2
  lupus vulgaris, in, 187
  myiasis, in, 205
  nasal fractures, from, 24
  non-allergic rhinitis, in, 219
  olfactory neuroblastoma, from, 363
  osteosarcoma of maxilla causing, 371
  phycomycoses, in, 201
  polypi causing, 228
  sarcoidosis, in, 189
  septal capillary haemangioma, from, 363
  septal deviation causing, 89
  septal haematoma, in, 83
  tumours causing, 365
  Wegener's granulomatosis causing, 351
Nasal processes, abnormal fusion of, 4
Nasal provocation tests, 213
Nasal pyramid,
  deviation of, with septal deviation, 87
  external assessment of, 109
  functional aspects of, 106
Nasal speculum, use of, 1
Nasal tip,
  abnormalities of, 61
  alteration of projection of, 119
  bifid, 54
  cleft, 74
  correction of position of, 119
  cosmetic surgery of, 49
  crooked, 54
  elevation of, 119
  hanging, treatment of, 52
  large bulbous, 53

Nasal tip (*continued*)
  operations on, cleft lip and palate, in, 55
  reshaping of, 116
  septo-rhinoplasty, in, 116
  supra saddling of, 131
Nasal vestibule,
  acute infections of, 13
  examination of, 5
  papilloma, 358
  squamous carcinoma of, 359
Nasolacrimal groove, cleft of, 56
Nasopharyngeal angiofibroma, 162
Nasopharyngeal leishmaniasis, 205
Nasopharyngeal tumours, 264
Nasopharyngitis, complicating common cold, 169
Nasopharynx,
  defence against common cold, 167
  examination in sinusitis of, 258
  scleroma, in, 191
Necrosis with atypical cellular exudate, 354
Neoplastic disease (*See* Tumours)
Nerve supply to nasal mucosa, 216
Nerve tumours, 364
Neuralgia, 398–413
  atypical, 394, 422
  cervical, 413
  confusing diagnosis of sinusitis, 260
  dental, 405
  edentulous jaw, in, 408
  galvanism causing, 409
  glossopharyngeal, 402
  multiple sclerosis, from, 403, 414
  nasal, 409
  peroidic migrainous, 420
  persistent maxillary, maxillary neurectomy for, 472
  post-extraction, 407
  post-herpetic, 391, 413
  primary, 398
  secondary, 403
  traumatic, 412
  trigeminal (*See* Trigeminal neuralgia)
Neuroblastoma, olfactory, 363
Neurofibroma, 365
Neurofibrosarcoma, 367
Non-healing granuloma, 351–356
Nose,
  absence of, 74
  anatomy and embryology, 73
  blood vessel pathology of, 154
  examination of, 1
    adults, in, 4
    airway, 6
    floor, 8
    fossae, 6
    infants, in, 2
    probing, 8
    radiography, 8
    septum, 7
    turbinates, 6, 7
    under anaesthesia, 9
    vestibule, 5
  laterally displaced, 59

Nose (*continued*)
  loss of cover, 65
    restoration of, 68
  shape of, 4
  vascular anatomy of, 148
Nostrils, valvular, 54
Nutrition, coryza and, 164

Odours, primary, 238
Oestrogens, epistaxis and, 161
Olfactory nerve lesions, abnormalities of smell and,
    236, 240
Olfactory neuroblastoma, 363
Olfactory reference syndrome, 241
Open-roof syndrome, 124
Ophthalmoplegia following trans-ethmoidal hypo-
    physectomy, 439
Optic neuritis, 340
Oral-antral fistula, 343
Orbit,
  abscess, 231, 317
  apex syndrome, 340
  cellulitis, complicating sinusitis, 316, 332, 333,
    342
    ethmoiditis, from, 318
  complications of ethmoid operations, 298
  floor,
    blow-out, fracture of, 39
    collapse of, 42
  haematoma, 231
    facial fractures, in, 45
    fractures of maxilla, in, 32
  infection of, 143
  involvement in fibro-osseous disease of maxilla,
    370
  involvement in sphenoidal sinus osteoma, 369
Osler's disease,
  epistaxis in, 161
  septal perforation in, 134
Osteitis, sclerosing, complicating sinusitis, 332
Osteoma of sinuses, 308, 367
Osteomyelitis, complicating sinusitis, 328
    bacteriology of, 331
    management of, 335
    radiology of, 334, 339
    symptoms and signs of, 332, 338
    treatment of, 340
  frontal bone, of, 317
  maxilla, of, children, in, 339
Osteoplastic frontal sinus operation, 304
Otitis media complicating common cold, 170
Otorrhoea, sinusitis and, 280

Paget's disease, 371
Pain,
  acupuncture and, 423
  anxiety and, 396
  central pathways of, 386
  fast and slow, 389
  gate-control theory of, 390
  iatrogenic disease and, 397
  influence of reticular system in, 387

Pain (*continued*)
  nerve fibres conducting, 388
  receptors of, 388
Palatal fenestrations, 381
Palatal swelling in sinus carcinoma, 375
Palate,
  cleft (*See* Cleft lip and palate)
  haematoma of, 32
  perforations of, 185
  split, 33, 37
  ulceration of, 181
Papillomata, 6, 19
Parotid enlargement, 190
Parrot beak deformity, 126, 127, 128
Patterson's operation, 233, 308
Peenash, 205
Peer's operation, 92, 94
Peri-apical abscess, sinusitis from, 246
Periodic migrainous neuralgia, 420
Periodontal abscess, sinusitis from, 246
Periodontal infections, 405
Periodontitis, sinusitis and, 246
Peripheral nerve tumours, 364
Pertussis, 173
Petrosal neuralgia, 420
Petrosal neurectomy, 456
  indications for, 473
Pharyngeal artery, 452
Pharyngeal hypophysis, 442
Pharyngitis, acute sinusitis and, 348
Pharyngotympanic salpingitis complicating
    common cold, 170
Pharynx,
  examination of sinusitis, in, 258, 282
  infection, sinusitis from, 245
  leishmaniasis, in, 205
  ulceration of, 181
Phycomycoses, 201
Pigmented naevus, 66
Pipe stem neck, 343
Pituitary ablation, 439
  ultrasonic, 441
Pituitary gland,
  cryosurgery of, 441
  exposure of, 434
  heavy particle irradiation of, 440
  interstitial irradiation of, 440
  removal of (*See* Trans-ethmoidal hypo-
    physectomy)
  tele-radiation, 439
Plasmacytoma, 366
Plastic surgery, 47
Polly (parrot beak) deformity, 126, 127, 128
Polypectomy, 286
Polypi, 7, 8, 225–234, 310
  clinical features of, 228
  infection and, 226
  loss of smell from, 240
  neoplastic disease and, 228, 234
  pathogenesis of, 225
  pathology of, 226
  radiology of, 229
  recurrent, Vidian neurectomy for, 474
  rhinitis in, 181

Polypi (*continued*)
  rhinosporidiosis, in, 200, 201
  sinusitis caused by, 255
  treatment of, 229
Posterior choanal atresia, 76–80
Posterior inferior cerebellar artery, thrombosis of,
    414
Posterior rhinoscopy, 282
Post-nasal drip in sinusitis, 279
Post-nasal inlay, 65
Pott's puffy tumour, 332
Proboscis lateralis, 74
Proptosis, in facial fracture, 40
Prostate, carcinoma of, 431
Psychiatric syndromes, facial pain and, 394
Pterygoid canal, 449
Pterygo-palatine fossa,
  arteries of, 451
  fat in, 453
  surgery of, 447–481 (*See also* Vidian neurectomy,
      Maxillary neurectomy etc.)
    classic trans-antral route, 464
    indications for, 469
    practical considerations, 464
  surgical anatomy of, 447
  transverse plane of nerves, 449
  veins of, 452
Pulp space infections, 405
Purpura, 162
Pyocoeles, complicating sinusitis, 332, 341

Quinsy, cavernous sinus thrombophlebitis in, 343

Radioallergosorbent test, 213
Radiofrequency gangliolysis, 402
Reid index, 276
Renal cell carcinoma, 382
Respiratory air currents, nasal tip and, 106, 107,
    108
Respiratory obstruction in fractures of maxilla, 33
Respiratory tract symptoms of sinusitis, 280
Respiratory viruses, sinusitis and, 253
Rhabdomyosarcoma, 367
Rhinitis,
  acute infective, 163
    sinusitis from, 244
  acute nasal diphtheria, in, 174
  allergic (extrinsic), 209, 279
    hyposensitization in, 213
    loss of smell in, 240
    perennial, 211
    predisposing factors, 211
    seasonal, 210
    sinusitis and, 251
    special tests for, 212
    treatment of, 213
  anthrax, in, 175
  atrophic, 176
    aetiology of, 176
    clinical picture of, 177
    diagnosis of, 184

Rhinitis (*continued*)
  atrophic (*continued*)
    investigations in, 179
    leprosy, in, 196
    lupus vulgaris, in, 188
    nasal injury, from, 30
    pathology of, 177
    syphilis, in, 183
    treatment of, 179
    types of, 177
  candidiasis, in, 175
  caseosa, 180
  chronic diphtheritic, 191
  chronic hypertrophic, 220
  chronic infective, 176
  coryza, in (*See under* Coryza)
  definition of, 209
  erysipelas, in, 174
  exanthems, of, 173
  fibrinous, 191
  glanders, in, 174, 199
  gonorrhoea, in, 175
  hypertrophic, 176
  infective, loss of smell in, 240
  influenzal, 172
  local irritants and trauma causing, 175
  non-allergic (intrinsic), 215
    clinical picture of, 219
    contributing factors in, 218
    differential diagnosis of, 220
    examination in, 220
    management of, 221
  posterior choanal atresia, after, 79
  sicca, 180
  specific, 174
  syphilis, in, 174, 179, 182, 185
  tuberculous, 186
  vasomotor, 209–224, 458
    anosmia in, 10
    classification of, 459
Rhinocerebral phycomycosis, 202
Rhinoliths, 144
  definition of, 143
  management of, 146
Rhinopathy,
  secreto-motor, 461
    clinical features of, 461
    neural mechanisms of, 462
    Vidian neurectomy for, 463, 473, 478
  vasomotor, 461
Rhinopharyngitis mutilans, 181
Rhinophycomycosis, 201
Rhinophyma, 4, 18, 66
Rhinoplasty, 106 (*See also* Septo-rhinoplasty)
  augmentation, 131
  cosmetic, 48
    post-operative treatment of, 52
  Italian, 71
  reduction, 124
Rhinorrhoea, 460
  non-allergic rhinitis, in, 219, 220
  polypi, in, 228
  senile, Vidian neurectomy for, 472
  vestibulitis, causing, 15

Rhinorrhoea (*continued*)
    Vidian neurectomy for, 460
Rhinoscleroma, 191
    clinical picture of, 193
    pathology of, 191
    treatment of, 194
Rhinosporidiosis, 200, 227
Rhinotomy, lateral, 379
Rhinoviruses, 165
Ringertz tumour, 358
Rodent ulcers, 19
    treatment of, 67
Rosacea, 66
Russell bodies, 192

Saddle nose, 63
Sarcoidosis, 184, 188–190
    aetiology of, 189
    clinical picture of, 189
    diagnosis of, 190
    incidence of, 189
    treatment of, 190
Scarlet fever, 173
Schwannoma, 363
Scleroma, 183, 191
Sebaceous cysts, 4
Sellotomy, exploratory, 431
Septal impactions, pain from, 412
Septoplasty, 95
    combined with rhinoplasty, 97
    exposure in, 97
    fixation in, 102
    incision for, 96
    mobilization and straightening in, 99
Septo-rhinoplasty, 105–124
    anaesthesia for, 115
    assessment of external nasal pyramid in, 109
    biometric analysis and, 109
    correction of nasal tip position in, 119
    exposure of alar cartilages in, 120, 123
    functional examination in, 106
    nasal tip in, 116
    operative technique of, 115
    physical and psychological contraindications, 112
    pre-operative planning of, 112
Septum, 83–139
    abscess of, 7, 84
    bleeding polypus of, 227, 363
    bone graft for, 61
    bony and cartilaginous dorsum, surgery of, 124
    capillary haemangioma of, 363
    classic submucous resection operation of, 102–105
    destruction of, 5
    deviation of, 85–105
        aetiology of, 85
        birth moulding theory of, 85
        cartilaginous, 87
        effects of, 88
        pain in, 89
        pathological anatomy of, 85
        sinusitis and, 250
        submucous operations, 90
        symptoms and signs of, 89

Septum (*continued*)
    dislocations of, 86
        newborn, in 105
    examination of, 7
    fracture of cartilage of, 83
    haematoma of, 7, 29, 83, 102
        complications of, 84
        symptoms and signs of, 83
        treatment of, 84
    injuries to, 21, 83
    leishmaniasis, in, 205
    loss of support of, 61, 63
    lupus vulgaris, in, 186, 188
    malignant melanoma of, 361
    perforation of, 7, 133
        causes of, 134
        closure with obturators of, 136
        diagnosis of, 135
        leprosy, in, 195
        lupus vulgaris, in, 188
        occupational causes of, 134
        operative closure of, 137
        sarcoidosis, in, 189
        symptoms and signs of, 135
        syphilis, in, 184
        treatment of, 135
        Wegener's granulomatosis, in, 352
    squamous carcinoma of, 359
    submucosal removal operation of, 90, 286
    surgery of (*See also* Septoplasty *and* Septo-rhinoplasty)
        anaesthesia for, 95
        bony and cartilaginous dorsum of, 124
        development of, 90
            growing nose, in, 104
        principles of, 94
    syphilis, in, 183
    ulceration of, 133
        symptoms and signs, 135
        treatment of, 135
Shape of nose, 4
Sinobronchial syndrome, 312
Sinus barotrauma, 269
Sinus disease, 8
Sinuses,
    adenocarcinoma of, 374
    carcinoma of, 372
    development of, 243
    infection of, polypi causing, 228
    involved in nasal fractures, 20
    malignant lymphoma, 366
    metastatic tumours of, 382
    neoplasia of, 265
    opaque, 259
    osteoma of, 367
    sounding or puncturing of, 283
    tuberculosis, of, 270
    tumours of, 367–382
        aetiology of, 373
        classification of, 373
        diagnosis, of, 375
        nerve compression in, 404
        pain from, 411
        surgical procedures in, 379

Sinuses (*continued*)
  tumours of (*continued*)
    symptoms of, 375
    treatment of, 377
Sinusitis,
  acute, 243–271
    aetiology of, 244
    anterior rhinoscopy in, 257
    antibiotics in, 266
    associated chest conditions in, 251
    bacteriology of, 252
    barotrauma and, 249
    children, in, 268
    clinical features of, 255
    complications (*See under* Sinusitis,
      complications)
    contributory and predisposing factors of, 249
    decongestants in, 266
    dental infection causing, 245
    differential diagnosis of, 260
    examination in, 258
    exposure to cold and, 250
    fluid level in, 259
    foreign bodies and, 249
    fracture of sinuses and, 249
    maxillary, 245
    pathology of, 254
    pharyngeal infection causing, 245
    poor environment and, 249
    prophylaxis of, 265
    radiology in, 258
    rhinitis causing, 244
    surgical treatment of, 267
    swimming and diving and, 248
    symptoms of, 255
    teeth extraction and, 247
    traumatic causes of, 248
    treatment of, 265
    virus infection and, 253
  asthma and, 251, 348
  atrophic, 274
  barotrauma and, 269
  baro-, 411
  blood changes in, 277
  bronchiectasis and, 252, 347
    children, in, 268, 311
  bronchitis and, 347
  chronic, 273–313
    aetiology of, 273
    anterior rhinoscopy in, 281
    antibiotics in, 288
    bacteriology of, 273, 285
    children, in, 311
    choice of treatment, 309
    clinical features of, 278
    complications (*See under* Sinusitis, compli-
      cations)
    conservative treatment of, 287
    decongestants in, 287
    diagnosis and assessment of, 285
    digestive tract symptoms, 281
    displacement therapy of, 288
    ear symptoms of, 280
    enzymes and mucolytic drugs in, 288

Sinusitis (*continued*)
  chronic (*continued*)
    examinations in, 282
    eye symptoms of, 280
    headache in, 280, 285
    inhalants in, 287
    minor surgical procedures in, 289
    mucosal reaction in, 276
    operative treatment of, 293
    pathology of, 274
    physiopathology of, 278
    posterior rhinoscopy in, 282
    Reid index in, 276
    respiratory tract symptoms of, 280
    shortwave diathermy in, 289
    sounding or puncturing in, 283
    symptoms of, 279
    therapeutic options, 287
    transillumination in, 282
    treatment of, 286
  chronic bronchitis and, 251
  chronic hypertrophic papillary, 347
  complicating common cold, 170
  complications of, 315–349
    anterior group, 315
    cavernous sinus thrombophlebitis, 342
    cellulitis of orbit, 342
    fistulae, 325
    intracranial, 326
    mucocoele, 320, 341
    orbital cellulitis, 332
    oro-antral fistula, 344
    osteomyelitis, 328
    pyocoele, 322, 341
    sclerosing osteitis, 332
  congenital factors, 252
  environment and, 289
  eosinophilia in, 275
  focal sepsis and, 348
  foreign bodies causing, 143
  fungal infection causing, 269
  goblet-cell hyperplasia in, 277
  hypertrophic or polypoid, 274
  incidence of, 243
  leprosy and, 270
  malignant disease and, 347, 373
  mental illness and, 281
  mucosal lining in, 259
  nasal injury, from, 30
  pain from, 410, 411
  papillary hypertrophic, 274
  physiopathology of, 255
  polypi and, 228
  rhinitis caseosa, in, 181
  sarcoidosis, in, 189
  secondary effects of, 347–348
  secretions and cilia in, 277
  syphilis and, 270
  wax keratosis and, 252
Sinus operations, 293
  choice of treatment, 310
Skin grafts to nose, 68
Skin pain, afferent fibres in, 389
Skull, fractures of base, 32

Sluder's lower-half headache, 420
Smallpox, 173
Smell,
  abnormalities of, 235–241
    causes of, 236, 240
    chronic sinusitis, in, 279
    classification of, 235
    psychogenic disorders causing, 241
Smell, loss of, (*See* Anosmia)
  primary odours, 238
  testing of, 236
Sneezing, 460
  aspergillosis, in, 202
  foreign bodies causing, 143
Snoring, 77
Snuffles, 185, 186
Soft palate, haematoma of, 32
Sphenoidal sinus,
  catheterizing, 284
  irrigating, 285
  operations on, 303, 311
  osteoma, 369
  pain from, 411
  Patterson's operation in, 308
Sphenoidal sinusitis,
  complications of, 339
    intracranial, 342
  fluid level in, 260
  pain in, 257
  radiology of, 282
  treatment of, 303
Spheno-palatine artery, 216
Spheno-palatine bundle, 451
Spheno-palatine ganglion, 449, 454
Spheno-palatine ganglionectomy, 467
  indications for, 472
Spheno-palatine neuralgia, 420
Spinal injury, headache following, 413
Sporotrichosis, 204
Squamous-cell carcinoma, 19, 359
Stellate ganglion block, atrophic rhinitis, in, 180
Steroids, polypi and, 230
Straus's reaction, 199
Styloid process, elongated, 404
Subdural empyema, 327
Sublabial fistula, 346
Supra-orbital nerve, pain in, sinusitis and, 256
Swimming, sinusitis and, 248
Synechiae, nasal injury, following, 31
Syphilis, 17
  congenital, 18
  diagnosis of, 182, 183
  differential diagnosis of, 184
  fistula from, 347
  hereditary or congenital, 185
  loss of airway lining in, 65
  nasal, 182
  primary, 182
  rhinitis in, 174, 179, 183
  secondary, 182
  septal perforation in, 134, 135
  sinusitis and, 270
  tertiary, 182
  treatment of, 185

Tears, crocodile, Vidian neurectomy for, 474
Teeth,
  extraction of,
    oro-antral fistula following, 344
    pain following, 407
    sinusitis and, 247
  infections of,
    osteomyelitis from, 337
    sinusitis caused by, 245
  pulp space infections of, 405
  unerupted, impacted, 406
Temporal arteritis, 263, 421
Temporal lobe epilepsy, loss of smell in, 241
Temporo-mandibular joint disorders, pain from, 417
Temporo-mandibular neuralgia, 263
Thalamic lesions, facial pain from, 414
Thrombophlebitis,
  complicating sinusitis, 316, 317
  furuncles, from, 14
Thrush, 204
Tic douloureux (*See* Trigeminal neuralgia)
Tongue, pain, in, 415
Tonsillitis,
  complicating common cold, 170
  sinusitis and, 245, 280
Tracheobronchitis, acute sinusitis and, 347
Tracheostomy in fractures of maxilla, 33
Transantral ethmoidectomy, 308
Trans-ethmoidal hypophysectomy, 425–445
  complications of, 438
  exposure and removal of gland in, 434, 435
  history of, 425
  indications for, 426
  maintenance therapy after, 437
  post-operative care, 437
  pre-operative assessment for, 431
  technique for, 432
Trauma,
  deformities from, 59
  examination of, 4
Trigeminal nerve, 217, 386
  lesions, 45, 264
  pressure involvement of, 404
Trigeminal neuralgia, 280, 399–402
  diagnosis, 263, 400
  maxillary neurectomy for, 471
  treatment of, 400
Trigeminal pathways, intracranial decompression of, 401
Trismus, fracture in, 40
Tuberculosis,
  diagnosis of, 184
  rhinitis in, 186
  septal perforation in, 134
  sinuses, of, 270
Tumours, 357–384 (*See also under type and region*)
  benign epithelial, 367
  cartilaginous, 364
  epithelial, 358
  incidence of, 357, 358
  metastatic, 382
  nasopharyngeal, 264
  non-epithelial, 363

Tumours (*continued*)
  polypi and, 228, 234
  sinusitis and, 251
  vascular, 363
Turbinates,
  blood vessels of, 148, 149, 152
  diathermy of, in non-allergic rhinitis, 221
  examination of, 6
  hypertrophy of, 7
    septum deviation and, 86
  inferior, examination of, 7
  leprosy, in, 195, 196
  lupus vulgaris, in, 188
  middle, examination of, 7
  non-allergic rhinitis, in, 220
  oedema of, 8
  rhinitis, in, 177
  superior, examination of, 8
  surgical reduction of, 222
Tympanic membrane, pain in, 390
Typhoid fever, 264
Typhus, 173

Ultrasonics in pituitary ablation, 441
Urine, melanin in, 362

Vaccines,
  common cold, for, 171
  influenzal, 173
Valvular nostrils, 54
Vascular pain, 420
Vasoconstrictors, rhinitis caused by, 218
Vestibulitis, 15
  chronic sinusitis, in, 279
Vidian artery, anatomy of, 452
Vidian nerve, 455
  adrenergic and cholinergic fibres of, 457

Vidian nerve (*continued*)
  anatomy of, 449
  autonomic efferents of, 457
  parasympathetic and sympathetic effects of, 456
Vidian neuralgia, 420
Vidian neurectomy, 222, 451
  alternative methods of, 475
  complications of, 478
  histologic changes, 479
  indications for, 465, 473
  nasal effects of, 479
  ocular effects of, 480
  rationale of, 463
  results of, 478
  trans-antral subperiostial route for, 476
  trans-nasal approaches for, 476
  trans-palatal approach for, 477
Viruses in common cold, 165
Visual impairment following trans-ethmoidal hypophysectomy, 438
Vitamin deficiency, common colds and, 164
Vomerine spurs, removal of, 100
Vomiting, 327

Waldenstrom's macroglobulinaemia, 162
Wax keratitis, 252, 347
Wegener's granulomatosis, 134, 351–354, 355
  aetiology of, 352
  septal perforation in, 135
  treatment of, 353
Wolff grafts, 68
Worms in nose, 145, 205

Yaws, 181, 184, 197–199
Yeasts, infections from, 200

Zygomatic arch, fractures of, 39, 41, 43